Bioeth

Jones and Bartlett Series in Philosophy
Robert Ginsberg, General Editor

A.J. Ayer, 1994 reissue with new introduction by Thomas Magnell, Drew University, *Metaphysics and Common Sense*

Francis J. Beckwith, University of Nevada, Las Vegas, Editor, *Do the Right Thing: A Philosophical Dialogue on the Moral and Social Issues of Our Time*

Anne H. Bishop and John R. Scudder, Jr., Lynchburg College, *Nursing Ethics: Therapeutic Caring Presence*

Peter Caws, The George Washington University, *Ethics from Experience*

Joseph P. DeMarco, Cleveland State University, *Moral Theory: A Contemporary Overview*

Bernard Gert et al., Dartmouth College, *Morality and the New Genetics*

Michael Gorr, Illinois State University, and Sterling Harwood, San Jose State University, Editors, *Crime and Punishment: Philosophic Explorations*

Joram Graf Haber, Bergen Community College, Interviewer, *Ethics in the 90's*, A 26-part Video Series

Sterling Harwood, San Jose State University, Editor, *Business as Ethical and Business as Usual: Text, Readings, and Cases*

John Heil, Davidson College, *First Order Logic: A Concise Introduction*

Gary Jason, San Diego State University, *Introduction to Logic*

John LaPuma, Lutheran General Hospital, and David Schiedermayer, Medical College of Wisconsin, *Ethics Consultation: A Practical Guide*

Brendan Minogue, Youngstown State University, *Bioethics: A Committee Approach*

Linus Pauling and Ikeda Diasaku, Richard L. Gage, Translator and Editor, *A Lifelong Quest for Peace: A Dialogue*

Louis P. Pojman, The University of Mississippi, and Francis Beckwith, University of Nevada, Las Vegas, Editors, *The Abortion Controversy: A Reader*

Louis P. Pojman, The University of Mississippi, *Life and Death: Grappling with the Moral Dilemmas of Our Time*

Louis P. Pojman, The University of Mississippi, *Environmental Ethics: Readings in Theory and Application*

Holmes Rolston III, Colorado State University, Editor, *Biology, Ethics, and the Origins of Life*

Melville Stewart, Bethel College, *Philosophy of Religion: An Anthology of Contemporary Views*

Dabney Townsend, The University of Texas at Arlington, Editor, *Aesthetics: Classic Readings from the Western Tradition*

Robert M. Veatch, Georgetown University, Editor, *Medical Ethics, Second Edition*

Robert M. Veatch, Georgetown University, Editor, *Cross-Cultural Perspectives in Medical Ethics*

D.P. Verene, Emory University, Editor, *Sexual Love and Western Morality*, A Philosophical Anthology, *Second Edition*

Clifford Williams, Trinity College, Editor, *On Love and Friendship: Philosophical Readings*

Bioethics

An Introduction to the History, Methods, and Practice

NANCY S. JECKER, PH.D.
University of Washington
School of Medicine
Department of Medical History and Ethics

ALBERT R. JONSEN, PH.D.
University of Washington
School of Medicine
Department of Medical History and Ethics

ROBERT A. PEARLMAN, M.D., M.P.H.
University of Washington
School of Medicine
Department of Medicine
and Seattle V.A. Medical Center

Jones and Bartlett Publishers
Sudbury, Massachusetts
Boston   London   Singapore

Editorial, Sales, and Customer Service Offices
Jones and Bartlett Publishers
40 Tall Pine Drive
Sudbury, MA 01776
508-443-5000
info@jbpub.com
http://www.jbpub.com

Jones and Bartlett Publishers International
Barb House, Barb Mews
London W6 7PA
UK

Library of Congress Cataloging-in-Publication Data

Bioethics : an introduction to the history, methods, and practice /
  [edited by] Nancy S. Jecker, Albert R. Jonsen, Robert A. Pearlman.
     p.   cm.
  Includes bibliographical references and index.
  ISBN 0-7637-0228-5
  1. Medical ethics. 2. Bioethics. I. Jecker, Nancy Ann
Silbergeld. II. Jonsen, Albert R. III. Pearlman, Robert A.
  [DNLM: 1. Ethics, Medical. W 50 B6142 1997]
R724.B4583   1997
174'.2—dc20
DNLM/DLC
for Library of Congress   96-44667
                                                                      CIP

Vice President, Editorial: Joseph E. Burns
Sr. Production Administrator: Mary Sanger
Manufacturing Manager: Dana L. Cerrito
Editorial Production Service: Colophon
Typesetting: Modern Graphics
Cover Design: Hannus Design Associates
Printing and Binding: Edwards Brothers, Inc.
Cover Printing: Coral Graphic Services, Inc.

Printed in the United States of America
01 00 99 98 97   10 9 8 7 6 5 4 3 2 1

Contents

v

PART II   THE METHODS OF BIOETHICS

Preface

Textbooks are often generated out of teachers' experience with their students. We, the three editors of this textbook, teach bioethics students at four levels: college undergraduates, medical students, graduate students, and health care professionals in continuing education. We have found that the many existing textbooks in bioethics serve well enough for one or perhaps two of these groups, but do not address the needs of the others. We wondered if we could design a text that we could recommend to all of our students. *Bioethics: An Introduction to the History, Methods, and Practice* is the result.

We have also found that several aspects of modern bioethics are treated less than adequately by other textbooks. The strengths of these texts lie in the exposition of ethical theory and the review of standard problems that bioethics has treated. They reveal little of the history of the field, rarely explain the methodologies used to analyze ethical issues, and hardly mention the techniques for carrying ethical analyses into the various settings in which health care is practiced. We have tried to address those omissions in this book. If it is necessary to provide a fuller survey of the standard bioethical problems, we recommend *Medical Ethics, Second Edition* by Robert M. Veatch (Jones and Bartlett, 1997) also published in this series.

As the title suggests, *Bioethics: An Introduction to the History, Methods, and Practice* offers insight into the field of bioethics by exploring its history, methods, and practice with a critical eye. It teaches students: (1) how the field of bioethics originated; (2) what methods ethicists use to define and analyze ethical issues; and (3) how ethics is actually practiced by doctors, nurses, ethicists, and others in the clinical setting. This text also shows how social and cultural forces shape the historical development of bioethics and influence its methods and practice.

Part I: The History of Bioethics surveys the development of bioethics as a field of scholarly inquiry during the latter half of the twentieth century. It furnishes students with a sense of the historical development of specific bioethics topics, while introducing students to some of the field's most prominent founders. Students gain an appreciation of how bioethics first found a practical role for itself in hospitals and other health care settings.

Part II: The Methods of Bioethics presents and critically discusses deductive and inductive methods of ethical analysis, including principlism, casuistry, narrative ethics, and feminist approaches. It also discusses the role of empirical research in bioethical analysis by exploring the contributions of both quantitative and qualitative empirical methods.

Part III: The Practice of Bioethics explores how bioethics currently functions in the clinical setting through the workings of ethics committees and ethics consultation services. It explains how clinical ethics policies develop at federal, state, professional association, and health care institution levels.

Among the text's notable features are feminist critiques that challenge students to reflect on the assumptions implicit in the methods and practice of bioethics. The articles selected express diverse viewpoints and come from scholars representing a range of disciplinary perspectives including anthropology, history, theology, philosophy, and literature. Cross-cultural comparisons heighten students' awareness of social and cultural assumptions that are often taken for granted in Western philosophy, ethics, and medicine.

To assist teachers and students, each of the book's three main parts (History, Methods, and Practice) begins with an introduction in which we encapsulate the most critical issues raised, and then place them in a broader context. In addition, each of the sections within the parts is followed by discussion questions, which review important points. The index helps readers to locate historical, methodological, and practical aspects of specific ethical topics.

Having explained where *Bioethics* came from and what we hope it will accomplish, let us tell you something about ourselves. The three of us are colleagues at the University of Washington School of Medicine, Seattle.

Nancy S. Jecker is a philosopher who entered the field of bioethics during the 1980s. She is an Associate Professor at the University of Washington School of Medicine, Department of Medical History and Ethics, and adjunct Associate Professor at the University of Washington Department of Philosophy and School of Law. She is the author of *Aging and Ethics* (Humana Press, 1991) and (with Lawrence J. Schneiderman) of *Wrong Medicine: Doctors, Patients, and Futile Treatment* (Johns Hopkins University Press, 1995).

Albert R. Jonsen is Professor of Ethics in Medicine and Chairman of the Department of Medical History and Ethics at the University of Washington. A senior scholar in ethics, Dr. Jonsen was one of the pioneers in the field of bioethics during the 1970s. He served as Commissioner on the National Commission for the Protection of Human Subjects of Biomedical and Behavioral Research, and on the President's Commission for the Study of Ethical Problems in Medicine and Biomedical and Behavioral Research. Dr. Jonsen is the author (with Mark Siegler and William Winslade) of *Clinical Ethics, Third Edition* (McGraw-Hill, 1992); *The New Medicine and the Old Ethics* (Harvard University Press, 1990); and (with Stephen Toulmin) *The Abuse of Casuistry* (University of California Press, 1988).

Robert A. Pearlman is Associate Professor of Medicine at the University of Washington School of Medicine, where he practices geriatric and internal medicine. Dr. Pearlman has contributed to journals addressing clinical bioethics topics and recently authored *Your Life, Your Choices* (Department of Veterans Affairs, 1997), a workbook to assist patients and families with health care decisions.

PART I

The History of Bioethics

Introduction to the History of Bioethics

Albert R. Jonsen

The Early History

The work of healing, from time immemorial and in all cultures, has been wrapped in moral and religious meanings. The power of the healer has been considered a divine gift. Prayers and rituals accompanied the acts of healing. In the temples of gods associated with healing, such as Asklepios in the Greek and Roman civilizations, where physicians were priests, votive tablets attested to the patients' pleas and gratitude. Yet one of those Asklepiads, the Greek physician Hippocrates (fourth century B.C.) insisted that healing should be a scientific activity, based upon observation of nature and the natural effects of attempts to cure illness. He drew medicine away from religion but not from its moral origins. "Love of the medical art," he wrote, "is the love of humankind." The physician must enter the patient's house, he admonished, with the intent to bring benefit and to avoid all harm and injustice.

In the Western tradition, those maxims have guided physicians who tried to carry out their work in a moral manner. In the Judaic and Christian traditions, physicians were depicted as agents of God's own healing. They were to be competent and dedicated, caring for the sick poor and even for strangers and enemies. Organizations of physicians, from medieval guilds to the modern American Medical Association, have preserved that image of the physician as trustworthy, reputable, and competent. Thus, medical ethics, throughout the centuries and in very different social and cultural settings, has consisted of a somewhat stable set of moral admonitions and ideals.[1]

The New Biology

By the middle of the twentieth century, the medical treatment with which this traditional medical morality was associated bore little resemblance to the healing practices of prior centuries. During the previous one hundred years, scientific discoveries in physiology and bacteriology had radically changed the understanding of health and disease and had begun to improve the ability of physicians to diagnose and treat their patients. Immunization prevented the deadly epidemics that had devastated populations for centuries; anesthesia and aseptic surgery enabled direct attack on diseased organs. In 1921, insulin was discovered and quickly applied to forstall the lethal effects of diabetes; in the late 1940s the first antibiotics cured infections that had often been fatal. New mind-altering drugs attacked the most serious mental disorders. Other drugs provided new control over human reproduction. Radiology viewed the body's interior. Dramatic improvements in surgical technique, stimulated by military medicine during World War II, emboldened surgeons to enter the brain and the heart. In the 1950s, kidneys were transplanted, opening the era of organ transplantation. Over the decades 1930–1960, clinical medicine, based on a stream of scientific advances and armed with powerful diagnostic and therapeutic capacities, flourished.

Clinical medicine, which had changed so radically in the course of a century, is destined to change even more radically. In 1956, James Watson and James Crick announced that they had discerned the "secret of life," the double helical structure of the DNA molecule. This discovery opened the possibility of learning the most basic lessons about how biological organisms develop, how defects enter that development, and how scientists might deliberately modify (and even improve) it. Consequent research in the biochemistry of life gradually infiltrated clinical medicine, making possible genetic diagnosis and screening for genetic diseases and even holding out the promise of gene therapy as well as "improvement" of human traits. These developments stimulated serious commentary in the 1970s among scientists and other scholars. A selection from several early commentators on these issues is included in this anthology (Kass, 1971).

The new clinical medicine brought life and health to millions. At the same time, its power challenged the adequacy of the traditional medical morality. The old maxims ordering the physician to act for the benefit of the patient and not to do harm remained imperative. However, it was no longer always clear what constituted benefit and harm. The new treatments that often saved life sometimes left the person alive but damaged. The ability to accomplish changes in the patient's biological and physiological state and to measure these changes with accuracy did not always signal improvements in health. The effects of medical intervention, now achievable more predictably than ever before, did not always benefit the patient.

One of the remarkable advances was the invention of chronic hemodialysis. Certain diseases totally impair the ability of the kidneys to rid the body of the toxins produced by natural metabolism. In the 1940s, a machine that could substitute for damaged kidneys had been invented, but its use was limited by the difficulty of attaching the patient to the machine. In 1961, Dr. Belding Scribner invented a plastic tube that could be inserted permanently into the vein and artery of the forearm, by which the patient could be "plugged into" the dialysis machine several times a week for a lifetime. Thus, persons who were doomed to die within weeks of diagnosis lived for years. This technique was among the first true life-sustaining technologies of modern medicine.

The clinicians who devised this technique and applied it to their patients were elated. At the same time, the more thoughtful among them glimpsed problems in the offing. First among these problems was the selection of patients for this very scarce and expensive resource, but other troubling issues, such as the overt termination of treatment, soon appeared. In his 1964 presidential address to the Society for Artificial Organs, Dr. Scribner predicted that the ethical problems that his renal dialysis program had encountered "will recur again and again as other new, complicated, expensive, life-saving techniques are developed."[2] Commentators from philosophy, theology, and the law began to scrutinize the problem of selection for a scarce medical resource. One of these commentaries is included in this anthology (Childress, 1970).

Similar issues were raised by another dramatic innovation, the transplantation of organs from one person to another. The cornea of the eye had been successfully transplanted for some time, but skin grafting was plagued by the recipient body's rejection of foreign tissue. Intense investigations into the body's immune system revealed the mechanisms of rejection and improved the clinical ability to match tissues that would less likely be rejected. This led to the first bold attempt, in 1954, to transplant a kidney. Kidney transplants soon became a common clinical procedure for irreversible renal failure. The procedure, however, remained highly risky until the invention of dialysis provided a backup in the event of rejection. In 1969, the most startling surgical innovation, transplantation of a heart from cadaver to patient, was performed for the first time. Although the first patient and several sucessive ones died soon after the transplantation, surgeons throughout the world began to experiment, often with tragic results. The scientific excitement stimulated by transplantation, the hope of life for those doomed to death by organ failure, and the worldwide public interest coalesced to make organ transplantation one of the earliest topics for ethical reflection in the new medicine. Its great risks in the face of great hope, the scarcity of human organs, and, above all, the need to seek an organ from one person, living or dead, in order to help another—a situation unique in the history of medicine—called for serious ethical reflection. Kenneth Vaux, a theologian working at the University of Texas Medical Center in Houston, provided an early sample of that reflection (Vaux, 1968).

Experimentation with Human Subjects

The clinical advances of the 1950s and '60s, then, created clinical problems that the traditional medical morality had not imagined. Clinicians now had unprecedented skills to save life, but they were uncertain when and where to apply those skills. There were many more patients awaiting their help than they could accept into services: how should patients be selected? Once admitted, patients' lives might be salvaged but at great price to the quality of their remaining days: should this dismal expectation justify refraining from saving life? The application of these technologies was costly: should expense be taken into account in deciding to apply them? If not, who should pay? The technologies did not spring into existence perfectly efficacious: they needed to be tried, tested, and improved. Which patients would undergo this testing? How would medical advances appear without experimentation on human subjects? The traditional medical morality had not contemplated these questions, and its maxims did not address them. Thoughtful modern clinicians realized that and raised the questions in hopes that someone could help answer them. Answers to these difficult problems were hard to come by, but in the late '60s and early '70s, scholars from outside science and medicine joined in the inquiry. A distinct scholarly literature, which soon came to be called *bioethics*, appeared. An essay by Dan Callahan, one of the most influential figures in this emerging discipline, appears in this anthology (Callahan, 1973).

One of the most obvious candidates for exploration was experimentation with human beings. "Experimental medicine," in the sense of designed and controlled observation of the effects of disease and of medicine on living humans, was a creation of the medical scientists of the nineteenth century. Although earlier clinicians, such as Thomas Sydenham, had advocated and pioneered this approach, the exciting progress of physiology under such scientists as Claude Bernard made it an ideal. Bernard, author of the classic *An Introduction to the Study of Experimental Medicine* (1865), stated the ethics that should govern such work: "It is our duty and right to experiment on man whenever it can save his life, cure him, or gain him some personal benefit. The principle of medical and surgical morality, therefore, consists in never performing on man an experiment which might be harmful to him to any extent, even though the result might be highly advantageous to science, that is, to the health of others."[3]

Bernard's rigid rule, though noble, was unrealistic, for all experimentation is a journey into the unknown and poses some risk. The most famous experiments of that era, Walter Reed's attempts to determine the source of yellow fever, clearly exposed healthy persons, volunteers though they were, to the danger of death. The prospect of saving millions made it difficult to abide by Barnard's maxim. Even moral scientists pressed its limits; immoral scientists ignored it. The ultimate horrors of medical experimentation were revealed in the "scientific" work done by Nazi doctors in the concentration camps of World War II. Although Americans could hardly believe that such things would happen here, they learned that, indeed, similar things—perhaps less horrific but still unethical—did happen in American hospitals. The distinguished Harvard professor of anesthesiology, Henry Beecher, exposed twenty-two clinical investigations that he branded unethical. His article is printed in this anthology. If these studies, done by leading scientists and published in reputable journals, could be so branded, Beecher wondered how many other studies were being performed that were equally or more reprehensible? (Beecher, 1966).

Beecher's article was a specific indictment cast into an already growing stream of concern about the ethics of clinical research. The National Institutes of Health, beneficiary of Congressional largess, had grown from a tiny federal agency to a powerful engine of scientific research. It dispensed millions each year to investigators working in the nation's laboratories and hospitals and pushed the leading edge of clinical investigation in its own clinical center in Bethesda, Maryland. Although NIH imposed no special ethical rules on its extramural investigators, relying instead on the ethical probity of physicians to guard against abuse, its administrators began to worry about the absence of internal standards in their own hospital, where the experimental subjects were sometimes healthy volunteers and were often asked to expose themselves to undefinable risks. In 1963, the confidence of NIH administrators in their grantees' probity was shaken by reports that clinical investigators had injected cancer cells into unknowing elderly patients in a New York geriatric hospital. The beginnings of a regulatory system emerged; it was forced forward by the news that, from 1931 onward, the U.S Public Health Service has sponsored a study in which impoverished rural African Americans living in Tuskeegee, Alabama, were unknowingly deprived of treatment for syphylis in order to study the course of untreated disease.

The ethics of clinical research grew from concern and outrage over experiments that showed scientists and clinicians treating their patients with less than respect for their rights and welfare. One remedy for this failure would be to exhort clinician scientists to be more respectful and, indeed, this was the approach taken by many commentators, including Dr. Beecher himself. Another approach would be the creation of a set of stringent regulations that would legally bind researchers. Yet another approach would be to deepen understanding of what constitutes respect in the context of clinical investigation and attempt to create around that deeper understanding a new culture of research. At this point, sincere clinicial scientists could invite philosophers and theologians to participate in the discussion. The nature of respect and, indeed, the nature of experimentation—not as a scientific practice but as a social enterprise—were appropriate topics for those trained in the disciplines of theology and philosophy.

Conferences on the ethics of human experimentation began to be held in the mid-1960s and philosophers and theologians were invited. At one such conference, a prominent philosopher, Hans Jonas, presented a paper that would become a classical statement of the moral standing of biomedical research. This anthology presents a brief selection from that paper. A theologian, John Fletcher, was admitted to the inner sanctum of the NIH Clinical Center as a graduate student studying the ethics of human experimentation. An article resulting from that experience is reprinted in this anthology (Fletcher, 1973). Fletcher was later invited to join the NIH staff permanently as assistant to the director for bioethics, a position in which he provided consultation to all clinical researchers on the ethical design of their work.

The discussion of the ethics of clinical investigation provided an opening event for the development of clinical ethics. Although scientific research in clinical settings is relatively uncommon, it is not rare. Most clinicians are not researchers and most patients are not experimental subjects, yet many hospitals— particularly those affiliated with medical schools—do sponsor clinical research, and many patients are invited to participate. In the early 1970s, the discussion of the ethics of research moved to a new plane. Congress, impelled to action by the revelations of the Tuskeegee experiments and several other federally funded examples of ethically questionable research, established the National Commission for the Protection of Human Subjects of Biomedical and Behavioral Research. This body, which joined scientists, legal scholars, and ethicists, was charged with developing "the ethical principles that should govern research with human subjects" and with "recommending regulations that would protect the rights and welfare of human subjects of research." As it performed these tasks from 1974 to 1978, the Commission invited scholars from many fields to contribute their analyses of topics such as "Consent," "The Benefit-Risk Ratio," "Respect or Autonomy," and "Children as Research Subjects." This endeavor contributed greatly to the field of bioethics, bringing into it many scholars who had not previously engaged in the study of such topics and producing a literature of considerable merit. In addition, many clinicians encountered bioethics for the first time when they were invited to sit on the institutional review boards of their hospitals, now required by the new federal regulations on research with human subjects.

To Save or Let Die

The common activities of clinical care contain many subtle ethical dimensions, such as the obligation of informing the patient frankly and honestly about his or her condition and treatment, the duty of faithful attendance, and the strictures of confidentiality. But nothing is as common and as agonizing as the confrontation with death. Physicians are trained to save life, yet their skills and technologies are limited. This has always been a hard truth of medicine and humility before the inevitability of death has been inculcated as a medical virtue throughout the centuries. As mentioned above, the advent of modern technologies gave physicians the power to produce effects that might not always be counted as benefits by the patient, to save life that was severely limited, to save some lives at the expense of others. Thus, the clinical problem of deciding whether to save or let die became, as Richard McCormick wrote in the article included in this anthology, the "dilemma of modern medicine" (McCormick, 1974).

By chance, the dilemma appeared dramatically in a short film that recorded the agonizing decision to allow an infant with Down's syndrome to die. The film, made at Johns Hopkins Hospital in 1971, was distributed by the Joseph P. Kennedy Foundation. It stimulated responses from several ethicists and became the focus of discussion in many incipient medical ethics courses in many medical schools. Two years later, Drs. Raymond Duff and A.G.M. Campbell published the article reprinted in this anthology that reported their own clinical experience with allowing babies to die in the special-care nursery (Duff and Campbell, 1973). Theologian Richard McCormick's essay attempted to analyze the ethical issues raised by this now-acknowledged practice. In an influential article, philosopher James Rachels asked whether the "allowing to die" that many ethicists now found acceptable differed in any morally relevant way from killing—a question that lingered in discussions of clinical ethics (Rachels, 1975).

The focus shifted from the intensive care nursery to the adult intensive care unit as hospitals realized that the technique of cardiopulmonary resuscitation developed during the 1960s was being applied to patients whose death was imminent from lethal disease. In 1976, the ethical and legal problem of allowing to die had leapt to public attention as the media covered the first case of this sort ever to reach an American court, the story of Karen Ann Quinlan. In the New Jersey Supreme Court's judgment, which granted to Ms. Quinlan's father the power to have her life support discontinued, the opinions of theologians and ethicists were cited. Theologian Paul Ramsey's commentary on the case is reprinted in this anthology (Ramsey, 1976). In the wake of that case, the idea of preparing a statement of one's wishes regarding care at the end of life was much discussed; the State of California passed legislation making such statements legally recognized documents.

Bioethics as a Discipline

The original topics of bioethics, then, were the new biology and its genetic implications, organ transplantation and experimentation with human subjects. These topics touched issues that were clinical, insofar as, in each of these endeavors, physicians interacted with patients. However, most physicians were not researchers, relatively few dealt with genetic disease, and very few were transplanters of organs. Still, once interest in the ethical dimensions of modern medicine had been kindled, it spread into the activities in which many practitioners engaged regularly. In 1979, Mark Siegler, an internist at the University of Chicago, coined the term *clinical ethics*, in an editorial inaugurating a series entitled, "Clinical Ethics" in the *Archives of Internal Medicine*. He wrote, "Clinical ethics, which focuses on issues that confront the physician in his daily interactions with patients, is to be contrasted with biomedical ethics, which is greatly concerned with public policy issues . . . Changes in modern medicine . . . have created an unanticipated range of ethical dilemmas that demand creative and reflective clinical response."[4]

Early issues such as genetic engineering and experimentation were somewhat remote from the activities of most physicians. The problems of caring for the seriously ill and dying patient is an intimate part of a physician's experience. Moral questions arise in daily practice for which the clinician inevitably has direct responsibility. Guidelines might be formulated, but their application requires discretion exercised in the ever-changing circumstances of cases. Callahan, writing in 1973, had suggested that "one important test of the acceptance of bioethics as a discipline will be the extent to which it is called upon by scientists and physicians. This means that it should be developed inductively, working at least initially from the kinds of problems scientists and physicians believe they face and need assistance on," and this problem will often involve "Mrs. Jones in ward 5 at 4:10 in the afternoon."[5] In 1975, Dan Clouser, the first philosopher to be appointed to a medical faculty in recent times, attempted to clarify the relation between medical ethicists and clinicians; his essay is included in this anthology (Clouser, 1975). Clearly, as he points out, persons trained in the language, methods, and topics of philosophy would view a clinical problem very differently than would physicians. Still, philosophers can help "structure the issues . . .

showing where various arguments and actions lead, what facts would be relevant, what concepts are crucial, and what moral principles are at issue and probably in conflict."[6]

During the 1970s, a few ethicists trained in philosophy or in theology became more involved in the world of clinical medicine. They moved from participation in the fascinating but somewhat abstract world of interdisciplinary discussion and analysis of bioethical issues into the daily activities of hospitals. Many were appointed to faculties of medical schools to teach medical ethics, and most of these engaged from time to time in the clinical rounds that are intrinsic to medical education. As they observed doctors at close range, they learned some of the esoteric language of clinical medicine and, more importantly, experienced something of the moral complexity of real cases. Although few of these ethicists were physicians, they became companions of physicians, finding collaborative ways and words to participate in the process of thinking through the ethical dimensions of a clinical decision about the care of a patient. The essay by Stephen Toulmin suggests some of the ways in which this collaboration revitalized moral philosophy itself (Toulmin, 1982).

No single systematic theory of ethics presided over this development of a new discipline: various philosophers and theologians utilized concepts and arguments from various approaches to morality. In their important 1979 text, *Principles of Biomedical Ethics*, Tom Beauchamp and James Childress showed how a range of theory and principle could be applied to the problems of biomedical ethics. If any one principle could be singled out as centrally influential in the early period of bioethics, it would be the principle of respect for autonomy. The prominence of this principle stems in large part from the debates over the ethics of human experimentation, in which the free and voluntary consent of the research subject is crucially important. In addition, a concern over an excessive paternalism of physicians in their relation to patients encouraged attention to the choices of patients regarding their care.[7]

The early history of clinical ethics can end here. It has shown the origins of the field of bioethics in the new biology and the new medicine of the post–World War II era. The revolution in genetics, the expansion of human experimentation, and especially the advent of organ transplanation, stirred interest in the moral dimensions of the medical world (psychopharmacology and reproduction, which we have not reviewed here, did so as well). All these innovations clearly had moral dimensions that dwarfed the medical morality of tradition. Each of them seemed to use human beings or change human nature in ways that had never been contemplated within the moral reflections of either philosophers or physicians. Thus, bioethics came into being.

Although moral concerns over these new practices often arose in the clinical situations in which they were used, the discussion frequently left the clinical situation and moved to the realm of abstract analysis and policy guidelines. However, in the 1970s, bioethics moved back into the clinical setting, enticed particularly by the ethical complexities of dealing with death under the conditions of the new medicine. The excerpts reproduced in the first section of this anthology represent some of the early efforts to merge the thinking and language of ethicists with that of clinicians.

References

1. Beauchamp, T., Childress, J. *Principles of Biomedical Ethics.* New York: Oxford University Press, 1st edition, 1979.
2. Bernard, C. *An Introduction to the Study of Experimental Medicine.* Ch. 2, iii, p. 101.
3. Callahan, D. "Bioethics as a discipline." *Hastings Center Report* 1973; 1: p. 73.
4. Clouser, K.D. Medical ethics: some uses, abuses, and limitations. *New England Journal of Medicine* 1975; p. 385.
4a. "Medical ethics, history of," In Reich, W. (ed.) *Encyclopedia of Bioethics.* 2d ed. New York: Macmillan, 1995.
5. Scribner, B. "Ethical problems of using artificial organs to sustain life." *Proceedings of the American Society of Artificial Internal Organs,* 1964.
6. Siegler, M. "Clinical ethics." *Archives of Internal Medicine* 1979; p. 915.

MORAL QUESTIONS AND THE "NEW BIOLOGY"

ॐ

The New Biology
What Price Relieving Man's Estate?

Leon R. Kass

Leon R. Kass is a physician with a strong philosophical bent. Beginning his career as a research scientist at the National Institutes of Health, he is now professor of humanities at the University of Chicago. His book *The New Biology* collects many of his trenchant essays on bioethics and the philosophy of medicine.

This essay represents one of the first sweeping reviews of the ethical implications of the "new biology" that was published in a leading scientific journal. The excerpts are but the opening paragraphs and one other section of a long article that presages many of the major questions bioethicists will ponder over the next several decades.

Recent advances in biology and medicine suggest that we may be rapidly acquiring the power to modify and control the capacities and activities of men by direct intervention and manipulation of their bodies and minds. Certain means are already in use or at hand, others await the solution of relatively minor technical problems, while yet others, those offering perhaps the most precise kind of control, depend upon further basic research. Biologists who have considered these matters disagree on the question of how much how soon, but all agree that the power for "human engineering," to borrow from the jargon, is coming and that it will probably have profound social consequences.

Leon R. Kass. "The New Biology: What Price Relieving Man's Estate?" Abridged from *Science* 1971, Volume 174, pp.779–790. Copyright © 1971 American Association for the Advancement of Science. Reprinted by permission.

These developments have been viewed both with enthusiasm and with alarm; they are only just beginning to receive serious attention. Several biologists have undertaken to inform the public about the technical possibilities, present and future. Practitioners of social science "futurology" are attempting to predict and describe the likely social consequences of and public responses to the new technologies. Lawyers and legislators are exploring institutional innovations for assessing new technologies. All of these activities are based upon the hope that we can harness the new technology of man for the betterment of mankind.

Yet this commendable aspiration points to another set of questions, which are, in my view, sorely neglected—questions that inquire into the meaning of phrases such as the "betterment of mankind." A *full* understanding of the new technology of man requires an exploration of ends, values, standards. What ends will or should the new techniques serve? What values should guide society's adjustments? By what standards should agencies assess? Behind these questions lie others: what is a good man, what is a good life for man, what is a good community? This article is an attempt to provoke discussion of these neglected and important questions.

While these questions about ends and ultimate ends are never unimportant or irrelevant, they have rarely been more important or more relevant. That this is so can be seen once we recognize that we are dealing here with a group of technologies that are in a decisive respect unique: the object upon which they operate is man himself. The technologies of energy or food production, of communication, of manufacture, and of motion greatly alter the implements available to man and the conditions in which he uses them. In contrast, the biomedical technology works to change the user himself. To be sure, the printing press, the automobile, the television, and the jet airplane have greatly altered the conditions under which and the way in which men live; but men as biological beings have remained largely unchanged. They have been, and remain, able to accept or reject, to use and abuse these technologies; they choose, whether wisely or foolishly, the ends to which these technologies are means. Biomedical technology may make it possible to change the inherent capacity for choice itself. Indeed, both those who welcome and those who fear the advent of "human engineering" ground their hopes and fears in the same prospect: *that man can for the first time recreate himself.* . . .

After this cursory review of the powers now and soon to be at our disposal, I turn to the questions concerning the use of these powers. First, we must recognize that questions of use of science and technology are always moral and political questions, never simply technical ones. All private or public decisions to develop or to use biomedical technology—and decisions *not* to do so—inevitably contain judgments about value. This is true even if the values guiding those decisions are not articulated or made clear, as indeed they often are not. Secondly, the value judgments cannot be derived from biomedical science. This is true even if scientists themselves make the decisions.

These important points are often overlooked for at least three reasons.

1) They are obscured by those who like to speak of "the control of nature by science." It is men who control, not that abstraction "science." Science may provide the means, but men choose the ends; the choice of ends comes from beyond science.

2) Introduction of new technologies often appears to be the result of no decision whatsoever, or of the culmination of decisions too small or unconscious to be recognized as such. What can be done is done. However, someone is deciding on the basis of some notions of desirability, no matter how self-serving or altruistic.

3) Desires to gain or keep money and power no doubt influence much of what happens, but these desires can also be formulated as reasons and then discussed and debated.

Insofar as our society has tried to deliberate about questions of use, how has it done so? Pragmatists that we are, we prefer a utilitarian calculus: we weigh "benefits" against "risks," and we weigh them for both the individual and "society." We often ignore the fact that the very definitions of "a benefit" and "a risk" are themselves based upon judgments about value. In the biomedical areas just reviewed, the benefits are considered to be self-evident: prolongation of life, control of fertility and of population size, treatment and prevention of genetic disease, the reduction of anxiety and aggressiveness, and the enhancement of memory, intelligence, and pleasure. The assessment of risk is, in general, simply pragmatic—will the technique work effectively and reliably, how much will it cost, will it do detectable bodily harm, and who will complain if we proceed with development? As these questions are familiar and congenial, there is no need to belabor them.

The very pragmatism that makes us sensitive to considerations of economic cost often blinds us to the larger social costs exacted by biomedical advances. For one thing, we seem to be unaware that we may not be able to maximize all the benefits, that several of the goals we are promoting conflict with each other. On the one hand, we seek to control population growth by lowering fertility; on the other hand, we develop techniques to enable every infertile woman to bear a child. On the one hand, we try to extend the lives of individuals with genetic disease; on the other, we wish to eliminate deleterious genes from the human population. I am not urging that we resolve these conflicts in favor of one side or the other, but simply that we recognize that such conflicts exist. Once we do, we are more likely to appreciate that most "progress" is heavily paid for in terms not generally included in the simple utilitarian calculus.

The Heart Transplant: Ethical Dimensions

Kenneth Vaux

When he wrote "The Heart Transplant," Kenneth Vaux was a Presbytrian professor of ethics at The Institute of Religion, Texas Medical Center, Houston. He had studied ethics with the German theologian, Helmut Thielicke, one of the first European scholars to write extensively on ethical issues in modern technological medicine. Hence, Vaux was prepared both by his training and by his presence in one of the pioneer transplant institutions to respond to the questions raised by this new technology. From 1979 until 1993, Vaux was professor of bioethics and director of the program in Medical Humanities at the School of Medicine, University of Illinois in Chicago.

In December, 1967, Dr. Christiaan Barnard performed the first human-to-human heart transplant in Cape Town, South Africa. This feat, which was replicated one month later, aroused worldwide admiration and considerable uneasiness about its ethics. Vaux describes the major ethical problems that were discussed and puts them into a context of the religious beliefs of the major Western religions.

The Judeo-Christian tradition which informs Western culture views the heart of man as the locus of the emotions that structure his life. Anger and hostility, love and compassion are all thought of as proceeding from the heart. Witness not only our common speech but also our poetry and art, our religion and philosophy. Thus Erich Fromm, in his recent book *The Heart of Man*, writes of the ambiguity of the impulses that proceed from the "heart," impulses at once creative and destructive. Fromm of course is speaking symbolically. But translated into physiological terms this view seems rather primitive. The fact is, however, that recent medical discoveries support the notion that the heart is the center of life. A human body can survive for years with very low-grade cerebral activity, in a complete coma. But without the presence of the pulsating heart life is soon extinguished. As *Time* magazine put it (issue of December 15, 1967, page 71): " . . . the heart is essential to life in a more immediate temporal sense than any other organ, even the brain.". . .

The Time and Meaning of Death

Our first problem of ethical significance concerns the time and meaning of death. When Denise Darvall arrived at the Cape Town hospital she was at the threshold of death. Although the electroencephalograph showed lingering impulses in her body, her heart had stopped. Dr. Marius Barnard (as quoted in the same issue of *Time* magazine, page 64) explained how his brother, Dr. Christiaan N. Barnard, and the surgical team made their decision to remove her heart. "I know," he said, "in some places they consider the patient dead when the electroencephalogram shows no more brain function. We are on the conservative side, and consider a patient dead when the heart is no longer working and there are no longer any complexes on the electrocardiogram."

What is the correct index to determine the time of death? Is it heart or brain function? Is there a distinction between existence and life? Is sustained physiological activity without any relational capacity really human life? When a man has lost the capacity to respond to both external and existential environment, is he still a man? Are we justified in hastening natural death? Are we justified in extending life through extraordinary measures? Our culture is now being forced to grapple with these extremely difficult questions.

In heart transplantation it is urgently necessary that the donated heart be as fresh as possible. This necessity raises the profound ethical problem of who decides—and how—whether and when a person is dead. The case of Clive Haupt, the second of the South African heart donors, points up this question. After his stroke on the beach he was immediately treated as a potential heart donor rather than as a present stroke victim—a fact that raises the shocking specter of a future day of corpse snatching. *Newsweek* (December 18, 1967, page 87) quotes a public health official in Washington: "I have a horrible vision of ghouls hovering over an accident victim with long knives unsheathed, waiting to take out his organs as soon as he is pronounced dead." Here perhaps is the ethical issue on which heart transplantation focuses. As Dr. Michael DeBakey—a pioneer in the field of heart surgery—notes in an article soon to be published: "The controversy has resumed on this point, with proposals for a new criterion of death based, for example, on electroencephalographic findings and other demonstrable evidence of cessation of vital cellular function. The legal, moral, and theologic aspects of this problem are intricate and formidable, but not impenetrable." . . .

The Question of Consent

Our second ethical problem area concerns the question of consent by donor and recipient. In the Cape Town case, to be sure, the problem hardly arose. Louis Washkansky, Dr. Barnard's patient, needed only two minutes to make a decision that he could have taken two hours for. He agreed at once to have his heart cut out and replaced with a donor's. Edward Darvall, Denise's father, also made a decision immediately. When the doctors told him, "There is no hope for her. You can do us and humanity a great favor if you let us transplant your daughter's heart," Darvall answered: "If there is no hope for her, then try to save this man's life."

But the problem of consent is frequently much more complex. What, for instance, if neither the donor nor recipient is able to decide for himself—which member of his family has the power of decision? The Clive Haupt case illustrates this problem. His bride of three months collapsed when she was asked to permit removal of his heart. His mother finally consented to the removal. . . .

There is also the identity problem which may arise on the side of both donor and recipient. Thus Philip Blaiberg, Dr. Barnard's second transplant recipient, said he felt like a different person, and he appeared so to his daughter when she flew to his bedside from her studies in Israel. And to Louis Washkansky's death Mr. Darvall reacted pathetically: "I have nothing left to live for. My daughter lived on for a while; now all is gone."

Who Decides Who Shall Receive?

But the most difficult question in this matter is that of which among the many persons who need it is to receive one of the few available hearts. Perhaps some day there will be organ banks and a multitude of card-carrying donors. Not so at present. Moreover, in a "Face the Nation" television interview on December 24, 1967, Dr. Barnard revealed a medical attitude that compounds this problem. "My duty as a doctor," he said, "is to treat my patient. The donor I could treat no longer. I had only one way to treat my patient: transplant. To me that's not immoral." Of course he is absolutely right. The genius of the medical profession is the single-minded devotion of the physician to an individual patient. Yet when there are hundreds of thousands of desperately ill coronary patients, who decides who shall be given a new heart? What are the criteria of this decision? Will the transplant technique be available only to people who have money or connections? In other words, there is a social-ethical issue here. The physician's devotion to his patient must be augmented by social concern. . . .

Let us now look at this whole problem in the light of the three ethical options that shape our culture: the Jewish-humanitarian, the situation-ethic, and the Roman Catholic natural-law options.

Rabbi Immanuel Jacobovits, chief rabbi of the British Commonwealth, has said (according to the issue of *Newsweek* cited above) that the most profound ethical question regarding heart transplantation is the termination of the life of the donor. He holds that even the minutest fraction of life is precious and that morally speaking, we have no right to terminate life, though only minimal hope exists or none at all. . . .

Christian theology also emphasizes the sanctity of life. Opposed to the fatalism of "When your number's up, it's up," Christianity declares that man must struggle for life incessantly. As Dietrich Bonhoeffer has put it: "It is only when one loves life and the earth so much that without them everything else would seem lost and gone, that one can believe in the resurrection of the dead."

Our second option, that of situation ethics, holds that each particular person, each particular instance is unique and must be evaluated in its uniqueness. The remarks by Christiaan Barnard cited above emphasize the high humanism of a decision motivated by concern for a specific person in a specific situation. Dr.

Barnard's posture shows freedom from legalistic norms, along with compassion springing from deep ethical principles. . . .

At this point the situationist could refer to what both Christianity and other world religions consider the highest ethical act man is capable of; namely, the sacrifice of his own life for another's. Christians believe that this principle was personified in Jesus Christ, who said, "Greater love hath no man than this, that a man lay down his life for his friend" (John 15:13). Thus the situationist in ethics would say that the decision to transplant a heart, though fraught with dangerous concessions all the way, is one that basically affirms the preciousness of human life, and at the same time opens an opportunity for the highest form of self-sacrifice.

We turn now to the Roman Catholic option, which, because it is organized around a single principle, offers the most systematic moral theory in regard to our problem. That principle, simply stated, is that any violation or abrogation of the natural process is wrong; for such intervention strikes at the mysterious beauty of that divinely instituted and directed process, the origin and development of life.

Bringing this principle to bear on the question of heart transplants, the Vatican newspaper, *L'Osservatore Romano*, declared that the heart is a physiological organ with a purely mechanical function. This view has been echoed by Dr. Thomas O'Donnell, former lecturer in medical ethics at Georgetown University School of Medicine, a Jesuit institution. O'Donnell (as cited in the issue of *Newsweek* mentioned above) regards the heart as "an efficient pump with no intrinsic moral significance." In other words, the natural-law position would consider radical techniques justified when they enrich and extend the life of man, provided that there is no moral violation at any other point. Specifically, the requirements are approval from the next of kin and the assurance that the donor is medically dead. . . .

We must admit, however, that so far as heart transplantation is concerned, no clear moral directive issues from any one or all of these positions. This is not surprising. Such directives have never been easily arrived at; in our complex society they are almost always ambiguous. The one thing that is clear in our time is this: technology can be used for the benefit of the individual and of society, or it can be used for destructive and dehumanizing ends. We must continually affirm the goodness of science when it works for the welfare of mankind; and we must continually be on guard lest science, however noble its professions, violate human dignity. With Robert Oppenheimer we must remember that what is technically desirable is not necessarily good.

Who Shall Live When Not All Can Live?

James F. Childress

James F. Childress began his teaching career in the Department of Religion, University of Virginia; he later taught at Georgetown University before returning to the University of Virginia as the Kornfeld Professor of Biomedical Ethics. He is the co-author, with Tom Beauchamp, of *Principles of Biomedical Ethics*, first published in 1979. This volume, in its fourth edition, is the leading exposition of the philosophical underpinnings and the practical application of biomedical ethics.

"Who Shall Live" comments on the problem of selecting patients for a scarce life-saving resource, as exemplified by the Seattle Selection Committee's policy of using "social worth" criteria to choose patients for dialysis. That policy had been strongly criticized by two law professors, David Sanders and Jesse Dukeminier, in their article, "Medical Advance and Legal Lag: Hemodialysis and Kidney Transplantation" (*UCLA Law Review* 1968; 15: 366–380) and implicitly defended by philosopher Nicholas Rescher in one of the earliest philosophical contributions to the field of bioethics, "The Allocation of Exotic Medical Lifesaving Therapy," (*Ethics* 1969; 79: 173–186). Childress agrees with the broad criticism made by Sanders and Dukeminier and attempts to craft an ethical position contrary to the utilitarianism of Rescher.

Who shall live when not all can live? Although this question has been urgently forced upon us by the dramatic use of artificial internal organs and organ transplantations, it is hardly new.

A significant example of the distribution of scarce medical resources is seen in the use of penicillin shortly after its discovery. Military officers had to determine which soldiers would be treated—those with venereal disease or those wounded in combat.[1] In many respects such decisions have become routine in medical circles. Day after day physicians and others make judgments and decisions "about allocations of medical care to various segments of our population, to various types of hospitalized patients, and to specific individuals,"[2] for example, whether mental illness or cancer will receive the higher proportion of available funds. Nevertheless, the dramatic forms of "Scarce Life-Saving Medical Resources" (hereafter abbreviated as SLMR) such as hemodialysis and kidney and heart transplants have compelled us to examine the moral questions that have been concealed in many routine decisions. . . .

Just as current SLMR decisions are not totally discontinuous with other medical decisions, so we must ask whether some other cases might, at least by analogy, help us develop the needed criteria and procedures. Some have looked at the principles at work in our responses to abortion, euthanasia, and artificial

James F. Childress. "Who Shall Live When Not All Can Live." Abridged from *Soundings*, Volume 53, 1970, pp. 339–355. Reprinted by permission.

insemination.[3] Usually they have concluded that these cases do not cast light on the selection of patients for artificial and transplanted organs. The reason is evident: in abortion, euthanasia, and artificial insemination, there is no conflict of life with life for limited but indispensable resources (with the possible exception of therapeutic abortion). In current SLMR decisions, such a conflict is inescapable, and it makes them so morally perplexing and fascinating. If analogous cases are to be found, I think that we shall locate them in moral conflict situations.

Analogous Conflict Situations

An especially interesting and pertinent one is *U.S. v. Holmes*.[4] In 1841 an American ship, the *William Brown*, which was near Newfoundland on a trip from Liverpool to Philadelphia, struck an iceberg. The crew and half the passengers were able to escape in the two available vessels. One of these, a longboat, carrying too many passengers and leaking seriously, began to founder in the turbulent sea after about twenty-four hours. In a desperate attempt to keep it from sinking, the crew threw overboard fourteen men. Two sisters of one of the men either jumped overboard to join their brother in death or instructed the crew to throw them over. The criteria for determining who should live were "not to part man and wife, and not to throw over any women." Several hours later the others were rescued. Returning to Philadelphia, most of the crew disappeared, but one, Holmes, who had acted upon orders from the mate, was indicted, tried, and convicted on the charge of "unlawful homicide."

We are interested in this case from a moral rather than a legal standpoint, and there are several possible responses to and judgments about it. Without attempting to be exhaustive I shall sketch a few of these. The judge contended that lots should have been cast, for in such conflict situations, there is no other procedure "so consonant both to humanity and to justice." Counsel for Holmes, on the other hand, maintained that the "sailors adopted the only principle of selection which was possible in an emergency like theirs—a principle more humane than lots."

Another version of selection might extend and systematize the maxims of the sailors in the direction of "utility"; those are saved who will contribute to the greatest good for the greatest number. . . .

There are several significant differences between the *Holmes* and SLMR cases, a major one being that the former involves *direct* killing of another person, while the latter involve only *permitting* a person to die when it is not possible to save all. Furthermore, in extreme situations such as *Holmes*, the restraints of civilization have been stripped away, and something approximating a state of nature prevails, in which life is "solitary, poor, nasty, brutish and short." The state of nature does not mean that moral standards are irrelevant and that might should prevail, but it does suggest that much of the matrix which normally supports morality has been removed. Also, the necessary but unfortunate decisions about who shall live and die are made by men who are existentially and personally involved in the outcome. Their survival too is at stake. Even though the institutional role of sailors seems to require greater sacrificial actions, there is obviously no assurance that they will adequately assess the number of sailors required to man the vessel or that they will impartially and objectively weigh the common good at stake. As the judge insisted in his defense of casting lots in the *Holmes* case: "In no other way than this [casting lots] or some like way are those having equal rights put upon an equal footing, and in no other way is it possible to guard against partiality and oppression, violence, and conflict." This difference should not be exaggerated since self-interest, professional pride, and the like obviously affect the outcome of many medical decisions. Nor do the remaining differences cancel *Holmes'* instructiveness.

Criteria of Selection for SLMR

Which set of arrangements should be adopted for SLMR? Two questions are involved: Which standards and criteria should be used? and, Who should make the decision? The first question is basic, since the debate about implementation, e.g., whether by a lay committee or physician, makes little progress until the criteria are determined.

We need two sets of criteria which will be applied at two different stages in the selection of recipients of SLMR. First, medical criteria should be used to exclude those who are not "medically acceptable." Second, from this group of "medically acceptable" applicants, the final selection can be made. Occasionally in current American medical practice, the first stage is omitted, but such an omission is unwarranted. Ethical and social responsibility would seem to require distributing these SLMR only to those who have some reasonable prospect of responding to the treatment. Furthermore, in transplants such medical tests as tissue and blood typing are necessary, although they are hardly fully developed. . . .

The most significant moral questions emerge when we turn to the final selection. Once the pool of medically acceptable applicants has been defined and still the number is larger than the resources, what other criteria should be used? How should the final selection be made? First, I shall examine some of the difficulties that stem from efforts to make the final selection in terms of social value; these difficulties raise serious doubts about the feasibility and justifiability of the utilitarian approach. Then I shall consider the possible justification for random selection or chance.

Occasionally criteria of social worth focus on past contributions but most often they are primarily future-oriented. The patient's potential and probable contribution to the society is stressed, although this obviously cannot be abstracted from his present web of relationships (e.g., dependents) and occupational activities (e.g., nuclear physicist). Indeed, the magnitude of his contribution to society (as an abstraction) is measured in terms of these social roles, relations, and functions. Enough has already been said to suggest the tremendous range of factors that affect social value or worth.[5] Here we encounter the first major difficulty of this approach: How do we determine the relevant criteria of social value?

The difficulties of quantifying various social needs are only too obvious. How does one quantify and compare the needs of the spirit (e.g., education, art, religion), political life, economic activity, technological development? . . . I am not convinced that we can ever quantify values, or that we should attempt to do so. But even if the various social and human needs, in principle, could be quantified, how do we determine how much weight we will give to each one? Which will have priority in case of conflict? Or even more basically, in the light of which values and principles do we recognize social "needs"?

One possible way of determining the values which should be emphasized in selection has been proposed by Leo Shatin.[6] He insists that our medical decisions about allocating resources are already based on an unconscious scale of values (usually dominated by material worth). Since there is really no way of escaping this, we should be self-conscious and critical about it. How should we proceed? He recommends that we discover the values that most people in our society hold and then use them as criteria for distributing SLMR. These values can be discovered by attitude or opinion surveys. Presumably if fifty-one percent in this testing period put a greater premium on military needs than technological development, military men would have a greater claim on our SLMR than experimental researchers. But valuations of what is significant change, and the student revolutionary who was denied SLMR in 1970 might be celebrated in 1990 as the greatest American hero since George Washington.

Shatin presumably is seeking criteria that could be applied nationally, but at the present, regional and local as well as individual prejudices tincture the criteria of social value that are used in selection. Nowhere is this more evident than in the deliberations and decisions of the anonymous selection committee of the Seattle Artificial Kidney Center where such factors as church membership and Scout leadership have been deemed significant for determining who shall live.[7] As two critics conclude after examining these criteria and procedures, they rule out "creative nonconformists, who rub the bourgeoisie the wrong way but who historically have contributed so much to the making of America. The Pacific Northwest is no place for a Henry David Thoreau with bad kidneys."[8]

Closely connected to this first problem of determining social values is a second one. Not only is it difficult if not impossible to reach agreement on social values, but it is also rarely easy to predict what our needs will be in a few years and what the consequences of present actions will be. Furthermore it is difficult to predict which persons will fulfill their potential function in society. Admissions committees in colleges and universities experience the frustrations of predicting realization of potential. For these reasons, as someone has indicated, God might be a utilitarian, but we cannot be. We simply lack the capacity to predict very accurately the consequences which we then must evaluate. Our incapacity is never more evident than when we think in societal terms.

Other difficulties make us even less confident that such an approach to

SLMR is advisable. Many critics raise the spectre of abuse, but this should not be overemphasized. The fundamental difficulty appears on another level: the utilitarian approach would in effect reduce the person to his social role, relations, and functions. Ultimately it dulls and perhaps even eliminates the sense of the person's transcendence, his dignity as a person which cannot be reduced to his past or future contribution to society. It is not at all clear that we are willing to live with these implications of utilitarian selection. Wilhelm Kolff, who invented the artificial kidney, has asked: "Do we really subscribe to the principle that social standing should determine selection? Do we allow patients to be treated with dialysis only when they are married, go to church, have children, have a job, a good income and give to the Community Chest?"[9] . . .

The Values of Random Selection

My proposal is that we use some form of randomness or chance (either natural, such as "first come, first served," or artificial, such as a lottery) to determine who shall be saved. Many reject randomness as a surrender to non-rationality when responsible and rational judgments can and must be made. Edmond Cahn criticizes "Holmes' judge" who recommended the casting of lots because, as Cahn puts it, "the crisis involves stakes too high for gambling and responsibilities too deep for destiny."[10] Similarly, other critics see randomness as a surrender to "non-human" forces which necessarily vitiates human values. Sometimes these values are identified with the process of decision-making (e.g., it is important to have persons rather than impersonal forces determining who shall live). Sometimes they are identified with the outcome of the process (e.g., the features such as creativity and fullness of being which make human life what it is are to be considered and respected in the decision). Regarding the former, it must be admitted that the use of chance seems cold and impersonal. But presumably the defenders of utilitarian criteria in SLMR want to make their application as objective and impersonal as possible so that subjective bias does not determine who shall live.

Such criticisms, however, ignore the moral and nonmoral values which might be supported by selection by randomness or chance. A more important criticism is that the procedure that I develop draws the relevant moral context too narrowly. That context, so the argument might run, includes the society and its future and not merely the individual with his illness and claim upon SLMR. But my contention is that the values and principles at work in the narrower context may well take precedence over those operative in the broader context both because of their weight and significance and because of the weaknesses of selection in terms of social worth. As Paul Freund rightly insists, "The more nearly total is the estimate to be made of an individual, and the more nearly the consequence determines life and death, the more unfit the judgment becomes for human reckoning. . . . Randomness as a moral principle deserves serious study."[11] Serious study would, I think, point toward its implementation in certain conflict situations, primarily because it preserves a significant degree of *personal dignity* by providing *equality* of opportunity. Thus it cannot be dismissed as a "non-rational" and "non-human" procedure without an inquiry into the reasons, including human values, which might justify it. Paul Ramsey stresses this point about the *Holmes* case:

> Instead of fixing our attention upon "gambling" as the solution—with all the frivolous and often corrupt associations the word raises in our minds—we should think rather of *equality* of opportunity as the ethical substance of the relations of those individuals to one another that might have been guarded and expressed by casting lots.[12]

The individual's personal and transcendent dignity, which on the utilitarian approach would be submerged in his social role and function, can be protected and witnessed to by a recognition of his equal right to be saved. Such a right is best preserved by procedures which establish equality of opportunity. Thus selection by chance more closely approximates the requirements established by human dignity than does utilitarian calculation. It is not infallibly just, but it is preferable to the alternatives of letting all die or saving only those who have the greatest social responsibilities and potential contribution.

This argument can be extended by examining values other than individual dignity and equality of opportunity. Another basic value in the medical sphere is the relationship of trust between physician and patient. Which selection criteria are most in accord with this relationship of trust? Which will maintain, extend, and deepen it? My contention is that selection by randomness or chance is preferable from this standpoint too.

Trust, which is inextricably bound to respect for human dignity, is an attitude of expectation about another. It is not simply the expectation that another will perform a particular act, but more specifically that another will act toward him in certain ways—which will respect him as a person. . . . This trust cannot be preserved in life-and-death situations when a person expects decisions about him to be made in terms of his social worth, for such decisions violate his status as a person. An applicant rejected on grounds of inadequacy in social value or virtue would have reason for feeling that his "trust" had been betrayed. Indeed, the sense that one is being viewed not as an end in himself but as a means in medical progress or the achievement of a greater social good is incompatible with attitudes and relationships of trust. We recognize this in the billboard which was erected after the first heart transplants: "Drive Carefully. Christiaan Barnard Is Watching You." The relationship of trust between the physician and patient is not only an instrumental value in the sense of being an important factor in the patient's treatment. It is also to be endorsed because of its intrinsic worth as a relationship.

Thus the related values of individual dignity and trust are best maintained in selection by chance. But other factors also buttress the argument for this approach. Which criteria and procedures would men agree upon? We have to suppose a hypothetical situation in which several men are going to determine for themselves and their families the criteria and procedures by which they would want to be admitted to and excluded from SLMR if the need arose.[13] We need to assume two restrictions and then ask which set of criteria and procedures would be chosen as the most rational and, indeed, the fairest. The restrictions are these: (1) The men are *self-interested.* They are interested in their own welfare (and that of members of their families), and this, of course, includes survival. Basically, they are not motivated by altruism. (2) Furthermore, they are *ignorant* of their own talents, abilities, potential, and probable contribution to the social good. They do not know how they would fare in a competitive situation, e.g., the competition for SLMR in terms of social contribution. Under these conditions which institution would be chosen—letting all die, utilitarian selection, or the use of chance? Which would seem the most rational? the fairest? By which set of criteria would they want to be included in or excluded from the list of those who will be saved? The rational choice in this setting (assuming self-interest and ignorance of one's competitive success) would be random selection or chance since this alone provides equality of opportunity. A possible response is that one would prefer to take a "risk" and therefore choose the utilitarian approach. But I think not, especially since I added that the participants in this hypothetical situation are choosing for their children as well as for themselves; random selection or chance could be more easily justified to the children. It would make more sense for men who are self-interested but uncertain about their relative contribution to society to elect a set of criteria which would build in equality of opportunity. They would consider selection by chance as relatively just and fair.[14]

An important psychological point supplements earlier arguments for using chance or random selection. The psychological stress and strain among those who are rejected would be greater if the rejection is based on insufficient social worth than if it is based on chance. Obviously stress and strain cannot be eliminated in these borderline situations, but they would almost certainly be increased by the opprobrium of being judged relatively "unfit" by society's agents using society's values. . . .

In the framework that I have delineated, are the decrees of chance to be taken without exception? If we recognize exceptions, would we not open Pandora's box again just after we had succeeded in getting it closed? The direction of my argument has been against any exceptions, and I would defend this as the proper way to go. But let me indicate one possible way of admitting exceptions while at the same time circumscribing them so narrowly that they would be very rare indeed.

An obvious advantage of the utilitarian approach is that occasionally circumstances arise which make it necessary to say that one man is practically indispensable for a society in view of a particular set of problems it faces (e.g., the President when the nation is waging a war for survival). Certainly the argument to this point has stressed that the burden of proof would fall on those who think that the social danger in this instance is so great that they simply cannot abide by the outcome of a lottery or a first come, first served policy. Also, the reason must be negative rather than positive; that is, we depart from chance in this instance not because we want to take advantage of this person's potential contribution to the improvement of our society, but because his immediate loss would possibly (even probably) be disastrous (again, the President in a grave national emergency). Finally, social value (in the negative sense) should be used as a standard of exception in dialysis, for example, only if it would provide a reason strong enough to warrant removing another person from a kidney machine if all machines were taken. Assuming this strong reluctance to remove anyone once the commitment has been made for him, we would be willing to put this patient ahead of another applicant for a vacant machine only if we would be willing (in circumstances in which all machines are being used) to vacate a machine by removing someone from it. These restrictions would make an exception almost impossible.

While I do not recommend this procedure of recognizing exceptions, I think that one can defend it while accepting my general thesis about selection by randomness or chance. If it is used, a lay committee (perhaps advisory, perhaps even stronger) would be called upon to deal with the alleged exceptions since the doctors or others would in effect be appealing the outcome of chance (either natural or artificial). This lay committee would determine whether this patient was so indispensable at this time and place that he had to be saved even by sacrificing the values preserved by random selection. It would make it quite clear that exception is warranted, if at all, only as the "lesser of two evils." Such a defense would be recognized only rarely, if ever, primarily because chance and randomness preserve so many important moral and nonmoral values in SLMR cases.[15]

Notes

1. Henry K. Beecher, "Scarce Resources and Medical Advancement," *Daedalus* (Spring 1969), pp. 279–280.
2. Leo Shatin, "Medical Care and the Social Worth of a Man," *American Journal of Orthopsychiatry*, 36 (1967), 97.
3. Harry S. Abram and Walter Wadlington, "Selection of Patients for Artificial and Transplanted Organs," *Annals of Internal Medicine*, 69 (September 1968), 615–620.
4. *United States v. Holmes* 26 Fed. Cas. 360 (C.C.E.D. Pa. 1842). All references are to the text of the trial as reprinted in Philip E. Davis, ed., *Moral Duty and Legal Responsibility: A Philosophical-Legal Casebook* (New York, 1966), pp. 102–118.
5. I am excluding from consideration the question of the ability to pay because most of the people involved have to secure funds from other sources, public or private, anyway.
6. Leo Shatin, op. cit., pp. 96–101.
7. For a discussion of the Seattle selection committee, see Shana Alexander, "They Decide Who Lives, Who Dies," *Life*, 53 (Nov. 9, 1962), 102. For an examination of general selection practices in dialysis see "Scarce Medical Resources," *Columbia Law Review*, 69:620 (1969) and Harry S. Abram and Walter Wadlington, op cit.
8. David Sanders and Jesse Dukeminier, Jr., "Medical Advance and Legal Lag:

Hemodialysis and Kidney Transplantation." *UCLA Law Review* 15:367 (1968) 378.

9. "Letters and Comments," *Annals of Internal Medicine*, 61 (Aug. 1964), 360. Dr. G. E. Schreiner contends that "if you really believe in the right of society to make decisions on medical availability on these criteria you should be logical and say that when a man stops going to church or is divorced or loses his job, he ought to be removed from the programme and somebody else who fulfills these criteria substituted. Obviously no one faces up to this logical consequence" (G.E.W. Wolstenholme and Maeve O'Connor, eds. *Ethics in Medical Progress: With Special Reference to Transplantation.* A Ciba Foundation Symposium [Boston, 1966], p. 127).

10. Cahn, op. cit., p. 71.

11. Paul Freund, "Introduction," *Daedalus* (Spring 1969), xiii.

12. Paul Ramsey, *Nine Modern Moralists* (Englewood Cliffs, N.J., 1962), p. 245.

13. My argument is greatly dependent on John Rawls's version of justice as fairness, which is a reinterpretation of social contract theory. Rawls, however, would probably not apply his ideas to "borderline situations." See "Distributive Justice: Some Addenda," *Natural Law Forum*, 13 (1968), 53. For Rawls's general theory, see "Justice as Fairness," *Philosophy, Politics and Society* (Second Series), ed. by Peter Laslett and W. G. Runciman (Oxford, 1962), pp. 132–157 and Rawls's other essays on aspects of this topic.

14. Occasionally someone contends that random selection may reward vice. Leo Shatin (op. cit., p. 100) insists that random selection "would reward socially disvalued qualities by giving their bearers the same special medical care opportunities as those received by the bearers of socially valued qualities. Personally I do not favor such a method." Obviously society must engender certain qualities in its members, but not all of its institutions must be devoted to that purpose. Furthermore, there are strong reasons, I have contended, for exempting SLMR from that sort of function.

15. I read a draft of this paper in a seminar on "Social Implications of Advances in Biomedical Science and Technology: Artificial and Transplanted Internal Organs," sponsored by the Center for the Study of Science, Technology, and Public Policy of the University of Virginia, Spring 1970. I am indebted to the participants in that seminar, and especially to its leaders, Mason Willrich, Professor of Law, and Dr. Harry Abram, Associate Professor of Psychiatry, for criticisms which helped me to sharpen these ideas. Good discussions of the legal questions raised by selection (e.g., equal protection of the law and due process) which I have not considered can be found in "Scarce Medical Resources," *Columbia Law Review*, 69:620 (1969); "Patient Selection for Artificial and Transplanted Organs," *Harvard Law Review*, 82:1322 (1969); and Sanders and Dukeminier, op. cit.

Questions for Discussion
Part I, Section 1

1. Why should advances of undeniable benefit for deeper understanding of human health and development and for treatment of diseases be viewed with the suspicion shown by Kass?

2. According to Vaux, what were the central ethical concerns that attended the first human-to-human heart transplant in 1967? Do these concerns remain valid for new and innovative treatments today?

3. Do you agree with Childress's contention that patient selection for scarce resources should be based on some form of randomness, or chance, once medical selection criteria are exhausted?

EXPERIMENTATION AND HUMAN SUBJECTS

ầ

Ethics and Clinical Research*

Henry K. Beecher

Henry Beecher was Dorr Professor of Research in Anaesthesia at Harvard Medical School. He began to write about the ethical problems in experimentation with human subjects in the mid-1960s, and in "Ethics and Clinical Research" he offers in evidence twenty-two articles, written by prominent researchers and published in leading medical journals, in which patients were subjected to significant risk without adequate consent or any consent. Beecher had great difficulty having this article published and was severely criticized by many of his colleagues, but the article became a centerpiece in the evidence that biomedical research as practiced in the 1960s was an area ripe for ethical scrutiny.

Human experimentation since World War II has created some difficult problems with the increasing employment of patients as experimental subjects when it must be apparent that they would not have been available if they had been truly aware of the uses that would be made of them. Evidence is at hand that many of the patients in the examples to follow never had the risk satisfactorily explained to them, and it seems obvious that further hundreds have not known that they were the subjects of an experiment although grave consequences have been suffered as a direct result of experiments described here. There is a belief prevalent in some sophisticated circles that attention to

Henry K. Beecher. "Ethics and Clinical Research." Reprinted from *The New England Journal of Medicine* , Volume 274, 1966, pp. 1354–1360. Reprinted by permission of the *New England Journal of Medicine*. Copyright © 1966, *Massachusetts Medical Society*.

*From the Anaesthesia Laboratory of the Harvard Medical School at the Massachusetts General Hospital

these matters would "block progress." But, according to Pope Pius XII,[1] ". . . science is not the highest value to which all other orders of values . . . should be subordinated."

I am aware that these are troubling charges. They have grown out of troubling practices. They can be documented, as I propose to do, by examples from leading medical schools, university hospitals, private hospitals, governmental military departments (the Army, the Navy and the Air Force), governmental institutes (the National Institutes of Health), Veterans Administration hospitals and industry. The basis for the charges is broad.‡

I should like to affirm that American medicine is sound, and most progress in it soundly attained. There is, however, a reason for concern in certain areas, and I believe the type of activities to be mentioned will do great harm to medicine unless soon corrected. It will certainly be charged that any mention of these matters does a disservice to medicine, but not one so great, I believe, as a continuation of the practices to be cited.

Experimentation in man takes place in several areas: in self-experimentation; in patient volunteers and normal subjects; in therapy; and in the different areas of *experimentation on a patient not for his benefit but for that, at least in theory, of patients in general.* The present study is limited to this last category.

Reasons for Urgency of Study

Ethical errors are increasing not only in numbers but in variety—for example, in the recently added problems arising in transplantation of organs.

There are a number of reasons why serious attention to the general problem is urgent.

Of transcendent importance is the enormous and continuing increase in available funds, as shown below.

Money Available for Research Each Year

Massachusetts General Hospital		National Institutes of Health*	
1945	$ 500,000†	$ 701,800
1955	2,222,816	36,063,200
1965	8,384,342	436,600,000

*National Institutes of Health figures based upon decade averages, excluding funds for construction, kindly supplied by Dr. John Sherman, of National Institutes of Health.

†Approximation, supplied by Mr. David C. Crockett, of Massachusetts General Hospital.

---

‡At the Brook Lodge Conference on "Problems and Complexities of Clinical Research" I commented that "what seem to be breaches of ethical conduct in experimentation are by no means rare, but are almost, one fears, universal." I thought it was obvious that I was by "universal" referring to the fact that examples could easily be found in *all* categories where research in man takes place to any significant extent. Judging by press comments, that was not obvious: hence, this note.

Since World War II the annual expenditure for research (in large part in man) in the Massachusetts General Hospital has increased a remarkable 17-fold. At the National Institutes of Health, the increase has been a gigantic 624-fold. This "national" rate of increase is over 36 times that of the Massachusetts General Hospital. These data, rough as they are, illustrate vast opportunities and concomitantly expanded responsibilities.

Taking into account the sound and increasing emphasis of recent years that experimentation in man must precede general application of new procedures in therapy, plus the great sums of money available, there is reason to fear that these requirements and these resources may be greater than the supply of responsible investigators. All this heightens the problems under discussion.

Medical schools and university hospitals are increasingly dominated by investigators. Every young man knows that he will never be promoted to a tenure post, to a professorship in a major medical school, unless he has proved himself as an investigator. If the ready availability of money for conducting research is added to this fact, one can see how great the pressures are on ambitious young physicians.

Implementation of the recommendations of the President's Commission on Heart Disease, Cancer and Stroke means that further astronomical sums of money will become available for research in man.

In addition to the foregoing three practical points there are others that Sir Robert Platt[2] has pointed out: a general awakening of social conscience; greater power for good or harm in new remedies, new operations and new investigative procedures than was formerly the case; new methods of preventive treatment with their advantages and dangers that are now applied to communities as a whole as well as to individuals, with multiplication of the possibilities for injury; medical science has shown how valuable human experimentation can be in solving problems of disease and its treatment; one can therefore anticipate an increase in experimentation; and the newly developed concept of clinical research as a profession (for example, clinical pharmacology)—and this, of course, can lead to unfortunate separation between the interests of science and the interests of the patient.

Frequency of Unethical or Questionably Ethical Procedures

Nearly everyone agrees that ethical violations do occur. The practical question is, how often? A preliminary examination of the matter was based on 17 examples, which were easily increased to 50. These 50 studies contained references to 186 further likely examples, on the average 3.7 leads per study; they at times overlapped from paper to paper, but this figure indicates how conveniently one can proceed in a search for such material. The data are suggestive of widespread problems, but there is need for another kind of information, which was obtained by examination of 100 consecutive human studies published in 1964, in an excellent journal; 12 of these seemed to be unethical. If only one quarter of them is truly unethical, this still indicates the existence of a serious situation. Pappworth,[3] in England, has collected, he says, more than 500 papers based upon unethical experimentation. It is evident from such observations that unethical or questionably ethical procedures are not uncommon.

The Problem of Consent

All so-called codes are based on the bland assumption that meaningful or informed consent is readily available for the asking. As pointed out elsewhere,[4] this is very often not the case. Consent in any fully informed sense may not be obtainable. Nevertheless, except, possibly, in the most trivial situations, it remains a goal toward which one must strive for sociologic, ethical and clear-cut legal reasons. There is no choice in the matter.

If suitably approached, patients will accede, on the basis of trust, to about any request their physician may make. At the same time, every experienced clinician investigator knows that patients will often submit to inconvenience and some discomfort, if they do not last very long, but the usual patient will never agree to jeopardize seriously his health or his life for the sake of "science."

In only 2 of the 50* examples originally compiled for this study was consent mentioned. Actually, it should be emphasized in all cases for obvious moral and legal reasons, but it would be unrealistic to place much dependence on it. In any precise sense statements regarding consent are meaningless unless one knows how fully the patient was informed of all risks, and if these are not known, that fact should also be made clear. A far more dependable safeguard than consent is the presence of a truly *responsible* investigator.

Examples of Unethical or Questionably Ethical Studies

These examples are not cited for the condemnation of individuals; they are recorded to call attention to a variety of ethical problems found in experimental medicine, for it is hoped that calling attention to them will help to correct abuses present. During ten years of study of these matters it has become apparent that thoughtlessness and carelessness, not a willful disregard of the patient's rights, account for most of the cases encountered. Nonetheless, it is evident that in many of the examples presented, the investigators have risked the health or the life of their subjects. No attempt has been made to present the "worst" possible examples; rather, the aim has been to show the variety of problems encountered.

References to the examples presented are not given, for there is no intention of pointing to individuals, but rather, a wish to call attention to widespread practices. All, however, are documented to the satisfaction of the editors of the *[New England] Journal [of Medicine]*.

---

*Reduced here to 22 for reasons of space.

Known Effective Treatment Withheld

Example 1. It is known that rheumatic fever can usually be prevented by adequate treatment of streptococcal respiratory infections by the parenteral administration of penicillin. Nevertheless, definitive treatment was withheld, and placebos were given to a group of 109 men in service, while benzathine penicillin G was given to others.

The therapy that each patient received was determined automatically by his military serial number arranged so that more men received penicillin than received placebo. In the small group of patients studied 2 cases of acute rheumatic fever and 1 of acute nephritis developed in the control patients, whereas these complications did not occur among those who received the benzathine penicillin G.

Example 2. The sulfonamides were for many years the only antibacterial drugs effective in shortening the duration of acute streptococcal pharyngitis and in reducing its suppurative complications. The investigators in this study undertook to determine if the occurrence of the serious nonsuppurative complications, rheumatic fever and acute glomerulonephritis, would be reduced by this treatment. This study was made despite the general experience that certain antibiotics, including penicillin, will prevent the development of rheumatic fever.

The subjects were a large group of hospital patients; a control group of approximately the same size, also with exudative Group A streptococcus, was included. The latter group received only non-specific therapy (no sulfadiazine). The total group denied the effective penicillin comprised over 500 men.

Rheumatic fever was diagnosed in 5.4 per cent of those treated with sulfadiazine. In the control group rheumatic fever developed in 4.2 per cent.

In reference to this study a medical officer stated in writing that the subjects were not informed, did not consent and were not aware that they had been involved in an experiment, and yet admittedly 25 acquired rheumatic fever. According to this same medical officer *more than 70* who had had known definitive treatment withheld were on the wards with rheumatic fever when he was there.

Example 3. This involved a study of the relapse rate in typhoid fever treated in two ways. In an earlier study by the present investigators chloramphenicol had been recognized as an effective treatment for typhoid fever, being attended by half the mortality that was experienced when this agent was not used. Others had made the same observations, indicating that to withhold this effective remedy can be a life-or-death decision. The present study was carried out to determine the relapse rate under the two methods of treatment; of 408 charity patients 251 were treated with chloramphenicol, of whom 20, or 7.97 per cent, died. Symptomatic treatment was given, but chloramphenicol was withheld in 157, of whom 36, or 22.9 per cent, died. According to the data presented, 23 patients died in the course of this study who would not have been expected to succumb if they had received specific therapy.

Study of Therapy

Example 4. TriA (triacetyloleandomycin) was originally introduced for the treatment of infection with gram-positive organisms. Spotty evidence of hepatic dysfunction emerged, especially in children, and so the present study was undertaken on 50 patients, including mental defectives or juvenile delinquents who were inmates of a children's center. No disease other than acne was present; the drug was given for treatment of this. The ages of the subjects ranged from thirteen to thirty-nine years. "By the time half the patients had received the drug for four weeks, the high incidence of significant hepatic dysfunction . . . led to the discontinuation of administration to the remainder of the group at three weeks." (However, only two weeks after the start of the administration of the drug, 54 per cent of the patients showed abnormal excretion of bromsulfalein.) Eight patients with marked hepatic dysfunction were transferred to the hospital "for more intensive study." Liver biopsy was carried out in these 8 patients and repeated in 4 of them. Liver damage was evident. Four of these hospitalized patients, after their liver-function tests returned to normal limits, received a "challenge" dose of the drug. Within two days hepatic dysfunction was evident in 3 of the 4 patients. In 1 patient a second challenge dose was given after the first challenge and again led to evidence of abnormal liver function. Flocculation tests remained abnormal in some patients as long as five weeks after discontinuance of the drug.

Physiologic Studies

Example 5. In this controlled, double-blind study of the hematologic toxicity of chloramphenicol, it was recognized that chloramphenicol is "well known as a cause of aplastic anemia" and that there is a "prolonged morbidity and high mortality of aplastic anemia" and that ". . . chloramphenicol-induced aplastic anemia can be related to dose . . ." The aim of the study was "further definition of the toxicology of the drug. . . ."

Forty-one randomly chosen patients were given either 2 or 6 gm. of chloramphenicol per day; 12 control patients were used. "Toxic bone-marrow depression, predominantly affecting erythropoiesis, developed in 2 of 20 patients given 2.0 gm. and in 18 of 21 given 6 gm. of chloramphenicol daily." The smaller dose is recommended for routine use.

Example 6. In a study of the effect of thymectomy on the survival of skin homografts 18 children, three and a half months to eighteen years of age, about to undergo surgery for congenital heart disease, were selected. Eleven were to have total thymectomy as part of the operation, and 7 were to serve as controls. As part of the experiment, full-thickness skin homografts from an unrelated adult donor were sutured to the chest wall in each case. (Total thymectomy is occasionally, although not usually part of the primary cardiovascular surgery involved, and whereas it may not greatly add to the hazards of the necessary operation, its eventual effects in children are not known.) This work was proposed as part of a long-range study of "the growth and development of these children over the years." No difference in the survival of the skin homograft was observed in the 2 groups.

Example 7. This study of cyclopropane anesthesia and cardiac arrhythmias consisted of 31 patients. The average duration of the study was three hours, ranging from two to four and a half hours. "Minor surgical procedures" were carried out in all but 1 subject. Moderate to deep anesthesia, with endotracheal intubation and controlled respiration, was used. Carbon dioxide was injected into the closed respiratory system until cardiac arrhythmias appeared. Toxic levels of carbon dioxide were achieved and maintained for considerable periods. During the cyclopropane anesthesia a variety of pathologic cardiac arrhythmias occurred. When the carbon dioxide tension was elevated above normal, ventricular extrasystoles were more numerous than when the carbon dioxide tension was normal, ventricular arrhythmias being continuous in 1 subject for ninety minutes. (This can lead to fatal fibrillation.)

Example 8. Since the minimum blood-flow requirements of the cerebral circulation are not accurately known, this study was carried out to determine "cerebral hemodynamic and metabolic changes . . . before and during acute reductions in arterial pressure induced by drug administration and/or postural adjustments." Forty-four patients whose ages varied from the second to the tenth decade were involved. They included normotensive subjects, those with essential hypertension and finally a group with malignant hypertension. Fifteen had abnormal electrocardiograms. Few details about the reasons for hospitalization are given.

Signs of cerebral circulatory insufficiency, which were easily recognized, included confusion and in some cases a nonresponsive state. By alteration in the tilt of the patient "the clinical state of the subject could be changed in a matter of seconds from one of alertness to confusion, and for the remainder of the flow, the subject was maintained in the latter state." The femoral arteries were cannulated in all subjects, and the internal jugular veins in 14.

The mean arterial pressure fell in 37 subjects from 109 to 48 mm. of mercury, with signs of cerebral ischemia. "With the onset of collapse, cardiac output and right ventricular pressures decreased sharply."

Since signs of cerebral insufficiency developed without evidence of coronary insufficiency the authors concluded that "the brain may be more sensitive to acute hypotension than is the heart."

Example 9. This is a study of the adverse circulatory responses elicited by intra-abdominal maneuvers:

> When the peritoneal cavity was entered, a deliberate series of maneuvers was carried out [in 68 patients] to ascertain the effective stimuli and the areas responsible for development of the expected circulatory changes. Accordingly, the surgeon rubbed

localized areas of the parietal and visceral peritoneum with a small ball sponge as discretely as possible. Traction on the mesenteries, pressure in the area of the celiac plexus, traction on the gallbladder and stomach, and occlusion of the portal and caval veins were the other stimuli applied.

Thirty-four of the patients were sixty years of age or older; 11 were seventy or older. In 44 patients the hypotension produced by the deliberate stimulation was "moderate to marked." The maximum fall produced by manipulation was from 200 systolic, 105 diastolic, to 42 systolic, 20 diastolic; the average fall in mean pressure in 26 patients was 53 mm. of mercury.

Of the 50 patients studied, 17 showed either atrioventricular dissociation with nodal rhythm or nodal rhythm alone. A decrease in the amplitude of the T wave and elevation or depression of the ST segment were noted in 25 cases in association with manipulation and hypotension or, at other times, in the course of anesthesia and operation. In only 1 case was the change pronounced enough to suggest myocardial ischemia. No case of myocardial infarction was noted in the group studied although routine electrocardiograms were not taken after operation to detect silent infarcts. Two cases in which electrocardiograms were taken after operation showed T-wave and ST-segment changes that had not been present before.

These authors refer to a similar study in which more alarming electrocardiographic changes were observed. Four patients in the series sustained silent myocardial infarctions; most of their patients were undergoing gallbladder surgery because of associated heart disease. It can be added further that in the 34 patients referred to above as being sixty years of age or older, some doubtless had heart disease that could have made risky the maneuvers carried out. In any event, this possibility might have been a deterrent.

Example 10. Starling's law—"that the heart output per beat is directly proportional to the diastolic filling"—was studied in 30 adult patients with atrial fibrillation and mitral stenosis sufficiently severe to require valvulotomy. "Continuous alterations of the length of a segment of left ventricular muscle were recorded simultaneously in 13 of these patients by means of a mercury-filled resistance gauge sutured to the surface of the left ventricle." Pressures in the left ventricle were determined by direct puncture simultaneously with the segment length in 13 patients and without the segment length in an additional 13 patients. Four similar unanesthetized patients were studied through catheterization of the left side of the heart transeptally. In all 30 patients arterial pressure was measured through the catheterized brachial artery.

Example 11. To study the sequence of ventricular contraction in human bundle-branch block, simultaneous catheterization of both ventricles was performed in 22 subjects; catheterization of the right side of the heart was carried out in the usual manner; the left side was catheterized transbronchially. Extrasystoles were produced by tapping on the epicardium in subjects with normal myocardium while they were undergoing thoracotomy. Simultaneous pressures were measured in both ventricles through needle puncture in this group.

The purpose of this study was to gain increased insight into the physiology involved.

Example 12.   This investigation was carried out to examine the possible effect of vagal stimulation on cardiac arrest. The authors had in recent years transected the homolateral vagus nerve immediately below the origin of the recurrent laryngeal nerve as palliation against cough and pain in bronchogenic carcinoma. Having been impressed with the number of reports of cardiac arrest that seemed to follow vagal stimulation, they tested the effects of intrathoracic vagal stimulation during 30 of their surgical procedures, concluding, from these observations in patients under satisfactory anesthesia, that cardiac irregularities and cardiac arrest due to vagovagal reflex were less common than had previously been supposed.

Example 13.   This study presented a technic for determining portal circulation time and hepatic blood flow. It involved the transcutaneous injection of the spleen and catheterization of the hepatic vein. This was carried out in 43 subjects, of whom 14 were normal; 16 had cirrhosis (varying degrees), 9 acute hepatitis, and 4 hemolytic anemia.

No mention is made of what information was divulged to the subjects, some of whom were seriously ill. This study consisted in the development of a technic, not of therapy, in the 14 normal subjects.

Studies to Improve the Understanding of Disease

Example 14.   In this study of the syndrome of impending hepatic coma in patients with cirrhosis of the liver certain nitrogenous substances were administered to 9 patients with chronic alcoholism and advanced cirrhosis: ammonium chloride, di-ammonium citrate, urea or dietary protein. In all patients a reaction that included mental disturbances, a "flapping tremor" and electroencephalographic changes developed. Similar signs had occurred in only 1 of the patients before these substances were administered:

> The first sign noted was usually clouding of the consciousness. Three patients had a second or a third course of administration of a nitrogenous substance with the same results. It was concluded that marked resemblance between this reaction and impending hepatic coma, implied that the administration of these [nitrogenous] substances to patients with cirrhosis may be hazardous.

Example 15.   The relation of the effects of ingested ammonia to liver disease was investigated in 11 normal subjects, 6 with acute virus hepatitis, 26 with cirrhosis, and 8 miscellaneous patients. Ten of these patients had neurologic changes associated with either hepatitis or cirrhosis.

The hepatic and renal veins were cannulated. Ammonium chloride was administered by mouth. After this, a tremor that lasted for three days developed in 1 patient. When ammonium chloride was ingested by 4 cirrhotic patients with tremor and mental confusion the symptoms were exaggerated during the test. The same thing was true of a fifth patient in another group.

Example 16.   This study was directed toward determining the period of infectivity of infectious hepatitis. Artificial induction of hepatitis was carried out in an institution for mentally defective children in which a mild form of hepatitis was endemic. The parents gave consent for the intramuscular injection or oral administration of the virus, but nothing is said regarding what was told them concerning the appreciable hazards involved.

A resolution adopted by the World Medical Association states explicitly: "Under no circumstances is a doctor permitted to do anything which would weaken the physical or mental resistance of a human being except from strictly therapeutic or prophylactic indications imposed in the interest of the patient." There is no right to risk an injury to 1 person for the benefit of others.

Example 17.   Live cancer cells were injected into 22 human subjects as part of a study of immunity to cancer. According to a recent review, the subjects (hospitalized patients) were "merely told they would be receiving 'some cells' "— ". . . the word cancer was entirely omitted. . . ."

Example 18.   Melanoma was transplanted from a daughter to her volunteering and informed mother, "in the hope of gaining a little better understanding of cancer immunity and in the hope that the production of tumor antibodies might be helpful in the treatment of the cancer patient." Since the daughter died on the day after the transplantation of the tumor into her mother, the hope expressed seems to have been more theoretical than practical, and the daughter's condition was described as "terminal" at the time the mother volunteered to be a recipient. The primary implant was widely excised on the twenty-fourth day after it had been placed in the mother. She died from metastatic melanoma on the four hundred and fifty-first day after transplantation. The evidence that this patient died of diffuse melanoma that metastasized from a small piece of transplanted tumor was considered conclusive.

Technical Study of Disease

Example 19.   During bronchoscopy a special needle was inserted through a bronchus into the left atrium of the heart. This was done in an unspecified number of subjects, both with cardiac disease and with normal hearts.

The technic [sic] was a new approach whose hazards were at the beginning quite unknown. The subjects with normal hearts were used, not for their possible benefit but for that of patients in general.

Example 20. The percutaneous method of catheterization of the left side of the heart has, it is reported, led to 8 deaths (1.09 per cent death rate) and other serious accidents in 732 cases. There was, therefore, need for another method, the transbronchial approach, which was carried out in the present study in more than 500 cases, with no deaths.

Granted that a delicate problem arises regarding how much should be discussed with the patients involved in the use of a new method, nevertheless where the method is employed in a given patient for *his* benefit, the ethical problems are far less than when this potentially extremely dangerous method is used "in 15 patients with normal hearts, undergoing bronchoscopy for other reasons." Nothing was said about what was told any of the subjects, and nothing was said about the granting of permission, which was certainly indicated in the 15 normal subjects used.

Example 21. This was a study of the effect of exercise on cardiac output and pulmonary-artery pressure in 8 "normal" persons (that is, patients whose diseases were not related to the cardiovascular system), in 8 with congestive heart failure severe enough to have recently required complete bed rest, in 6 with hypertension, in 2 with aortic insufficiency, in 7 with mitral stenosis and in 5 with pulmonary emphysema.

Intracardiac catheterization was carried out, and the catheter then inserted into the right or left main branch of the pulmonary artery. The brachial artery was usually catheterized; sometimes, the radial or femoral arteries were catheterized. The subjects exercised in a supine position by pushing their feet against weighted pedals. "The ability of these patients to carry on sustained work was severely limited by weakness and dyspnea." Several were in severe failure. This was not a therapeutic attempt but rather a physiologic study.

Bizarre Study

Example 22. There is a question whether ureteral reflux can occur in the normal bladder. With this in mind, vesicourethrography was carried out on 26 normal babies less than forty-eight hours old. The infants were exposed to x-rays while the bladder was filling and during voiding. Multiple spot films were made to record the presence or absence of ureteral reflux. None was found in this group, and fortunately no infection followed the catheterization. What the results of the extensive x-ray exposure may be, no one can yet say.

Comment on Death Rates

In the foregoing examples a number of procedures, some with their own demonstrated death rates, were carried out. The following data were provided by 3 distinguished investigators in the field and represent widely held views.

Cardiac catheterization: right side of the heart, about 1 death per 1000 cases; left side, 5 deaths per 1000 cases. "Probably considerably higher in some places, depending on the portal of entry." (One investigator had 15 deaths in his first 150 cases.) It is possible that catheterization of a hepatic vein or the renal vein would have a lower death rate than that of catheterization of the right side of the heart, for if it is properly carried out, only the atrium is entered en route to the liver or the kidney, not the right ventricle, which can lead to serious cardiac irregularities. There is always the possibility, however, that the ventricle will be entered inadvertently. This occurs in at least half the cases, according to 1 expert—"but if properly done is too transient to be of importance."

Liver biopsy: the death rate here is estimated at 2 to 3 per 1000, depending in considerable part on the condition of the subject.

Anesthesia: the anesthesia death rate can be placed in general at about 1 death per 2000 cases. The hazard is doubtless higher when certain practices such as deliberate evocation of ventricular extrasystoles under cyclopropane are involved.

Publication

In the view of the British Medical Research Council[5] it is not enough to ensure that all investigation is carried out in an ethical manner: it must be made unmistakably clear in the publications that the proprieties have been observed. This implies editorial responsibility in addition to the investigator's. The question rises, then, about valuable data that have been improperly obtained.* It is my view that such material should not be published. There is a practical aspect to the matter: failure to obtain publication would discourage unethical experimentation. How many would carry out such experimentation if they *knew* its results would never be published? Even though suppression of such data (by not publishing it) would constitute a loss to medicine, in a specific localized sense, this loss, it seems, would be less important than the far reaching moral loss to medicine if the data thus obtained were to be published. Admittedly, there is room for debate. Others believe that such data, because of their intrinsic value, obtained at a cost of great risk or damage to the subjects, should not be wasted but should be published with stern editorial comment. This would have to be done with exceptional skill, to avoid an odor of hypocrisy.

Summary and Conclusions

The ethical approach to experimentation in man has several components; two are more important than the others, the first being informed consent. The

---

*As far as principle goes, a parallel can be seen in the recent Mapp decision by the United States Supreme Court. It was stated there that evidence unconstitutionally obtained cannot be used in any judicial decision, no matter how important the evidence is to the ends of justice.

difficulty of obtaining this is discussed in detail. But it is absolutely essential to *strive* for it for moral, sociologic and legal reasons. The statement that consent has been obtained has little meaning unless the subject or his guardian is capable of understanding what is to be undertaken and unless all hazards are made clear. If these are not known this, too, should be stated. In such a situation the subject at least knows that he is to be a participant in an experiment. Secondly, there is the more reliable safeguard provided by the presence of an intelligent, informed, conscientious, compassionate, responsible investigator.

Ordinary patients will not knowingly risk their health or their life for the sake of "science." Every experienced clinician investigator knows this. When such risks are taken and a considerable number of patients are involved, it may be assumed that informed consent has not been obtained in all cases.

The gain anticipated from an experiment must be commensurate with the risk involved.

An experiment is ethical or not at its inception; it does not become ethical *post hoc*—ends do not justify means. There is no ethical distinction between ends and means.

In the publication of experimental results it must be made unmistakably clear that the proprieties have been observed. It is debatable whether data obtained unethically should be published even with stern editorial comment.

References

1. Pope Pius XII. Address. Presented at First International Congress on Histopathology of Nervous System, Rome, Italy, September 14, 1952.
2. Platt (Sir Robert), Ist bart. *Doctor and patient: Ethics, morals, government.* 87 pp. London: Nuffield provincial hospitals trust, 1963. Pp. 62 and 63.
3. Pappworth, M. H. Personal communication.
4. Beecher, H. K. Consent in clinical experimentation: myth and reality. *J.A.M.A.* 195:34, 1966.
5. Great Britain, Medical Research Council. *Memorandum,* 1953

Philosophical Reflections on Experimenting with Human Subjects

Hans Jonas

Hans Jonas is Professor Emeritus of Philosophy at the New School for Social Research in New York City. As a philosopher of science, he became interested in the ethical implications of the new biology and was an early participant in the discussions at the Hastings Center. He was asked to contribute "Philosophical Reflections on Experimenting with Human Subjects" to a conference on ethical aspects of experimenting with human subjects, one of the first on this topic, that was held in Boston, on November 3–4, 1967.

This excerpt is from a long, profound essay in which Jonas reflects on the nature of experimenting with human beings, in which the subject is not an inanimate thing but a responsible human relationship. He proposes that a utilitarian ethics is inadequate to deal with the ethics of human experimentation, and points out the limitations of a "social contract" ethics. Research progress, desirable as it is, is a "melioristic goal," subordinate to moral obligations of respect for personal freedom and authenticity. Jonas suggests "identification" and "descending order" as rules for selection of subjects. This essay was a seminal exposition of the ethics of medical research.

Experimenting with human subjects is going on in many fields of scientific and technological progress. It is designed to replace the over-all instruction by natural, occasional experience with the selective information from artificial, systematic experiment which physical science has found so effective in dealing with inanimate nature. Of the new experimentation with man, medical is surely the most legitimate; psychological, the most dubious; biological (still to come), the most dangerous. I have chosen here to deal with the first only, where the case *for* it is strongest and the task of adjudicating conflicting claims hardest. . . .

Before going any further, we should give some more articulate voice to the resistance we feel against a merely utilitarian view of the matter. It has to do with a peculiarity of human experimentation quite independent of the question of possible injury to the subject. What is wrong with making a person an experimental subject is not so much that we make him thereby a means (which happens in social contexts of all kinds), as that we make him a thing—a passive thing merely to be acted on, and passive not even for real action, but for token

Hans Jonas. "Philosophical Reflections on Experimenting with Human Subjects." Abridged from *Dædulus*, Journal of the American Academy of Arts and Sciences, from the issue entitled, "Ethical Aspects of Experimentation with Human Subjects," Spring 1969, Volume 98, No. 2.

action whose token object he is. His being is reduced to that of a mere token or "sample." This is different from even the most exploitative situations of social life: there the business is real, not fictitious. The subject, however much abused, remains an agent and thus a "subject" in the other sense of the word. The soldier's case is instructive: Subject to most unilateral discipline, forced to risk mutilation and death, conscripted without, perhaps against, his will—he is still conscripted with his capacities to act, to hold his own or fail in situations, to meet real challenges for real stakes. Though a mere "number" to the High Command, he is not a token and not a thing. (Imagine what he would say if it turned out that the war was a game staged to sample observations on his endurance, courage, or cowardice.)

These compensations of personhood are denied to the subject of experimentation, who is acted upon for an extraneous end without being engaged in a real relation where he would be the counterpoint to the other or to circumstance. Mere "consent" (mostly amounting to no more than permission) does not right this reification. Only genuine authenticity of volunteering can possibly redeem the condition of "thinghood" to which the subject submits. . . .

"Individual Versus Society" as the Conceptual Framework

The setting for the conflict most consistently invoked in the literature is the polarity of individual versus society—the possible tension between the individual good and the common good, between private and public welfare. Thus, W. Wolfensberger speaks of "the tension between the long-range interests of society, science, and progress, on one hand, and the rights of the individual on the other.[1] Walsh McDermott says: "In essence, this is a problem of the rights of the individual versus the rights of society."[2] . . . We concede, as a matter of course, to the common good some pragmatically determined measure of precedence over the individual good. In terms of rights, we let some of the basic rights of the individual be overruled by the acknowledged rights of society—as a matter of right and moral justness and not of mere force or dire necessity (much as such necessity may be adduced in defense of that right). But in making that concession, we require a careful clarification of what the needs, interests, and rights of society are, for society—as distinct from any plurality of individuals—is an abstract and, as such, is subject to our definition, while the individual is the primary concrete, prior to all definition, and his basic good is more or less known. Thus the unknown in our problem is the so-called common or public good and its potentially superior claims, to which the individual good must or might sometimes be sacrificed, in circumstances that in turn must also be counted among the unknowns of our question. . . .

Health as a Public Good

The cause invoked is health and, in its more critical aspect, life itself—clearly superlative goods that the physician serves directly by curing and the researcher indirectly by the knowledge gained through his experiments. There is no question about the good served nor about the evil fought—disease and premature death. But a good to whom and an evil to whom? Here the issue tends to become somewhat clouded. In the attempt to give experimentation the proper dignity (on the problematic view that a value becomes greater by being "social" instead of merely individual), the health in question or the disease in question is somehow predicated on the social whole, as if it were society that, in the persons of its members, enjoyed the one and suffered the other. For the purposes of our problem, public interest can then be pitted against private interest, the common good against the individual good. Indeed, I have found health called a national resource, which of course it is, but surely not in the first place.

In trying to resolve some of the complexities and ambiguities lurking in these conceptualizations, I have pondered a particular statement, made in the form of a question, which I found in the *Proceedings* of the earlier *Dædalus* conference: "Can society afford to discard the tissues and organs of the hopelessly unconscious patient when they could be used to restore the otherwise hopelessly ill, but still salvageable individual?" And somewhat later: "A strong case can be made that society can ill afford to discard the tissues and organs of the hopelessly unconscious patient; they are greatly needed for study and experimental trial to help those who can be salvaged."[3] I hasten to add that any suspicion of callousness that the "commodity" language of these statements may suggest is immediately dispelled by the name of the speaker, Dr. Henry K. Beecher, for whose humanity and moral sensibility there can be nothing but admiration. But the use, in all innocence, of this language gives food for thought. Let me, for a moment, take the question literally. "Discarding" implies proprietary rights—nobody can discard what does not belong to him in the first place. Does society then own my body? "Salvaging" implies the same and, moreover, a use-value to the owner. Is the life-extension of certain individuals then a public interest? "Affording" implies a critically vital level of such an interest—that is, of the loss or gain involved. And "society" itself—what is it? When does a need, an aim, an obligation become social? Let us reflect on some of these terms.

What Society Can Afford

"Can Society afford . . . ?" Afford what? To let people die intact, thereby withholding something from other people who desperately need it, who in consequence will have to die too? These other, unfortunate people indeed cannot afford not to have a kidney, heart, or other organ of the dying patient, on which they depend for an extension of their lease on life; but does that give them a right to it? And does it oblige society to procure it for them? What is it that *society* can or cannot afford—leaving aside for the moment the question of what it has a *right* to ? It surely can afford to lose members through death; more than that, it is built on the balance of death and birth decreed by the order of life. This is too general, of course, for our question, but perhaps it is well to remember. The specific question seems to be whether society can afford to let some people die whose death might be deferred by particular means if these were authorized by society. Again, if it is merely a question of what society can or cannot afford, rather than of what it ought or ought not to do, the answer must be: Of course, it can. If cancer, heart disease, and other organic, noncontagious ills, especially those tending to strike the old more than the young, continue to exact their toll at the normal rate of incidence (including the toll of private anguish and misery), society can go on flourishing in every way.

Here, by contrast, are some examples of what, in sober truth, society cannot afford. It cannot afford to let an epidemic rage unchecked; a persistent excess of deaths over births, but neither—we must add—too great an excess of births over deaths; too low an average life expectancy even if demographically balanced by fertility, but neither too great a longevity with the necessitated correlative dearth of youth in the social body; a debilitating state of general health; and things of this kind. These are plain cases where the whole condition of society is critically affected, and the public interest can make its imperative claims. The Black Death of the Middle Ages was a *public* calamity of the acute kind; the life-sapping ravages of endemic malaria or sleeping sickness in certain areas are a public calamity of the chronic kind. Such situations a society as a whole can truly not "afford," and they may call for extraordinary remedies, including, perhaps, the invasion of private sacrosanctities.

This is not entirely a matter of numbers and numerical ratios. Society, in a subtler sense, cannot "afford" a single miscarriage of justice, a single inequity in the dispensation of its laws, the violation of the rights of even the tiniest minority, because these undermine the moral basis on which society's existence rests. Nor can it, for a similar reason, afford the absence or atrophy in its midst of compassion and of the effort to alleviate suffering—be it widespread or rare—one form of which is the effort to conquer disease of any kind, whether "socially" significant (by reason of number) or not. And in short, society cannot afford the absence among its members of *virtue* with its readiness for sacrifice beyond defined duty. Since its presence—that is to say, that of personal ideal-ism—is a matter of grace and not of decree, we have the paradox that society depends for its existence on intangibles of nothing less than a religious order, for which it can hope, but which it cannot enforce. All the more must it protect this most precious capital from abuse.

For what objectives connected with the medico-biological sphere should this reserve be drawn upon—for example, in the form of accepting, soliciting, perhaps even imposing the submission of human subjects to experimentation? We postulate that this must be not just a worthy cause, as any promotion of the health of anybody doubtlessly is, but a cause qualifying for transcendent social sanction. Here one thinks first of those cases critically affecting the whole condition, present and future, of the community we have illustrated. Something equivalent to what in the political sphere is called "clear and present danger" may be invoked and a state of emergency proclaimed, thereby suspending certain otherwise inviolable prohibitions and taboos. We may observe that averting a disaster always carries greater weight than promoting a good. Extraordinary danger excuses extraordinary means. This covers human experimentation, which we would like to count, as far as possible, among the extraordinary rather than the ordinary means of serving the common good under public auspices. Naturally, since foresight and responsibility for the future are of the essence of institutional society, averting disaster extends into long-term prevention, although the lesser urgency will warrant less sweeping licenses.

Society and the Cause of Progress

Much weaker is the case where it is a matter not of saving but of improving society. Much of medical research falls into this category. As stated before, a permanent death rate from heart failure or cancer does not threaten society. So long as certain statistical ratios are maintained, the incidence of disease and of disease-induced mortality is not (in the strict sense) a "social" misfortune. I hasten to add that it is not therefore less of a human misfortune, and the call for relief issuing with silent eloquence from each victim and all potential victims is of no lesser dignity. But it is misleading to equate the fundamentally human response to it with what is owed to society: it is owed by man to man—and it is thereby owed by society to the individuals as soon as the adequate ministering to these concerns outgrows (as it progressively does) the scope of private spontaneity and is made a public mandate. It is thus that society assumes responsibility for medical care, research, old age, and innumerable other things not originally of the public realm (in the original "social contract"), and they become duties toward "society" (rather than directly toward one's fellow man) by the fact that they are socially operated.

Indeed, we expect from organized society no longer mere protection against harm and the securing of the conditions of our preservation, but active and constant improvement in all the domains of life: the waging of the battle against nature, the enhancement of the human estate—in short, the promotion of progress. This is an expansive goal, one far surpassing the disaster norm of our previous reflections. It lacks the urgency of the latter, but has the nobility of the free, forward thrust. It surely is worth sacrifices. It is not at all a question of what society can afford, but of what it is committed to, beyond all necessity, by our mandate. Its trusteeship has become an established, ongoing, institutionalized business of the body politic. As eager beneficiaries of its gains, we now owe to "society," as its chief agent, our individual contributions toward its *continued pursuit*. I emphasize "continued pursuit." Maintaining the existing level requires no more than the orthodox means of taxation and enforcement of professional standards that raise no problems. The more optional goal of pushing forward is also more exacting. We have this syndrome: Progress is by our choosing an acknowledged interest of society, in which we have a stake in various degrees; science is a necessary instrument of progress; research is a necessary instrument of science; and in medical science experimentation on human subjects is a necessary instrument of research. Therefore, human experimentation has come to be a societal interest.

The destination of research is essentially melioristic. It does not serve the preservation of the existing good from which I profit myself and to which I am obligated. Unless the present state is intolerable, the melioristic goal is in a sense gratuitous, and this not only from the vantage point of the present. Our descendants have a right to be left an unplundered planet; they do not have a right to new miracle cures. We have sinned against them, if by our doing we have destroyed their inheritance—which we are doing at full blast; we have not sinned against them, if by the time they come around arthritis has not yet been conquered (unless by sheer neglect). And generally, in the matter of progress, as humanity had no claim on a Newton, a Michelangelo, or a St. Francis to appear, and no right to the blessings of their unscheduled deeds, so progress, with all our methodical labor for it, cannot be budgeted in advance and its fruits received as a due. Its coming-about at all and its turning out for good (of which we can never be sure) must rather be regarded as something akin to grace.

The Melioristic Goal, Medical Research, and Individual Duty

Nowhere is the melioristic goal more inherent than in medicine. To the physician, it is not gratuitous. He is committed to curing and thus to improving the power to cure. Gratuitous we called it (outside disaster conditions) as a *social* goal, but noble at the same time. Both the nobility and the gratuitousness must influence the manner in which self-sacrifice for it is elicited, and even its free offer accepted. Freedom is certainly the first condition to be observed here. The surrender of one's body to medical experimentation is entirely outside the enforceable "social contract."

Or can it be construed to fall within its terms—namely, as repayment for benefits from past experimentation that I have enjoyed myself? But I am indebted for these benefits not to society, but to the past "martyrs," to whom society is indebted itself, and society has no right to call in my personal debt by way of adding new to its own. Moreover, gratitude is not an enforceable social obligation; it anyway does not mean that I must emulate the deed. Most of all, if it was wrong to exact such sacrifice in the first place, it does not become right to exact it again with the plea of the profit it has brought me. If, however, it was not exacted, but entirely free, as it ought to have been, then it should remain so, and its precedence must not be used as a social pressure on others for doing the same under the sign of duty.

Indeed, we must look outside the sphere of the social contract, outside the whole realm of public rights and duties, for the motivations and norms by which we can expect ever again the upwelling of a will to give what nobody—neither society, nor fellow man, nor posterity—is entitled to. There are such dimensions in man with trans-social wellsprings of conduct, and I have already pointed to the paradox, or mystery, that society cannot prosper without them, that it must draw on them, but cannot command them.

What about the moral law as such a transcendent motivation of conduct?

It goes considerably beyond the public law of the social contract. The latter, we saw, is founded on the rule of enlightened self-interest: *Do ut des*—I give so that I be given to. The law of individual conscience asks more. Under the Golden Rule, for example, I am required to give as I wish to be given to under like circumstances, but not in order that I be given to and not in expectation of return. Reciprocity, essential to the social law, is not a condition of the moral law. One subtle "expectation" and "self-interest," but of the moral order itself, may even then be in my mind: I prefer the environment of a moral society and can expect to contribute to the general morality by my own example. But even if I should always be the dupe, the Golden Rule holds. (If the social law breaks faith with me, I am released from its claim.) . . .

"Identification" as the Principle of Recruitment in General

If the properties we adduced as the particular qualifications of the members of the scientific fraternity itself are taken as general criteria of selection, then one should look for additional subjects where a maximum of identification, understanding, and spontaneity can be expected—that is, among the most highly motivated, the most highly educated, and the least "captive" members of the community. From this naturally scarce resource, a descending order of permissibility leads to greater abundance and ease of supply, whose use should become proportionately more hesitant as the exculpating criteria are relaxed. An inversion of normal "market" behavior is demanded here—namely, to accept the lowest quotation last (and excused only by the greatest pressure of need); to pay the highest price first.

The ruling principle in our considerations is that the "wrong" of reification can only be made "right" by such authentic identification with the cause that it is the subject's as well as the researcher's cause—whereby his role in its service is not just permitted by him, but *willed*. That sovereign will of his which embraces the end as his own restores his personhood to the otherwise depersonalizing context. To be valid it must be autonomous and informed. The latter condition can, outside the research community, only be fulfilled by degrees; but the higher the degree of the understanding regarding the purpose and the technique, the more valid becomes the endorsement of the will. A margin of mere trust inevitably remains. Ultimately, the appeal for volunteers should seek this free and generous endorsement, the appropriation of the research purpose into the person's own scheme of ends. Thus, the appeal is in truth addressed to the one, mysterious, and sacred source of any such generosity of the will—"devotion," whose forms and objects of commitment are various and may invest different motivations in different individuals. The following, for instance, may be responsive to the "call" we are discussing: compassion with human suffering, zeal for humanity, reverence for the Golden Rule, enthusiasm for progress, homage to the cause of knowledge, even longing for sacrificial justification (do not call that "masochism," please). On all these, I say, it is defensible and right to draw when the research objective is worthy enough; and it is a prime duty of the research community (especially in view of what we called the "margin of trust") to see that this sacred source is never abused for frivolous ends. For a less than adequate cause, not even the freest, unsolicited offer should be accepted.

The Rule of the "Descending Order" and Its Counter-Utility Sense

We have laid down what must seem to be a forbidding rule to the number-hungry research industry. Having faith in the transcendent potential of man, I do not fear that the "source" will ever fail a society that does not destroy it—and only such a one is worthy of the blessings of progress. But "elitistic" the rule is (as is the enterprise of progress itself), and elites are by nature small. The combined attribute of motivation and information, plus the absence of external pressures, tends to be socially so circumscribed that strict adherence to the rule might numerically starve the research process. This is why I spoke of a descending order of permissibility, which is itself permissive, but where the realization that it is a *descending* order is not without pragmatic import. Departing from the august norm, the appeal must needs shift from idealism to docility, from high-mindedness to compliance, from judgment to trust. Consent spreads over the whole spectrum. I will not go into the casuistics of this penumbral area. I merely indicate the principle of the order of preference: The poorer in knowledge, motivation, and freedom of decision (and that, alas, means the more readily available in terms of numbers and possible manipulation), the more sparingly and indeed reluctantly should the reservoir be used, and the more compelling must therefore become the countervailing justification.

Let us note that this is the opposite of a social utility standard, the reverse of the order by "availability and expendability": The most valuable and scarcest, the least expendable elements of the social organism, are to be the first candidates for risk and sacrifice. It is the standard of *noblesse oblige;* and with all its counter-utility and seeming "wastefulness," we feel a rightness about it and perhaps even a higher "utility," for the soul of the community lives by this spirit.[4] It is also the opposite of what the day-to-day interests of research clamor for, and for the scientific community to honor it will mean that it will have to fight a strong temptation to go by routine to the readiest sources of supply—the suggestible, the ignorant, the dependent, the "captive" in various senses.[5] I do not believe that heightened resistance here must cripple research, which cannot be permitted; but it may indeed slow it down by the smaller numbers fed into experimentation in consequence. This price—a possibly slower rate of progress—may have to be paid for the preservation of the most precious capital of higher communal life. . . .

No Experiments on Patients Unrelated to Their Own Disease

Although my ponderings have, on the whole, yielded points of view rather than definite prescriptions, premises rather than conclusions, they have led me to a few unequivocal yeses and noes. The first is the emphatic rule that patients should be experimented upon, if at all, *only* with reference to *their disease*. Never should there be added to the gratuitousness of the experiment as such the gratuitousness of service to an unrelated cause. This follows simply from what we have found to be the *only* excuse for infracting the special exemption of the sick at all—namely, that the scientific war on disease cannot accomplish its goal without drawing the sufferers from disease into the investigative process. If under this excuse they become subjects of experiment, they do so *because*, and only because, of *their* disease. . . .

. . . Let us not forget that progress is an optional goal, not an unconditional commitment, and that its tempo in particular, compulsive as it may become, has nothing sacred about it. Let us also remember that a slower progress in the conquest of disease would not threaten society, grievous as it is to those who have to deplore that their particular disease be not yet conquered, but that society would indeed be threatened by the erosion of those moral values whose loss, possibly caused by too ruthless a pursuit of scientific progress, would make its most dazzling triumphs not worth having.

References

1. Wolfensberger, "Ethical Issues in Research with Human Subjects," *Proceedings of the Conference on the Ethical Aspects of Experimentation on Human Subjects,* November 3–4, 1967 (Boston, Massachusetts; hereafter called *Proceedings*). p. 48.
2. *Proceedings*, p. 29.
3. *Proceedings*, pp. 50–51.
4. Socially, everyone is expendable relatively—that is, in different degrees; religiously, no one is expendable absolutely: The "image of God" is in all. If it can be enhanced, then not by anyone being expended, but by someone expending himself.
5. This refers to captives of circumstance, not of justice. Prison inmates are, with respect to our problem, in a special class. If we hold to some idea of guilt, and to the supposition that our judicial system is not entirely at fault, they may be held to stand in a special debt to society, and their offer to serve—from whatever motive—may be accepted with a minimum of qualms as a means of reparation.

Realities of Patient Consent to Medical Research

John Fletcher

John Fletcher, a graduate student in theological ethics at Union Theological Seminary of New York, gained admission to the Clinical Center at National Institutes of Health to do research on his doctoral dissertation on the ethics of medical research. Fletcher was later appointed special assistant for bioethics to the director of the Clinical Center, a position in which he provided consultation to the researchers of that institution. He is currently professor of medical ethics, School of Medicine, University of Virginia.

"Realities of Patient Consent" first appeared as "Human Experimentation: Ethics in the Consent Situation" in *Law and Contemporary Problems* (1967: 34:620–649). In this report of his research at NIH, Fletcher combines an ethical analysis of what it means to be "treated as a person" with an empirical study of the interaction of researchers and research subjects in several clinical investigations.

The theme of coercion and freedom is at the center of moral concern about the ethics of medical research in human beings. Intense efforts by groups in government, medical societies, and related professions have produced interpretations, codes and regulations in the conduct of research.[1] Among the many valued objectives clustered around the discussion of morality in medical research, obtaining informed consent from the subject in an experiment is emphasized most. The literature on the principles of informed consent is enormous. Ninety-nine percent of it considers what ought to be; only a small fraction contains reports of what *happens* when consent is given by patient to investigator. A handful of studies by Renée Fox, Henry K. Beecher, and Fellner and Marshall expose the fragility of the consent contract and lay bare many "myths" about the supposed freedom and rationality in informed consent.[2] Due to the considerable doubts about the possibility of obtaining informed consent in many circumstances, a fresh treatment of the actualities of giving consent in medical experiments is in order.

The most rewarding inquiry in ethics takes place between the "ought" and the "is." The dangers in the debate on informed consent are a too legalistic approach from the side of those who uphold the law and a too secretive approach from those who practice. H. Richard Niebuhr[3] noted that the two purposes of ethics are self-understanding and guidance in the concrete problems of using our freedom. Researchers need to know more about the ways they and their subjects actually make decisions, and those who are charged with regulating research need to keep rules within the reach of obedience. . . .

John Fletcher. "Realities of Patient Consent to Medical Research." Abridged from *Hasting Center Studies*, Volume 1, 1973, pp. 39–49. Reprinted by permission.

When consent is being sought for medical research, a human encounter involving decisions to take risks occurs between an investigator and a subject. I assume that in the majority of these encounters little discussion of whether the investigator is *really* justified in pursuing his study takes place. Usually, he has already had to justify his plan with a group of his peers. Further, I assume that it would be rare, if ever, that a question would be raised by either party as to whether the subject were *really* free to choose to participate, or whether there is an authentic condition called "freedom" anyway. As Henry D. Aiken, a moral philosopher, pointed out, these sorts of questions usually occur some distance from practice and are occasioned by changing social conditions or a severe conflict of rules.[4] I am not claiming that the raw materials for such questions are not present in the consent encounter, for wherever one self puts a claim on another and risk is a factor, ethical and theological questions are implicit. I am claiming that one observing the consent process would seldom hear self-conscious discussions of the ethics of consent.

I did assume, however, in approaching a field study of the consent process, that patient-volunteers in medical research would be able to reflect upon their impressions of the possibilities and limits of their freedom of choice. Since individualism or the sense of autonomy is the primary value orientation within which these patients might be expected to speak of their sense of freedom,[5] one might expect that when the patient reflects on his sense of being a "person" or being denied such a status, the issue of his freedom would be to the forefront. Thus, as an ethicist studying the issue of freedom in research, my research was designed to test the hypothesis that the conduct of the consent situation was decisive for the patient's sense of being treated as a "person."

Reading and interviews had convinced me that many investigators and administrators maintained a ritualistic attitude towards informed consent. That is, working from the assumption that a sick person will do almost anything a physician suggests, and feeling that the signing of a consent form entailed a ritual which covered over the impossibility of informed consent, many investigators went about their practice having despaired of attaining genuine informed consent from their patients. Several early interviews had opened with an investigator remarking that patients are so dependent on physicians that they would not be seriously affected by anything the physician did in his explanation of a study. These interviews were also spiced with a heavy antipathy to the legal profession and administrators who, according to several physicians interviewed, were interested only in protecting the reputation of the institution.

In short, it appeared to me that many people supposed that patients who entered the research situation left their sense of personhood behind, having surrendered their autonomy to the "white coat" world. From a deep professional interest in inquiring into dependency relations between "laymen" and experts who control valuable yet risky techniques, I expected that these patients would give signs, gestures, and verbal expression to how their experience in a risk-taking study reflected on their sense of having the status of a "person." I assumed, with those who have labored on the concept of informed consent, that the real meaning of the rule was to protect the status of personhood which is enshrined in the traditions of law, morality, and religion surrounding the concept of consent. . . .

What does the "sense of being treated as a person" mean? Three norms were accepted which nourish the basis of the symbolic status of "person."

1. The patient might perceive himself as a being who was addressable as "never merely as means. . . . but at the same time as ends in themselves."[6] To use more religious terms to describe this sense, one may perceive himself as a "thou and not an it"; as Buber stated: ". . . without *It* man cannot live. But he who lives with It alone is not a man."[7]

2. He might give signs of perceiving himself as a responsible being, capable of choice, exercising some control over his body and general welfare. To quote Tillich:

As a centered self and individual, man can respond in knowledge and action to the stimuli that reach him from the world to which he belongs; but because he also *confronts* his world, and in this sense is free from it, he can respond "responsibly," namely, after deliberation and decision rather than through a determined compulsion.[8]

3. The patient might give signs of including himself as a member of a community in which the transcendence of self-interest is an ever-present possibility. Both psychologist Jean Piaget and theologian Reinhold Niebuhr agree that social relations of cooperation, involving the transcendence of one's own interests, are the hallmark of personal life.[9]. . .

[An example] will illustrate my conclusion that patient-volunteers in this setting maintained their relation to personhood, but that several gave signs of having to defend themselves against their consent being "engineered" rather than "coerced." . . .

Study of Biogenic Amines. Dr. C. is a thirty-five year old neurologist. He works on several projects with patients who have diseases of the brain or disorders which affect the central nervous system. His interest lay in studying a group of chemicals, the biogenic amines, believed to play a central role in synaptic transmission in the brain. Dopamine is an example of one main subgroup of these chemicals, the catecholamines. He had designed a study, after a year of animal testing, to investigate the difference in the metabolism of dopamine in the brain as contrasted to its metabolism in the body. He explained that neurologists did not know if there were a difference; if there were, they will know more about dopamine's nature and the uses drug therapy can have in treating brain disease.

The following experiment was designed: patients with indwelling intraventricular catheters would be chosen as subjects. Some patients with brain tumors have such catheters to permit safer and easier treatment with chemotherapeutic agents. Radioactively labelled dopamine would be injected intravenously *or* intraventricularly in these patients, in a very small dose. By testing urine collections for four days following the injection, Dr. C. hoped to study the difference in metabolism.

He explained that the study carried no direct benefit to the patient-volunteer, although the potential information to be gained was within proportion to the risks. Animal tests showed no pharmacologic effect. The major risk of any injection, he stated, was infection, but every known precaution had been taken. Ninety-eight percent of injected radioactivity would be passed in the urine of each patient. His study had been approved by a group of his peers and by a radiation committee.

Dr. C. mentioned more than once the possibility that what transpires in the consent situation can be a "charade." He defined this term as the disappointment of society's expectation that the investigator will always obtain an informed consent, and that the patient will fully understand the risks and benefits. He frankly admitted that some patients are, through serious illness, unable to measure up to these expectations, even after serious attempts to communicate. In such cases, he stressed, he always sought third party consent.

Dr. C. had chosen two female patients, both of whom had had nursing educations, as participants in dopamine infusion. Both had come to the Center expecting research with treatment for brain tumor. Since they were roommates, he had met with them together several times prior to obtaining signed consent, six hours in all, and he showed he was very aware of their limitations. He had gradually unfolded his explanations for them, giving them ample time to discuss it. Dr. C. had noticed that Mrs. S., who was somewhat aphasic as a result of her brain tumor and had difficulty understanding others and expressing herself, had become very dependent upon Mrs. N. for interpretation and cues. Following the session in which both had signed forms, Dr. C. said that in his opinion Mrs. N. had given informed consent, but if strict standards were applied, Mrs. S. had not. "Her illness is so pronounced." He observed that "Mrs. N. really understands what is going on," but that Mrs. S. "kept looking at the other lady to find out what the right thing to do was." Under the circumstances, he concluded that Mrs. N. had given an authentic third-party consent for Mrs. S., and that the previous sessions had indicated to him that this was an acceptable route to follow.

It is seriously debatable as to whether one should choose a third party who is participating in the same experiment to authenticate the consent of another. In principle, such should never be the case. As the following interview shows, Mrs. S. gives dramatic signs that she felt treated humanely and as a person. Yet several hard questions should be raised here about the conclusion of Dr. C. that she could be included in the study on the basis of Mrs. N.'s consent. The two patient-volunteers made the following comments after each had already received an injection:

> **Q.:** You had met with the doctor several times before yesterday?
>
> **Mrs. N.:** Yes. He saw us four or five times, no . . . every day last week. Then one day he just sat down, for about an hour, and talked

and talked. He told us all about the project. He explained everything. He told us that this chemical he was studying was in the
body anyway, so it wouldn't put anything new into us.

Q.: How do you feel about Dr. C.?

Mrs. S.: He talks to you like you are a human being and not a glass. He
has a lot of warmth. He took our anxieties away. The doctor is
the most important thing in something like this. If he talks to
you then you know what is happening.

Q.: Then you liked that part of it?

Mrs. S.: Oh, yes. I like being told what is going on. It isn't that often a
doctor will talk to you that long. Dr. C. took his time and
answered all of our questions.

Q.: What do you understand about the purpose of this study?

Mrs. N.: Well, they are going to study how this chemical acts . . . maybe
they will be able to use it on others.

Q.: Will your participating in this study help you?

Mrs. N.: It won't help the illness I have. Maybe it will help someone else
someday, or the world of medicine.

Mrs. S.: At least we have contributed something. So much of the time
you are just like a robot; now you can do something, you can
give. Everyone is doing something for us all the time, now we
can repay them in this way.

Q.: Did any questions occur to you after we met yesterday?

Mrs. N.: No, no questions. We had them all answered before. Mainly,
we were concerned about how long it would last and if it would
do any harm. Since it was just a teeny bit of radioactivity, and
they would get that later, it didn't seem that it would do any
harm.

When the three norms of the presence of personhood discussed above are
applied, each appears clearly confirmed here. Being treated as an end and not
a means only is affirmed by Mrs. S. (the aphasic patient) as being a "human
being and not a glass." Her metaphor is possibly a more apt description of
personhood in this age than the "thou-it" terminology. Mrs. N. showed that
she understood the meaning of a non-therapeutic study, that she had had her
questions answered, and had exercised her capacity to choose. Mrs. N. also
answered all of the "technical" questions, showing the special role Dr. C. had
used with her. Mrs. S. perceived that she was a member of a community in
which the consuming self-interest of illness can be transcended; her use of the
term "robot" is especially compelling to describe the dehumanization of being
ill in a hospital. When contrasted with her "*now* you can give," a clear picture
of membership in a special community emerges.

When one contrasts Mrs. S.'s warm statements with the probability that
there is no firm basis for assuming that Dr. C. got consent in this case, he can
understand how complex a moral judgment there is to render in this case. First,
there is Dr. C.'s own estimate that Mrs. S. was too ill to speak for herself.

Secondly, Mrs. N. was never told that she was acting as a third party to consent for her roommate. Thirdly, even if Mrs. N. had been told, there is the likelihood that she was a poor choice, since she was a fellow-participant in the same study. In my opinion, a more independent third party consent should have been obtained by Dr. C. To the extent that I played that role unknowingly in discussion with Dr. C. about Mrs. S., I would have said "yes." Yet I must conclude that the wrong third party was used and that his choice did not constitute a sound basis for including Mrs. S. in the study. Dr. C.'s conduct of the consent situation was decisive for Mrs. S.'s sense of being treated as a person, but it was not sufficient to provide a firm moral basis for consent when studied by an independent party. Thus, the sense of "personhood" on the part of the patient is not sufficient evidence that all is well. A physician can be compassionate and extraordinarily informative, as was Dr. C., and his patient can feel quite free about his choices; yet each be found in serious legal and moral question. This case is an excellent prism for the problems of informed consent and a good illustration of the "finite freedom" of men. . . .

Many factors impinge on the patient-volunteer to limit or reduce his autonomy. First, serious illness is threatening and limiting. Patients tend to believe that the slightest change in the arrangements, such as the introduction of a tape recorder, will make them better. Almost everything that happens is filtered through illness, including consent to research. Bennett, a social worker in an experimental therapeutics ward of the Clinical Center, corroborated my findings in her study of twenty-three patients, and observed that "patients do not conceptualize the principal investigator as a scientist and equate treatment and research as one and the same."[10] Park and others reported on the same phenomenon in psychiatric patients.[11]

Secondly, the arrangements at an imposing institution like the Clinical Center tend to diminish the patient's willingness to complain or question. Surely the fact that treatment is free, and that each has a serious disease for which no cure has yet been found, limits a patient's freedom to question. Savard, also a social worker, reports for the whole social work staff: "One of the functions the social work staff sees for itself is to help the patient work through this conflict (guilt over being ungrateful when the wish to gripe crosses their minds). This could include second thoughts about continued participation in a research project."[12]

Thirdly, the expectations of the investigator for the subject are a strong force which may operate often to limit the subject's freedom. . . . Patients are also aware from the attitudes shown by investigators that they have much of their own prestige invested in studies. They are eager not to disappoint. The investigator's knowledge of human behavior has become as important for his work as his skill in carrying out his studies.

None of the three restrictions on freedom of the patient to question or withdraw mentioned above are comparable to outright examples of coercion. No investigator I observed ever used force, threat, or his authority to make a patient submit to research. Patients come to the Center knowing that they will be in studies, even though they tend to confuse research and treatment. The particular question of coercion and freedom in human studies revolves in part around the right of the patient to withdraw at any time. . . .

Coercion can be normally defined as the act of influencing others against their will. It has been said that the ultimate in coercion is manipulating another's emotions, "forcing him to will that which you will." If an entire will had to be created *ex nihilo* for the subject in research, this definition might hold; however, patients come prepared for research by cultural, medical, and institutional conditions. It is more true to say that a specific will to do a particular study has to be developed in the patient; he must be persuaded. A more capacious concept than "coercion" must be sought to describe the *pressure*, bordering on coercion, which some patients felt to accept research. I observed that some patients found an opportunity to defend themselves against their consent to research being "engineered," a term used by Cahn to describe the control of the conditions of consent by experts controlling information and technique.[13] . . .

I would attribute this sense of pressure to accept research "tied" to treatment, in these patients, as a result of institutional arrangements plus the unfinished business of a consent process. The patients entered an impressive research center for therapeutic and nontherapeutic studies. They knew that they had a right to withdraw, but they had not discussed it with their physician. One of the most important findings of the study, in my estimation, was the opportunity the presence of my inquiry gave to the physician and subject to maintain, build and repair their agreement. Savard and Bennett also report such effects. Although I did not present myself as an "ombudsman" or advocate for the patient to physicians, the implication of my position was similar. An intermediary person who has access to the consent process might function to enhance the freedom of patient and investigator to change the terms of an unfinished agreement. The range of options open to an individual constitutes his sphere of freedom. Whenever a third party enters, there may be new options available.

What is needed to remedy the possibility of coercion is not more exhortation, but more practical action within the consent process to insure a maximum number of options for improving qualitative consent between physician and patient. The addition of institutional review committees in grantee institutions funded by the government, obligated to assure the rights of subjects in research carried out by their own institutions, seems a creative step. . . .

. . . However, the time has arrived for all medical institutions which engage in human research to consider the step of designating one or more persons to bear the responsibility of advocating *for* the patient, to assure him and the public that consent is within the reach of obedience. Such steps definitely need to be taken wherever especially necessitous groups are involved in research such as prisoners, children and the mentally ill. The principal investigator in each human study is charged with the responsibility to be the final judge of the quality of consent obtained. My proposal would not shift that responsibility. It would help assure him that every step had been taken by providing maximum feedback between himself and the subject. The issue of informed consent has become too socially charged to relegate to the realm of goals alone. New moral initiatives should be taken by those responsible for regulating medical research to invent a flexible role for one working between what ought to be and what is in each research institution.

A proposal for a special representative of the subject in research may find its most productive work in the study done with poor or otherwise deprived persons who possess the least defenses for maintaining their moral status. As the history of human experimentation shows, the poor have been a "captive group" for medical experiments. A review of the policy of municipal hospitals in New York City cited evidence that research exploitation of the poor was a common occurrence known to city health officials.[14] A familiar method of exploitation is to make the receiving of continued treatment in outpatient clinics conditional upon participation in experimental drug trials.

Every moral resource in the religious traditions urges special attention to the needs of the sick, the defenseless, and the poor. Lying behind this moral concern is an ethic of universal responsibility, inhering in the double-love commandment. Yet, love has not yet become visible until it is embodied in concrete human relations which establish the "weighty matters" of justice and mercy. Now that the period of concern about the principle of informed consent has crested, and lest this concern be found to be mere sentimentality, more thorough steps to institutionalize and embody the value of personhood in medical research are required.

References

1. John Fletcher, "Human Experimentation Ethics in the Consent Situation," *Law and Contemporary Problems* 34:620–649, 1967, and "A Study of Ethics of Medical Research," Th.D. thesis. Union Theological Seminary, New York, 1969.
2. Renée C. Fox, *Experiment Perilous* (Glencoe, Illinois: The Free Press, 1959); Henry K. Beecher, "Ethics and Clinical Research," *New England Journal of Medicine* 274:1354–1360, 1966; and Beecher "Some Guiding Principles for Clinical Investigation," *Journal of the American Medical Association* 195:1135–1136, 1966; W. J. Curran and Henry K. Beecher, "Experimentation in Children," *Journal of the American Medical Association* 210:77–73, 1969; C. H. Fellner and J. R. Marshall, "Kidney Donors—The Myth of Informed Consent," *American Journal of Psychiatry* 126:1245–1251, 1970.
3. H. Richard Niebuhr, *The Responsible Self* (New York: Harper and Row, 1963), p. 48.
4. Henry D. Aiken, *Reason and Conduct* (New York: Knopf, 1962), p. 75.
5. C. Kluckholm, H. A. Murray and D. M. Schneider, *Personality in Nature, Society, and Culture* (New York: Knopf, 1964), p. 352.
6. I. Kant, "The Metaphysics of Morals," *Great Books of the Western World*, edited by R. M. Hutchins, Vol. 42 (Chicago: Encyclopedia Britannica, Inc., 1952), p. 274.
7. Martin Buber, *I and Thou* (New York: Scribner's Sons, 1958), p. 34.
8. Paul Tillich, *Morality and Beyond* (New York: Harper and Row, 1963), p. 19.
9. Jean Piaget, *The Moral Judgment of the Child* (Glencoe, Ill.: The Free Press,

1965), p. 395; Reinhold Niebuhr, *Man's Nature and His Communities* (New York: Scribner's Sons, 1965), p. 107.

10. C. M. Bennett, "Motivation, Expectations and Adjustment of Patients on an Experimental Therapeutics Service," 1970.

11. L. C. Park, *et al.*, "The Subjective Experience of the Research Patient," *Journal of Nervous and Mental Disease* 143:199–206, 1966.

12. R. J. Savard, "Serving Investigator, Patient and Community in Research Studies," *Annals of the New York Academy of Science* 169:429–434, 1970.

13. E. Cahn, "The Lawyer as Scientist and Scoundrel: Reflections on Francis Bacon's Quadricentennial," *New York University Law Review* 36:8, 1961.

14. R. Burlage, *New York City's Municipal Hospitals* (Washington DC). Institute for Policy Studies, 1967, p. 329.

Questions for Discussion
Part I, Section 2

1. What are some of the examples of uninformed consent to medical research that Beecher reports in his important article "Ethics and Clinical Research"?

2. Do you think that the kinds of practices that concerned Beecher in the 1960s still occur today?

3. Do you agree with the assertion (by Hans Jonas) that utilitarian philosophy provides an unsatisfactory account of the ethics governing biomedical research with human subjects?

4. Is there a moral obligation to seek knowledge from biomedical research? If so, what ethical limits does the requirement to treat human beings as persons (as developed by Fletcher) impose on biomedical research?

TO SAVE OR LET DIE

ॐ

Moral and Ethical Dilemmas in the Special-Care Nursery

Raymond S. Duff and A.G.M. Campbell

Raymond S. Duff and A.G.M. Campbell are pediatricians working in one of the most technically sophisticated areas of medicine: the new specialty of neonatology, which provided high-intensity care to premature infants. This care often saved the lives of infants who in an earlier time would certainly have died, but failed to prevent some of the severe consequences of prematurity (and of treatment), among which was often severe mental retardation. Duff and Campbell issued, in this article, the first forthright report of the practice of allowing some of these infants to die. The article aroused much debate and initiated thoughtful commentary on the ethics of care of the newborn.

B etween 1940 and 1970 there was a 58 per cent decrease in the infant death rate in the United States.[1] This reduction was related in part to the application of new knowledge to the care of infants. Neonatal mortality rates in hospitals having infant intensive-care units have been about ½ those reported in hospitals without such units.[2] There is now evidence that in many conditions of early infancy the long-term morbidity may also be reduced.[3] Survivors of these units may be healthy, and their parents grateful, but some infants continue to suffer from such conditions as chronic cardiopulmonary disease, short-bowel-syndrome or various manifestations of brain damage; others are severely handicapped by a myriad of congenital malformations that in previous times would have resulted in early death. Recently, both lay and professional persons have

Raymond S. Duff and A.G.M. Campbell. "Moral and Ethical Dilemmas in the Special-Care Nursery," *The New England Journal of Medicine*, Volume 289, 1973, pp. 890–894. Reprinted by permission of *The New England Journal of Medicine*. Copyright © 1973, *Massachusetts Medical Society*.

expressed increasing concern about the quality of life for these severely impaired survivors and their families.[4,5] Many pediatricians and others are distressed with the long-term results of pressing on and on to save life at all costs and in all circumstances. Eliot Slater[6] stated, "If this is one of the consequences of the sanctity-of-life ethic, perhaps our formulation of the principle should be revised."

The experiences described in this communication document some of the grave moral and ethical dilemmas now faced by physicians and families. They indicate some of the problems in a large special-care nursery where medical technology has prolonged life and where "informed" parents influence the management decisions concerning their infants.

Background and Methods

The special-care nursery of the Yale-New Haven Hospital not only serves an obstetric service for over 4000 live births annually but also acts as the principal referral center in Connecticut for infants with major problems of the newborn period. From January 1, 1970, through June 30, 1972, 1615 infants born at the Hospital were admitted, and 556 others were transferred for specialized care from community hospitals. During this interval, the average daily census was 26, with a range of 14 to 37.

For some years the unit has had a liberal policy for parental visiting, with the staff placing particular emphasis on helping parents adjust to and participate in the care of their infants with special problems. By encouraging visiting, attempting to create a relaxed atmosphere within the unit, exploring carefully the special needs of the infants, and familiarizing parents with various aspects of care, it was hoped to remove much of the apprehension—indeed, fear—with which parents at first view an intensive-care nursery.[7] At any time, parents may see and handle their babies. They commonly observe or participate in most routine aspects of care and are often present when some infant is critically ill or moribund. They may attend, as they choose, the death of their own infant. Since an average of two to three deaths occur each week and many infants are critically ill for long periods, it is obvious that the concentrated, intimate social interactions between personnel, infants and parents in an emotionally charged atmosphere often make the work of the staff very difficult and demanding. However, such participation and recognition of parents' rights to information about their infant appear to be the chief foundations of "informed consent" for treatment.

Each staff member must know how to cope with many questions and problems brought up by parents, and if he or she cannot help, they must have access to those who can. These requirements can be met only when staff members work closely with each other in all the varied circumstances from simple to complex, from triumph to tragedy. Formal and informal meetings take place regularly to discuss the technical and family aspects of care. As a given problem may require, some or all of several persons (including families, nurses, social workers, physicians, chaplains and others) may convene to exchange information and reach decisions. Thus, staff and parents function more or less as a small community in which a concerted attempt is made to ensure that each member may participate in and know about the major decisions that concern him or her. However, the physician takes appropriate initiative in final decision making, so that the family will not have to bear that heavy burden alone.

For several years, the responsibilities of attending pediatrician[s] have been assumed chiefly by ourselves, who, as a result, have become acquainted intimately with the problems of the infants, the staff, and the parents. Our almost constant availability to staff, private pediatricians and parents has resulted in the raising of more and more ethical questions about various aspects of intensive care for critically ill and congenitally deformed infants. The penetrating questions and challenges, particularly of knowledgeable parents (such as physicians, nurses, or lawyers), brought increasing doubts about the wisdom of many of the decisions that seemed to parents to be predicated chiefly on technical considerations. Some thought their child had a right to die since he could not live well or effectively. Others thought that society should pay the costs of care that may be so destructive to the family economy. Often, too, the parents' or siblings' rights to relief from the seemingly pointless, crushing burdens were important considerations. It seemed right to yield to parent wishes in several cases as physicians have done for generations. As a result, some treatments were withheld or stopped with the knowledge that earlier death and relief from suffering would result. Such options were explored with the less knowledgeable parents to ensure that their consent for treatment of their defective children was truly informed. As Eisenberg[8] pointed out regarding the application of technology, "At long last, we are beginning to ask, not *can* it be done, but *should* it be done?" In lengthy, frank discussions, the anguish of the parents was shared, and attempts were made to support fully the reasoned choices, whether for active treatment and rehabilitation or for an early death.

To determine the extent to which death resulted from withdrawing or withholding treatment, we examined the hospital records of all children who died from January 1, 1970, through June 30, 1972.

Results

In total, there were 299 deaths; each was classified in one of two categories; deaths in Category 1 resulted from pathologic conditions in spite of the treatment given; 256 (86 per cent) were in this category. Of these, 66 per cent were the result of respiratory problems or complications associated with extreme prematurity (birth weight under 1000 g). Congenital heart disease and other anomalies accounted for an additional 22 per cent (Table 1).

Deaths in Category 2 were associated with severe impairment, usually from congenital disorders (Table 2): 43 (14 per cent) were in this group. These deaths or their timing was associated with discontinuance or withdrawal of treatment. The mean duration of life in Category 2 (Table 3) was greater than that in Category 1. This was the result of a mean life of 55 days for eight infants who

TABLE 1   Problems Causing Death in Category 1

Problem	No. of Deaths	Percentage
Respiratory	108	42.2
Extreme prematurity	60	23.4
Heart disease	42	16.4
Multiple anomalies	14	5.5
Other	32	12.5
Totals	256	100.0

TABLE 2   Problems Associated with Death in Category 2

Problem	No. of Deaths	Percentage
Multiple anomalies	15	34.9
Trisomy	8	18.6
Cardiopulmonary	8	18.6
Meningomyelocele	7	16.3
Other central-nervous-system defects	3	7.0
Short-bowel syndrome	2	4.6
Totals	43	100.0

TABLE 3   Selected Comparisons of 256 Cases in Category 1 and 43 in Category 2

Attribute	Category 1	Category 2
Mean length of life	4.8 days	7.5 days
Standard deviation	8.8	34.3
Range	1–69	1–150
Portion living for < 2 days	50.0%	12.0%

became chronic cardiopulmonary cripples but for whom prolonged and intensive efforts were made in the hope of eventual recovery. They were infants who were dependent on oxygen, digoxin and diuretics, and most of them had been treated for the idiopathic respiratory-distress syndrome with high oxygen concentrations and positive-pressure ventilation.

Some examples of management choices in Category 2 illustrate the problems. An infant with Down's syndrome and intestinal atresia, like the much-publicized one at Johns Hopkins Hospital,[9] was not treated because his parents thought that surgery was wrong for their baby and themselves. He died seven days after birth. Another child had chronic pulmonary disease after positive-pressure ventilation with high oxygen concentrations for treatment of severe idiopathic respiratory-distress syndrome. By five months of age, he still required 40 per cent oxygen to survive, and even then, he was chronically dyspneic and cyanotic. He also suffered from cor pulmonale, which was difficult to control with digoxin and diuretics. The nurses, parents and physicians considered it cruel to continue, and yet difficult to stop. All were attached to this child, whose life they had tried so hard to make worthwhile. The family had endured high expenses (the hospital bill exceeding $15,000), and the strains of the illness were believed to be threatening the marriage bonds and to be causing sibling behavioral disturbances. Oxygen supplementation was stopped, and the child died in about three hours. The family settled down and 18 months later had another baby, who was healthy.

A third child had meningomyelocele, hydrocephalus and major anomalies of every organ in the pelvis. When the parents understood the limits of medical care and rehabilitation, they believed no treatment should be given. She died at five days of age.

We have maintained contact with most families of children in Category 2. Thus far, these families appear to have experienced a normal mourning for their losses. Although some have exhibited doubts that the choices were correct, all appear to be as effective in their lives as they were before this experience. Some claim that their profoundly moving experience has provided a deeper meaning in life, and from this they believe they have become more effective people.

Members of all religious faiths and atheists were participants as parents and as staff in these experiences. There appeared to be no relation between participation and a person's religion. Repeated participation in these troubling events did not appear to reduce the worry of the staff about the awesome nature of the decisions.

Discussion

That decisions are made not to treat severely defective infants may be no surprise to those familiar with special-care facilities. All laymen and professionals familiar with our nursery appeared to set some limits upon their application of treatment to extend life or to investigate a pathologic process. For example, an experienced nurse said about one child, "We lost him several weeks ago. Isn't it time to quit?" In another case, a house officer said to a physician investigating an aspect of a child's disease, "For this child, don't you think it's time to turn off your curiosity so you can turn on your kindness?" Like many others, these children eventually acquired the "right to die."

Arguments among staff members and families for and against such decisions were based on varied notions of the rights and interests of defective infants, their families, professionals and society. They were also related to varying ideas about prognosis. Regarding the infants, some contended that individuals should have a right to die in some circumstances such as anencephaly, hydranencephaly, and some severely deforming and incapacitating conditions. Such very defective individuals were considered to have little or no hope of achieving meaningful "humanhood."[10] For example, they have little or no capacity to love or be loved. They are often cared for in facilities that have been characterized as "hardly more than dying bins,"[11] an assessment with which, in our experience, knowledgeable parents (those who visited chronic-care facilities for placement of their children) agreed. With institutionalized well children, social participation may be essentially nonexistent, and maternal deprivation severe; this is known to have an adverse, usually disastrous, effect upon the child.[12] The situation for the defective child is probably worse, for he is restricted socially both by his need for care and by his defects. To escape "wrongful life,"[13] a fate rated as worse than death, seemed right. In this regard, Lasagna[14] notes, "We may, as a society, scorn the civilizations that slaughtered their infants, but our present treatment of the retarded is in some ways more cruel."

Others considered allowing a child to die wrong for several reasons. The person most involved, the infant, had no voice in the decision. Prognosis was not always exact, and a few children with extensive care might live for months, and occasionally years. Some might survive and function satisfactorily. To a few persons, withholding treatment and accepting death was condemned as criminal.

Families had strong but mixed feelings about management decisions. Living with the handicapped is clearly a family affair, and families of deformed infants thought there were limits to what they could bear or should be expected to bear. Most of them wanted maximal efforts to sustain life and to rehabilitate the handicapped; in such cases, they were supported fully. However, some families, especially those having children with severe defects, feared that they and their other children would become socially enslaved, economically deprived, and permanently stigmatized, all perhaps for a lost cause. Such a state of "chronic sorrow" until death has been described by Olshansky.[15] In some cases, families considered the death of the child right both for the child and for the family. They asked if that choice could be theirs or their doctors.

As Feifel has reported,[16] physicians on the whole are reluctant to deal with the issues. Some, particularly specialists based in the medical center, gave specific reasons for this disinclination. There was a feeling that to "give up" was disloyal to the cause of the profession. Since major research, teaching and patient-care efforts were being made, professionals expected to discover, transmit and apply knowledge and skills; patients and families were supposed to co-operate fully even if they were not always grateful. Some physicians recognized that the wishes of families went against their own, but they were resolute. They commonly agreed that if they were the parents of very defective children, with-holding treatment would be most desirable for them. However, they argued that aggressive management was indicated for others. Some believed that allowing death as a management option was euthanasia and must be stopped for fear of setting a "poor ethical example" or for fear of personal prosecution or damage to their clinical departments or to the medical center as a whole. Alexander's report on Nazi Germany[17] was cited in some cases as providing justification for pressing the effort to combat disease. Some persons were concerned about the loss through death of "teaching material." They feared the training of professionals for the care of defective children in the future and the advancing of the state of the art would be compromised. Some parents who became aware of this concern thought their children should not become experimental subjects.

Practicing pediatricians, general practitioners and obstetricians were often familiar with these families and were usually sympathetic with their views. However, since they were more distant from the special-care nursery than the specialists of the medical center, their influence was often minimal. As a result, families received little support from them, and tension in community-medical relations was a recurring problem.

Infants with severe types of meningomyelocele precipitated the most controversial decisions. Several decades ago, those who survived this condition beyond a few weeks usually became hydrocephalic and retarded, in addition to being crippled and deformed. Without modern treatment, they died earlier.[18] Some may have been killed or at least not resuscitated at birth.[19] From the early 1960's, the tendency has been to treat vigorously all infants with meningomyelocele. As advocated by Zachary[20] and Shurtleff,[21] aggressive management of these children became the rule in our unit as in many others. Infants were usually referred quickly. Parents routinely signed permits for operation though rarely had they seen their children's defects or had the nature of various management plans and their respective prognoses clearly explained to them. Some physicians believed that parents were too upset to understand the nature of the problems and the options for care. Since they believed informed consent had no meaning in these circumstances, they either ignored the parents or simply told them that the child needed an operation on the back as the first step in correcting several defects. As a result, parents often felt completely left out while the activities of care proceeded at a brisk pace.

Some physicians experienced in the care of these children and familiar with the impact of such conditions upon families had early reservations about this plan of care.[22] More recently, they were influenced by the pessimistic appraisal of vigorous management schemes in some cases.[5] Meningomyelocele, when treated vigorously, is associated with higher survival rates,[21] but the achievement of satisfactory rehabilitation is at best difficult and usually impossible for almost all who are severely affected. Knowing this, some physicians and some families[23] decide against treatment of the most severely affected. If treatment is not carried out, the child's condition will usually deteriorate from further brain damage, urinary-tract infections and orthopedic difficulties, and death can be expected much earlier. Two thirds may be dead by three months, and over 90 per cent by one year of age. However, the quality of life during that time is poor, and the strains on families are great, but not necessarily greater than with treatment.[24] Thus, both treatment and nontreatment constitute unsatisfactory dilemmas for everyone, especially for the child and his family. When maximum treatment was viewed as unacceptable by families and physicians in our unit, there was a growing tendency to seek early death as a management option, to avoid that cruel choice of gradual, often slow, but progressive deterioration of the child who was required under these circumstances in effect to kill himself. Parents and the staff then asked if his dying needed to be prolonged. If not, what were the most appropriate medical responses?

Is it possible that some physicians and some families may join in a conspiracy to deny the right of a defective child to live or to die? Either could occur. Prolongation of the dying process by resident physicians having a vested interest in their careers has been described by Sudnow.[25] On the other hand, from the fatigue of working long and hard some physicians may give up too soon, assuming that their cause is lost. Families, similarly, may have mixed motives. They may demand death to obtain relief from the high costs and the tensions inherent in suffering, but their sense of guilt in this thought may produce the opposite demand, perhaps in violation of the sick person's rights. Thus, the challenge of deciding what course to take can be most tormenting for the family and the physician. Unquestionably, not facing the issue would appear to be the easier course, at least temporarily; no doubt many patients, families, and physicians decline to join in an effort to solve the problems. They can readily assume that what is being done is right and sufficient and ask no questions. But pretending there is no decision to be made is an arbitrary and potentially devastating decision of default. Since families and patients must live with the problems one way or another in any case, the physician's failure to face the issues may constitute a victimizing abandonment of patients and their families in times of greatest need. As Lasagna[14] pointed out, "There is no place for the physician to hide."

Can families in the shock resulting from the birth of a defective child understand what faces them? Can they give truly "informed consent" for treatment or with-holding treatment? Some of our colleagues answer no to both questions. In our opinion, if families regardless of background are heard sympathetically and at length and are given information and answers to their questions in words they understand, the problems of their children as well as the expected benefits and limits of any proposed care can be understood clearly in practically all instances. Parents *are* able to understand the implications of such things as chronic dyspnea, oxygen dependency, incontinence, paralysis, contractures, sexual handicaps and mental retardation.

Another problem concerns who decides for a child. It may be acceptable for a person to reject treatment and bring about his own death. But it is quite a different situation when others are doing this for him. We do not know how often families and their physicians will make just decisions for severely handicapped children. Clearly, this issue is central in evaluation of the process of decision making that we have described. But we also ask, if these parties cannot make such decisions justly, who can?

We recognize great variability and often much uncertainty in prognoses and in family capacities to deal with defective newborn infants. We also acknowledge that there are limits of support that society can or will give to assist handicapped persons and their families. Severely deforming conditions that are associated with little or no hope of a functional existence pose painful dilemmas for the laymen and professionals who must decide how to cope with severe handicaps. We believe the burdens of decision making must be borne by families and their professional advisers because they are most familiar with the respective situations. Since families primarily must live with and are most affected by the decisions, it therefore appears that society and the health professions should provide only general guidelines for decision making. Moreover, since variations between situations are so great, and the situations themselves so complex, it follows that much latitude in decision making should be expected and tolerated. Otherwise, the rules of society or the policies most convenient for medical technologists may become cruel masters of human beings instead of their servants. Regarding any "allocation of death"[26] policy we readily acknowledge that the extreme excesses of Hegelian "rational utility" under dictatorships must be avoided.[17] Perhaps it is less recognized that the uncontrolled application of medical technology may be detrimental to individuals and families. In this regard, our views are similar to those of Waitzkin and Stoekle.[27] Physicians may hold excessive power over decision making by limiting or controlling the information made available to patients or families. It seems appropriate that the profession be held accountable for presenting fully all management options and their expected consequences. Also, the public should be aware that professionals often face conflicts of interest that may result in decisions against individual preferences.

What are the legal implications of actions like those described in this paper? Some persons may argue that the law has been broken, and others would contend otherwise. Perhaps more than anything else, the public and professional silence on a major social taboo and some common practices has been broken further. That seems appropriate, for out of the ensuing dialogue perhaps better choices for patients and families can be made. If working out these dilemmas in ways such as those we suggest is in violation of the law, we believe the law should be changed.

References

1. Wegman ME: Annual summary of vital statistics—1970. Pediatrics 48:979–983, 1971
2. Swyer PR: The regional organization of special care for the neonate. Pediatr Clin North Am 17:761–776, 1970
3. Rawlings G, Reynold EOR, Stewart A, et al: Changing prognosis for infants of very low birth weight. Lancet 1:516–519, 1971
4. Freeman E: The god committee New York Times Magazine, May 21, 1972, pp 84–90
5. Lorber J: Results of treatment of myelomeningocele. Dev Med Child Neurol 13:279–303, 1971
6. Slater E: Health service or sickness service. Br Med J 4:734–736, 1971
7. Klaus MH, Kennell JH: Mothers separated from their newborn infants. Pediatr Clin North Am 17:1015–1037, 1970
8. Eisenberg L: The human nature of human nature. Science 176:123–128, 1972
9. Report of the Joseph P. Kennedy Foundation International Symposium on

Human Rights, Retardation and Research. Washington, DC, The John F. Kennedy Center for the Performing Arts, October 16, 1971

10. Fletcher J: Indicators of humanhood: a tentative profile of man. The Hastings Center Report Vol 2, No 5. Hastings-on-Hudson, New York, Institute of Society, Ethics and the Life Sciences, November, 1972, pp 1–4

11. Freeman HE, Brim OG Jr, Williams G: New dimensions of dying, The Dying Patient. Edited by OG Brim Jr. New York, Russell Sage Foundation, 1970, pp xiii–xxvi

12. Spitz RA: Hospitalism: an inquiry into the genesis of psychiatric conditions in early childhood. Psychoanal Study Child 1: 53–74, 1945

13. Engelhardt HT Jr: Euthanasia and children: the injury of continued existence. J Pediatr 83:170–171, 1973

14. Lasagna L: Life, Death and the Doctor. New York, Alfred A Knopf, 1968

15. Olshansky S: Chronic sorrow: a response to having a mentally defective child. Soc Casework 43:190–193, 1962

16. Feifel H: Perception of death. Ann NY Acad Sci 164:669–677, 1969

17. Alexander L: Medical science under dictatorship. N Engl J Med 241:39–47, 1949

18. Laurence KM and Tew BJ: Natural history of spina bifida cystica and cranium bifidum cysticum: major central nervous system malformations in South Wales. Part IV. Arch Dis Child 46:127–138, 1971

19. Forrest DM: Modern trends in the treatment of spina bifida: early closure in spina bifida: results and problems. Proc R Soc Med 60:763–767, 1967

20. Zachary RB: Ethical and social aspects of treatment of spina bifida. Lancet 2:274–276. 1968

21. Shurtleff DB: Care of the myelodysplastic patient, Ambulatory Pediatrics. Edited by M Green, R Haggerty. Philadelphia, WB Saunders Company, 1968, pp 726–741

22. Matson DD: Surgical treatment of myelomeningocele. Pediatrics 42:225–227, 1968

23. MacKeith RC: A new look at spina bifida aperta. Dev Med Child Neurol 13:277–278, 1971

24. Hide DW, Williams HP, Ellis HL: The outlook for the child with a myelomeningocele for whom early surgery was considered inadvisable. Dev Med Child Neurol 14:304–307, 1972

25. Sudnow D: Passing On. Englewood Cliffs, New Jersey, Prentice Hall, 1967

26. Manning B: Legal and policy issues in the allocation of death, The Dying Patient. Edited by OG Brim Jr. New York, Russell Sage Foundation. 1970, pp 253–274

27. Waitzkin H. Stoeckle JD: The communication of information about illness. Adv Psychosom Med 8:180–215, 1972

To Save or Let Die
The Dilemma of Modern Medicine

Richard A. McCormick

Richard A. McCormick is a Jesuit theologian working in the Roman Catholic tradition of moral theology, which has a long history of interest in medical ethics. Father McCormick was Joseph P. Kennedy Professor of Medical Ethics at the Kennedy Institute for Ethics, Georgetown University, one of the earliest study centers in bioethics, and is now professor of moral theology at Notre Dame University.

"To Save or Let Die" was among the many responses to the ethical dilemmas posed by Duff and Campbell's revelations and by the paradigm case of a baby with Down's syndrome who was allowed to die at Johns Hopkins Hospital in 1971, a case widely publicized in a short film made by the Joseph P. Kennedy Foundation. In this article, Father McCormick develops a concept of "meaningful life" that, while rooted in theological ideas, can be translated into broadly acceptable secular terms and used as the basis for decisions to sustain newborn life or allow death to come.

. . . In a recent issue of the *New England Journal of Medicine*, Drs. Raymond S. Duff and A. G. M. Campbell[1] reported on 299 deaths in the special-care nursery of the Yale–New Haven Hospital between 1970 and 1972. Of these, 43 (14%) were associated with discontinuance of treatment for children with multiple anomalies, trisomy, cardiopulmonary crippling, meningomyelocele, and other central nervous system defects. After careful consideration of each of these 43 infants, parents and physicians in a group decision concluded that the prognosis for "meaningful life" was extremely poor or hopeless, and therefore rejected further treatment. . . .

In commenting on this study in the *Washington Post* (Oct. 28, 1973), Dr. Lawrence K. Pickett, chief-of-staff at the Yale–New Haven Hospital, admitted that allowing hopelessly ill patients to die "is accepted medical practice." He continued: "This is nothing new. It's just being talked about now."

It has been talked about, it is safe to say, at least since the publicity associated with the famous "Johns Hopkins Case"[2] some three years ago. In this instance, an infant was born with Down's syndrome and duodenal atresia. The blockage is reparable by relatively easy surgery. However, after consultation with spiritual

---

advisors, the parents refused permission for this corrective surgery, and the child died by starvation in the hospital after 15 days. For to feed him by mouth in this condition would have killed him. Nearly everyone who has commented on this case has disagreed with the decision.

It must be obvious that these instances—and they are frequent—raise the most agonizing and delicate moral problems. The problem is best seen in the ambiguity of the term "hopelessly ill." This used to and still may refer to lives that cannot be saved, that are irretrievably in the dying process. It may also refer to lives that can be saved and sustained, but in a wretched, painful, or deformed condition. With regard to infants, the problem is, which infants, if any, should be allowed to die? On what grounds or according to what criteria as determined by whom? Or again, is there a point at which a life that can be saved is not "meaningful life," as the medical community so often phrases the question. . . .

Thus far, the ethical discussion of these truly terrifying decisions has been less than fully satisfactory. Perhaps this is to be expected since the problems have only recently come to public attention. In a companion article to the Duff–Campbell report,[1] Dr. Anthony Shaw[3] of the Pediatric Division of the Department of Surgery, University of Virginia Medical Center, Charlottesville, speaks of solutions "based on the circumstances of each case rather than by means of a dogmatic formula approach." Are these really the only options available to us? Shaw's statement makes it appear that the ethical alternatives are narrowed to dogmatism (which imposes a formula that prescinds from circumstances) and pure concretism (which denies the possibility or usefulness of any guidelines). . . .

What has brought us to this position of awesome responsibility? Very simply, the sophistication of modern medicine. Contemporary resuscitation and life-sustaining devices have brought a remarkable change in the state of the question. Our duties toward the care and preservation of life have been traditionally stated in terms of the use of ordinary and extraordinary means. For the moment and for purposes of brevity, we may say that, morally speaking, ordinary means are those whose use does not entail grave hardships to the patient. Those that would involve such hardship are extraordinary. Granted the relativity of these terms and the frequent difficulty of their application, still the distinction has had an honored place in medical ethics and medical practice. Indeed, the distinction was recently reiterated by the House of Delegates of the American Medical Association (AMA) in a policy statement. After disowning intentional killing (mercy killing), the AMA statement continues: "The cessation of the employment of extraordinary means to prolong the life of the body when there is irrefutable evidence that biological death is imminent is the decision of the patient and/or his immediate family. The advice and judgment of the physician should be freely available to the patient and/or his immediate family" (*JAMA* 227:728, 1974).

This distinction can take us just so far—and thus the change in the state of the question. The contemporary problem is precisely that the question no longer concerns only those for whom "biological death is imminent" in the sense of the AMA statement. Many infants who would have died a decade ago, whose "biological death was imminent," can be saved. Yesterday's failures are today's successes. Contemporary medicine with its team approaches, staged surgical techniques, monitoring capabilities, ventilatory support systems, and other methods, can keep almost anyone alive. This has tended gradually to shift the problem from the means to reverse the dying process to the quality of the life sustained and preserved. The questions, "Is this means too hazardous or difficult to use" and "Does this measure only prolong the patient's dying," while still useful and valid, now often become "Granted that we can easily save the life, what kind of life are we saving?" This is a quality-of-life judgment. And we fear it. And certainly we should. But with increased power goes increased responsibility. Since we have the power, we must face the responsibility.

A Relative Good

In the past, the Judeo-Christian tradition has attempted to walk a balanced middle path between medical vitalism (that preserves life at any cost) and medical pessimism (that kills when life seems frustrating, burdensome, "useless"). Both of these extremes root in an identical idolatry of life—an attitude that, at least by inference, views death as an unmitigated, absolute evil, and life as the absolute good. The middle course that has structured Judeo-Christian attitudes is that life is indeed a basic and precious good, but a good to be preserved precisely as the condition of other values. It is these other values and possibilities that found the duty to preserve physical life and also dictate the limits of this duty. In other words, life is a relative good, and the duty to preserve it a limited one. These limits have always been stated in terms of the *means* required to sustain life. But if the implications of this middle position are unpacked a bit, they will allow us, perhaps, to adapt to the type of quality-of-life judgment we are now called on to make without tumbling into vitalism or a utilitarian pessimism.

A beginning can be made with a statement of Pope Pius XII[4] in an allocution to physicians delivered Nov. 24, 1957. After noting that we are normally obliged to use only ordinary means to preserve life, the Pontiff stated: "A more strict obligation would be too burdensome for most men and would render the attainment of the higher, more important good too difficult. Life, death, all temporal activities are in fact subordinated to spiritual ends." Here it would be helpful to ask two questions. First, what are these spiritual ends, this "higher, more important good"? Second, how is its attainment rendered too difficult by insisting on the use of extraordinary means to preserve life?

The first question must be answered in terms of love of God and neighbor. This sums up briefly the meaning, substance, and consummation of life from a Judeo-Christian perspective. What is or can easily be missed is that these two loves are not separable. . . . It is in others that God demands to be recognized and loved. If this is true, it means that, in Judeo-Christian perspective, the meaning, substance, and consummation of life is found in human *relationships*, and the qualities of justice, respect, concern, compassion, and support that surround them.

Second, how is the attainment of this "higher, more important (than life) good" rendered "too difficult" by life-supports that are gravely burdensome? One who must support his life with disproportionate effort focuses the time, attention, energy, and resources of himself and others not precisely on relationships, but on maintaining the condition of relationships. Such concentration easily becomes overconcentration and distorts one's view of and weakens one's pursuit of the very relational goods that define our growth and flourishing. The importance of relationships gets lost in the struggle for survival. The very Judeo-Christian meaning of life is seriously jeopardized when undue and unending effort must go into its maintenance.

I believe an analysis similar to this is implied in traditional treatises on preserving life. The illustrations of grave hardship (rendering the means to preserve life extraordinary and nonobligatory) are instructive, even if they are outdated in some of their particulars. Older moralists often referred to the hardship of moving to another climate or country. As the late Gerald Kelly[5] noted of this instance: "They (the classical moral theologians) spoke of other inconveniences, too: e.g., of moving to another climate or another country to preserve one's life. For people whose lives were, so to speak, rooted in the land, and whose native town or village was as dear as life itself, and for whom, moreover, travel was always difficult and often dangerous—for such people, moving to another country or climate was a truly great hardship, and more than God would demand as a 'reasonable' means of preserving one's health and life."

Similarly, if the financial cost of life-preserving care was crushing, that is, if it would create grave hardships for oneself or one's family, it was considered extraordinary and nonobligatory. Or again, the grave inconvenience of living with a badly mutilated body was viewed, along with other factors (such as pain in preanesthetic days, uncertainty of success), as constituting the means extraordinary. Even now, the contemporary moralist, M. Zalba,[6] states that no one is obliged to preserve his life when the cost is "a most oppressive convalescence" (*molestissima convalescentia*).

The Quality of Life

In all of these instances—instances where the life could be saved—the discussion is couched in terms of the means necessary to preserve life. But often enough it is the kind of, the quality of the life thus saved (painful, poverty-stricken and deprived, away from home and friends, oppressive) that establishes the means as extraordinary. *That* type of life would be an excessive hardship for the individual. It would distort and jeopardize his grasp on the overall meaning of life. Why? Because, it can be argued, human relationships—which are the very possibility of growth in love of God and neighbor—would be so threatened, strained, or submerged that they would no longer function as the heart and meaning of the individual's life as they should. Something other than the "higher, more important good" would occupy first place. Life, the condition of other values and achievements, would usurp the place of these and become itself the ultimate value. When that happens, the value of human life has been distorted out of context. . . .

Can these reflections be brought to bear on the grossly malformed infant? I believe so. Obviously there is a difference between having a terribly mutilated body as the result of surgery, and having a terribly mutilated body from birth. There is also a difference between a long, painful, oppressive convalescence resulting from surgery, and a life that is from birth one long, painful, oppressive convalescence. Similarly, there is a difference between being plunged into poverty by medical expenses and being poor without ever incurring such expenses. However, is there not also a similarity? Can not these conditions, whether caused by medical intervention or not, equally absorb attention and energies to the point where the "higher, more important good" is simply too difficult to attain? It would appear so. Indeed, is this not precisely why abject poverty (and the systems that support it) is such an enormous moral challenge to us? It simply dehumanizes.

Life's potentiality for other values is dependent on two factors, those external to the individual, and the very condition of the individual. The former we can and must change to maximize individual potential. That is what social justice is all about. The latter we sometimes cannot alter. It is neither inhuman nor unchristian to say that there comes a point where an individual's condition itself represents the negation of any truly human—i.e., relational—potential. When that point is reached, is not the best treatment no treatment? . . .

Human Relationships

If these reflections are valid, they point in the direction of a guideline that may help in decisions about sustaining the lives of grossly deformed and deprived infants. That guideline is the potential for human relationships associated with the infant's condition. If that potential is simply nonexistent or would be utterly submerged and undeveloped in the mere struggle to survive, that life has achieved its potential. There are those who will want to continue to say that some terribly deformed infants may be allowed to die *because* no extraordinary means need be used. Fair enough. But they should realize that the term "extraordinary" has been so relativized to the condition of the patient that it is this condition that is decisive. The means is extraordinary because the infant's condition is extraordinary. And if that is so, we must face this fact head-on—and discover the substantive standard that allows us to say this of some infants, but not of others.

Here several caveats are in order. First, this guideline is not a detailed rule that preempts decisions; for relational capacity is not subject to mathematical analysis but to human judgment. However, it is the task of physicians to provide some more concrete categories or presumptive biological symptoms for this human judgment. For instance, nearly all would very likely agree that the anencephalic infant is without relational potential. On the other hand, the same cannot be said of the mongoloid infant. The task ahead is to attach relational potential to presumptive biological symptoms for the gray area between such extremes. In other words, individual decisions will remain the anguishing onus of parents in consultation with physicians.

Second, because this guideline is precisely that, mistakes will be made. Some infants will be judged in all sincerity to be devoid of any meaningful relational potential when that is actually not quite the case. This risk of error should not lead to abandonment of decisions; for that is to walk away from the human scene. Risk of error means only that we must proceed with great humility, caution, and tentativeness. Concretely, it means that if err we must at times, it is better to err on the side of life—and therefore to tilt in that direction.

Third, it must be emphasized that allowing some infants to die does not imply that "some lives are valuable, others not" or that "there is such a thing as a life not worth living." Every human being, regardless of age or condition, is of incalculable worth. The point is not, therefore, whether this or that individual has value. Of course he has, or rather *is* a value. The only point is whether this undoubted value has any potential at all, in continuing physical survival, for attaining a share, even if reduced, in the "higher, more important good." This is not a question about the inherent value of the individual. It is a question about whether this worldly existence will offer such a valued individual any hope of sharing those values for which physical life is the fundamental condition. Is not the only alternative an attitude that supports mere physical life as long as possible with every means?

Fourth, this whole matter is further complicated by the fact that this decision is being made for someone else. Should not the decision on whether life is to be supported or not be left to the individual? Obviously, wherever possible. But there is nothing inherently objectionable in the fact that parents with physicians must make this decision at some point for infants. Parents must make many crucial decisions for children. The only concern is that the decision not be shaped out of the utilitarian perspectives so deeply sunk into the consciousness of the contemporary world. In a highly technological culture, an individual is always in danger of being valued for his function, what he can do, rather than for who he is. . . .

Were not those who disagreed with the Hopkins decision saying, in effect, that for the infant, involved human relationships were still within reach and would not be totally submerged by survival? If that is the case, it is potential for relationships that is at the heart of these agonizing decisions.

References

1. Duff, S., Campbell, A. G. M., Moral and ethical dilemmas in the special-care nursery. *N. Engl. J. Med.* 289:890–894, 1973.
2. Gustafson, J. M., Mongolism, parental desires, and the right to life. *Perspect. Biol. Med.* 16:529–559, 1973.

3. Shaw, A., Dilemmas of "informed" consent in children. *N. Engl. J. Med.* 289:885–890, 1973.
4. Pope Pius XII, *Acta Apostolicae Sedis.* 49:1031–1032, 1957.
5. Kelly, G., *Medico-Moral Problems.* St. Louis, Catholic Hospital Association of the United Stales and Canada, 1957, p. 132.
6. Zalba, M., *Theologiae Moralis Summa.* Madrid, La Editorial Catolica. 1957, vol. 2, p. 71.

Active and Passive Euthanasia

James Rachels

James Rachels, a professor of moral philosophy at University of Miami, offered a radical critique of a distinction that was common among medical ethicists, namely, that passive euthanasia, or allowing to die, was morally acceptable, while active euthanasia, equivalent to killing, was not. This paper did not notably change the prevalence of the received distinction at the time of its publication, but set in motion a skepticism about its viability as a useful ethical distinction that eventually gave credibility to the arguments for assisted suicide that appeared in the 1990s.

The distinction between active and passive euthanasia is thought to be crucial for medical ethics. The idea is that it is permissible, at least in some cases, to withhold treatment and allow a patient to die, but it is never permissible to take any direct action designed to kill the patient. This doctrine seems to be accepted by most doctors, and it is endorsed in a statement adopted by the House of Delegates of the American Medical Association on December 4, 1973:

> The intentional termination of the life of one human being by another—mercy killing—is contrary to that for which the medical profession stands and is contrary to the policy of the American Medical Association.
>
> The cessation of the employment of extraordinary means to prolong the life of the body when there is irrefutable evidence that biological death is imminent is the decision of the patient and/or his immediate family. The advice and judgment of the physician should be freely available to the patient and/or his immediate family.

However, a strong case can be made against this doctrine. In what follows I will set out some of the relevant arguments, and urge doctors to reconsider their views on this matter.

To begin with a familiar type of situation, a patient who is dying of incurable cancer of the throat is in terrible pain, which can no longer be satisfactorily alleviated. He is certain to die within a few days, even if present treatment is continued, but he does not want to go on living for those days since the pain is unbearable. So he asks the doctor for an end to it, and his family joins in the request.

Suppose the doctor agrees to withhold treatment, as the conventional doctrine says he may. The justification for his doing so is that the patient is in terrible agony, and since he is going to die anyway, it would be wrong to prolong his suffering needlessly. But now notice this. If one simply withholds treatment, it may take the patient longer to die, and so he may suffer more than he would if more direct action were taken and a lethal injection given. This fact provides strong reason for thinking that, once the initial decision not to prolong his agony has been made, active euthanasia is actually preferable to passive euthanasia, rather than the reverse. To say otherwise is to endorse the option that leads to more suffering rather than less, and is contrary to the humanitarian impulse that prompts the decision not to prolong his life in the first place.

Part of my point is that the process of being "allowed to die" can be relatively slow and painful, whereas being given a lethal injection is relatively quick and painless. Let me give a different sort of example. In the United States about one in 600 babies is born with Down's syndrome. Most of these babies are otherwise healthy—that is, with only the usual pediatric care, they will proceed to an otherwise normal infancy. Some, however, are born with congenital defects such as intestinal obstructions that require operations if they are to live. Sometimes, the parents and the doctor will decide not to operate, and let the infant die. Anthony Shaw describes what happens then:

> . . . When surgery is denied [the doctor] must try to keep the infant from suffering while natural forces sap the baby's life away. As a surgeon whose natural inclination is to use the scalpel to fight off death, standing by and watching a salvageable baby die is the most emotionally exhausting experience I know. It is easy at a conference, in a theoretical discussion, to decide that such infants should be allowed to die. It is altogether different to stand by in the nursery and watch as dehydration and infection wither a tiny being over hours and days. This is a terrible ordeal for me and the hospital staff—much more so than for the parents who never set foot in the nursery.*

I can understand why some people are opposed to all euthanasia, and insist that such infants must be allowed to live. I think I can also understand why other people favor destroying these babies quickly and painlessly. But why should anyone favor letting "dehydration and infection wither a tiny being over hours and days?" The doctrine that says that a baby may be allowed to dehydrate and wither, but may not be given an injection that would end its life without suffering, seems so patently cruel as to require no further refutation. The strong language is not intended to offend, but only to put the point in the clearest possible way.

My second argument is that the conventional doctrine leads to decisions concerning life and death made on irrelevant grounds.

Consider again the case of the infants with Down's syndrome who need

---

*Shaw A: 'Doctor, Do We Have a Choice?' The New York Times Magazine, January 30, 1972, p 54.

operations for congenital defects unrelated to the syndrome to live. Sometimes, there is no operation, and the baby dies, but when there is no such defect, the baby lives on. Now, an operation such as that to remove an intestinal obstruction is not prohibitively difficult. The reason why such operations are not performed in these cases is, clearly, that the child has Down's syndrome and the parents and doctor judge that because of that fact it is better for the child to die.

But notice that this situation is absurd, no matter what view one takes of the lives and potentials of such babies. If the life of such an infant is worth preserving, what does it matter if it needs a simple operation? Or, if one thinks it better that such a baby should not live on, what difference does it make that it happens to have an unobstructed intestinal tract? In either case, the matter of life and death is being decided on irrelevant grounds. It is the Down's syndrome, and not the intestines, that is the issue. The matter should be decided, if at all, on that basis, and not be allowed to depend on the essentially irrelevant question of whether the intestinal tract is blocked.

What makes this situation possible, of course, is the idea that when there is an intestinal blockage, one can "let the baby die," but when there is no such defect there is nothing that can be done, for one must not "kill" it. The fact that this idea leads to such results as deciding life or death on irrelevant grounds is another good reason why the doctrine should be rejected.

One reason why so many people think that there is an important moral difference between active and passive euthanasia is that they think killing someone is morally worse than letting someone die. But is it? Is killing, in itself, worse than letting die? To investigate this issue, two cases may be considered that are exactly alike except that one involves killing whereas the other involves letting someone die. Then, it can be asked whether this difference makes any difference to the moral assessments. It is important that the cases be exactly alike, except for this one difference, since otherwise one cannot be confident that it is this difference and not some other that accounts for any variation in the assessments of the two cases. So, let us consider this pair of cases:

In the first, Smith stands to gain a large inheritance if anything should happen to his six-year-old cousin. One evening while the child is taking his bath, Smith sneaks into the bathroom and drowns the child, and then arranges things so that it will look like an accident.

In the second, Jones also stands to gain if anything should happen to his six-year-old cousin. Like Smith, Jones sneaks in planning to drown the child in his bath. However, just as he enters the bathroom Jones sees the child slip and hit his head, and fall face down in the water. Jones is delighted; he stands by, ready to push the child's head back under if it is necessary, but it is not necessary. With only a little thrashing about, the child drowns all by himself, "accidentally," as Jones watches and does nothing.

Now Smith killed the child, whereas Jones "merely" let the child die. That is the only difference between them. Did either man behave better, from a moral point of view? If the difference between killing and letting die were in itself a morally important matter, one should say that Jones's behavior was less reprehensible than Smith's. But does one really want to say that? I think not. In the first place, both men acted from the same motive, personal gain, and both had exactly the same end in view when they acted. It may be inferred from Smith's conduct that he is a bad man, although that judgment may be withdrawn or modified if certain further facts are learned about him—for example, that he is mentally deranged. But would not the very same thing be inferred about Jones from his conduct? And would not the same further considerations also be relevant to any modification of this judgment? Moreover, suppose Jones pleaded, in his own defense, "After all, I didn't do anything except just stand there and watch the child drown. I didn't kill him; I only let him die." Again, if letting die were in itself less bad than killing, this defense should have at least some weight. But it does not. Such a "defense" can only be regarded as a grotesque perversion of moral reasoning. Morally speaking, it is no defense at all.

Now, it may be pointed out, quite properly, that the cases of euthanasia with which doctors are concerned are not like this at all. They do not involve personal gain or the destruction of normal healthy children. Doctors are concerned only with cases in which the patient's life is of no further use to him, or in which the patient's life has become or will soon become a terrible burden. However, the point is the same in these cases: the bare difference between killing and letting die does not, in itself, make a moral difference. If a doctor lets a patient die, for humane reasons, he is in the same moral position as if he had given the patient a lethal injection for humane reasons. If his decision was wrong—if, for example, the patient's illness was in fact curable—the decision would be equally regrettable no matter which method was used to carry it out. And if the doctor's decision was the right one, the method used is not in itself important.

The AMA policy statement isolates the crucial issue very well; the crucial issue is "the intentional termination of the life of one human being by another." But after identifying this issue, and forbidding "mercy killing," the statement goes on to deny that the cessation of treatment is the intentional termination of a life. This is where the mistake comes in, for what is the cessation of treatment, in these circumstances, if it is not "the intentional termination of the life of one human being by another?" Of course it is exactly that, and if it were not, there would be no point to it.

Many people will find this judgment hard to accept. One reason, I think, is that it is very easy to conflate the question of whether killing is, in itself, worse than letting die, with the very different question of whether most actual cases of killing are more reprehensible than most actual cases of letting die. Most actual cases of killing are clearly terrible (think, for example, of all the murders reported in the newspapers), and one hears of such cases every day. On the other hand, one hardly ever hears of a case of letting die, except for the actions of doctors who are motivated by humanitarian reasons. So one learns to think of killing in a much worse light than of letting die. But this does not mean that there is something about killing that makes it in itself worse than letting die, for it is not the bare difference between killing and letting die that makes the difference in these cases. Rather, the other factors—the murderer's motive of personal gain, for example, contrasted with the doctor's humanitarian motivation—account for different reactions to the different cases.

I have argued that killing is not in itself any worse than letting die; if my contention is right, it follows that active euthanasia is not any worse than passive euthanasia. What arguments can be given on the other side? The most common, I believe, is the following:

"The important difference between active and passive euthanasia is that, in passive euthanasia, the doctor does not do anything to bring about the patient's death. The doctor does nothing, and the patient dies of whatever ills already afflict him. In active euthanasia, however, the doctor does something to bring about the patient's death: he kills him. The doctor who gives the patient with cancer a lethal injection has himself caused his patient's death; whereas if he merely ceases treatment, the cancer is the cause of the death."

A number of points need to be made here. The first is that it is not exactly correct to say that in passive euthanasia the doctor does nothing, for he does do one thing that is very important: he lets the patient die. "Letting someone die" is certainly different, in some respects, from other types of action—mainly in that it is a kind of action that one may perform by way of not performing certain other actions. For example, one may let a patient die by way of not giving medication, just as one may insult someone by way of not shaking his hand. But for any purpose of moral assessment, it is a type of action nonetheless. The decision to let a patient die is subject to moral appraisal in the same way that a decision to kill him would be subject to moral appraisal: it may be assessed as wise or unwise, compassionate or sadistic, right or wrong. If a doctor deliberately let a patient die who was suffering from a routinely curable illness, the doctor would certainly be to blame for what he had done, just as he would be to blame if he had needlessly killed the patient. Charges against him would then be appropriate. If so, it would be no defense at all for him to insist that he didn't "do anything." He would have done something very serious indeed, for he let his patient die.

Fixing the cause of death may be very important from a legal point of view, for it may determine whether criminal charges are brought against the doctor. But I do not think that this notion can be used to show a moral difference between active and passive euthanasia. The reason why it is considered bad to be the cause of someone's death is that death is regarded as a great evil—and so it is. However, if it has been decided that euthanasia—even passive euthanasia—is desirable in a given case, it has also been decided that in this instance death is no greater an evil than the patient's continued existence. And if this is true, the usual reason for not wanting to be the cause of someone's death simply does not apply.

Finally, doctors may think that all of this is only of academic interest—the sort of thing that philosophers may worry about but that has no practical bearing on their own work. After all, doctors must be concerned about the legal consequences of what they do, and active euthanasia is clearly forbidden by the law.

But even so, doctors should also be concerned with the fact that the law is forcing upon them a moral doctrine that may well be indefensible, and has a considerable effect on their practices. Of course, most doctors are not now in the position of being coerced in this matter, for they do not regard themselves as merely going along with what the law requires. Rather, in statements such as the AMA policy statement that I have quoted, they are endorsing this doctrine as a central point of medical ethics. In that statement, active euthanasia is condemned not merely as illegal but as "contrary to that for which the medical profession stands," whereas passive euthanasia is approved. However, the preceding considerations suggest that there is really no moral difference between the two, considered in themselves (there may be important moral differences in some cases in their *consequences*, but, as I pointed out, these differences may make active euthanasia, and not passive euthanasia, the morally preferable option). So, whereas doctors may have to discriminate between active and passive euthanasia to satisfy the law, they should not do any more than that. In particular, they should not give the distinction any added authority and weight by writing it into official statements of medical ethics.

Prolonged Dying
Not Medically Indicated

Paul Ramsey

Paul Ramsey was Paine Professor of Religion at Princeton University when he wrote this article. Long considered a leading protestant theological ethicist, he turned his attention to medical ethics in the late 1960s and published a significant book, *Patient as Person*, in 1971. His work has been highly influential in bioethics.

"Prolonged Dying" is a short commentary, solicited by the Hastings Center Report, on the trial court's judgment in the case of Karen Ann Quinlan. Ramsey examines the language of "ordinary and extraordinary means" used in that case and widely among physicians and medical ethics. He, like Richard McCormick in "To Live and Let Die" (reprinted in this anthology), suggests that the distinction, while valuable in emphasizing the objective features of the patient's condition, should be reformulated to clarify the ethical issues at stake in the decision to allow a patient to die. His reformulation is more expansively developed in his later book, *On The Edges of Life*.

P ast moralists, in bringing principles to cases like this one [the case of Karen Anne Quinlan], used the term "ordinary means" to save life as an ethical category; it *meant* imperative means. They used the term "extraordinary means" as a term of moral permission; it *meant* electable or morally dispensable means. Like all other terms of moral approval or disapproval, these terms are, as classifications, incurably circular until filled with concrete or descriptive meaning. . . .

I suggest that the morally significant meaning of ordinary and extraordinary medical means can be reduced almost without remainder to two components. I further urge that the older language be abandoned, and that instead we should speak of (1) a comparison of treatments that are medically "indicated" and expected to be helpful, and those that are *not* medically indicated. In the case of the dying, that includes in all cases, or in most or many cases, a judgment that further curative treatment is *no longer* indicated.

Instead of the traditional language, still current among physicians, we should talk about (2) a patient's right to refuse treatment. Indeed, this entire language about ordinary and extraordinary means was developed by past moralists specifically to apply to conscious patients who are certainly not in the "process of

Paul Ramsey. "Prolonged Dying: Not Medically Indicated." Abridged from *Hastings Center Report*, Volume 6, 1976, pp. 14–16. Reprinted by permission.

dying." Thus they spoke of not leaving home and traveling great distances to obtain lifesaving treatment, of a justified revulsion of disfigurement, and so on.

Why do I say that the meaning of "ordinary/extraordinary" can be reduced "almost" without remainder to these two components? Why some hesitation in recommending that we drop the traditional language? Certainly not because of any doubt about the rightfulness of stopping further curative treatments in the case of the dying. Indeed, today we have commendably shifted debate about the meaning of those ancient terms to the case of the dying.

Still there was an important nuance in the older language that may be lost in these translations, especially in our contemporary talk about a patient's right to refuse treatment. The terms "ordinary/extraordinary"—however cumbersome, opaque, and unilluminating—directed the attention of physicians, patients, family, clergymen, and moralists to *objective* considerations of the patient's condition and the armamentarium of medicine's remedies which determined whether decisions to allow to die or to continue to try to save life were morally right or wrong decisions. . . .

We should now be prepared to see that this wording does not mislead. It rather directs attention to the objective condition of the patient, and not to the wishes of any of the parties concerned—not even the previously expressed opinion (as reported) of Karen Anne Quinlan. Treatment indicated or no further treatment indicated are not such by anyone's stipulation. Within whatever margin of error, these are objective medical determinations. That means that disagreement—for example, between physicians and the family of a comatose patient—may be *real* disagreements over an objective medical situation and about what should be done in a particular case.

At the same time, a comparison of treatments, or of treatment with no further curative treatments, is objectively relative to the patient's *present* condition—not to some notion of "standard medical care" in a physician's mind. A routinized understanding of "ordinary/extraordinary" is the "security blanket" of some physicians—who nevertheless have been known to call some ethicists "absolutists"!

The Karen Anne Quinlan case nicely—and tragically—illustrates most of these themes. Earlier there was some suggestion that she be declared legally dead. Medically that would have been a mistake. The thought behind taking the definitional route seemed to be that the sole reason for cutting off respirators is because the patient is already a corpse on which the face of life is maintained by machines alone. That assumption, in turn, is a moral mistake. In any case, to declare that a person has died means that treatment is no longer *possible*. That is different from saying that further treatment (of the still living) is counter-indicated.

Another reason for cutting off respirators, and a valid one, is because their continued use will affect the still living patient's condition in no significant respect except to prolong dying. Then trial curative treatments are no longer indicated, whether they be "standard" or "heroic" measures.

Karen's father, Joseph T. Quinlan, spoke nobly to the court about his family's desire to have "Karen returned to her natural state so that we could place her body and soul in the tender loving hands of the Lord." He wants her "taken from the machine and the tubes connected to her." Mr. Quinlan, however, expressed amazement when asked whether he wanted the apparatus for intravenous feeding removed, replying, "Oh no, that is her nourishment." So in the formation of the Quinlans' conscience there is a sharp distinction to be made between the IV and the respirator. One is ordinary (imperative) treatment, the other is extraordinary (dispensable) treatment.

I suggest that in a proper understanding of these terms (which are objectively relative to the patient's condition) the IV is as aimless as the respirator. It, too, is only prolonging Karen's dying. Surely it is not hunger that Karen feels now. To be on the safe side, perhaps we should say that she might experience dehydration. That is now the purpose of a glucose drip: to give the comfort of a cup of cool water to a patient who has entered upon her own particular dying. If a glucose drip prolongs this patient's dying, it is not given for that purpose, or as means in a continuing useless effort to save her life. More than five years ago, I learned that there are certain sugars which it might be possible to use in cases such as this to give water for hydration without metabolizing calories and prolonging the dying process.

The physicians in this case have a different formation of their professional conscience. To be sure, there is disagreement in the testimony as to whether they momentarily agreed to the Quinlans' request and then changed their minds. And before the case came to trial, suggestions were made that the physicians' primary motive was fear of malpractice suits or of criminal prosecution. I do not believe that this is true. The doctors (a neurologist, Dr. Robert Morse, and a pulmatory internist, Dr. Arshad Javed) are neither sadists nor automatons. They, too, are people of conscience, who said in open court that they would refuse to turn off the respirator even if ordered to do so. Their formation of professional conscience was shared by other physicians who testified—Dr. Sidney Diamond, neurologist at Mt. Sinai Hospital in New York, for example—and by the lawyer, Theodore Einhorn, for St. Clare's Hospital.

That professional judgment is remarkably similar to the Quinlans', however sharp the contrast materially and in the practical outcome. The truth is that neither the Quinlans nor the physicians have made the translation into "indicated" treatment and treatment "no longer indicated." As a consequence, they have opposed views of the meaning of "ordinary/extraordinary."

It is simply the case that for the physicians the respirator has become a "standard medical practice" equated with the IV as a lifesaving instrument. If there had been reliable information when Karen was brought to the hospital as to how she became comatose, how long she was in a state of respiratory distress, and what degree of anoxia her brain had suffered, Karen might not have been placed on a respirator. Under those circumstances, I ask, would not the IV for feeding have also been counter-indicated, and no life-sustaining treatments started? Having rightly begun curative treatment, the physicians now find they cannot in conscience stop. To do so would be for them a "quality of life" judgment, which the physicians (and the lawyers) declare they are not competent to make. Similarly, for Mr. Quinlan to ask to have the IV withdrawn would be to declare Karen's life to be not worth nourishing.

I suggest that both are wrong. Treatments that were potentially lifesaving (or reasonably believed to be so) when first begun have now become means for aimlessly prolonging Karen's dying. Is it not a routinized conscience which keeps physicians from determining when this point has come?

Questions for Discussion
Part I, Section 3

1. Consider the practice (reported by Duff and Campbell) of letting some infants with severe mental retardation die. Was this ethically humane? Would it be more or less humane to end the suffering of these infants by actively ending their lives?

2. What does it mean to have a "meaningful" life? Is it possible to develop criteria for a meaningful life and use these as a general basis for deciding whether to save or let die severely handicapped infants? Were early efforts by ethicists such as McCormick to provide such an analysis successful or unsuccessful?

3. Is there any ethical significance to the distinction between acting and omitting? How did Rachels's seminal paper attempt to dismiss such a distinction as ethically irrelevant?

4. Under what circumstances are life-sustaining treatments not medically indicated according to Ramsey?

BIOETHICS AS A DISCIPLINE

ટ**

Bioethics as a Discipline

Daniel Callahan

After Dan Callahan earned a Ph.D. in philosophy from Harvard University and worked briefly as an editor at the Catholic intellectual weekly *Commonwealth*, he turned his interests to the questions of the "new biology." In 1969, together with New York physician Willard Gaylin, he founded the Institute for Society, Ethics, and the Life Sciences, now known as the Hastings Center, with the purpose of encouraging scholarly study and public discussion of the ethical issues raised by scientific innovation.

"Bioethics as a Discipline" appeared in the Institute's publication, *Hastings Center Studies* (now known as *Hastings Center Report*). In this article, Callahan foresees the emergence of a discipline that he calls *bioethics* and reflects on what the role of the ethicist might be in the world of medicine and biology. He asserts that philosophers must learn about that world and adapt their standards of intellectual rigor to the nature of the problems arising in it. To serve the physicians and biologists responsible for making practical decisions, bioethics must define issues, methodological strategies, and decision procedures that are sensitive to specific cases in all the their complexity.

Just what is the role of the ethicist in trying to make a contribution to the ethical problems of medicine, biology, or population? I resisted, with utter panic, the idea of participating with the physicians in their actual decision. Who *me?* I much preferred the safety of the profound questions I pushed on them. But I also realized when faced with an actual case—and this is my excuse—that there was nothing whatever in my philosophical training which had prepared me to make a flat, clear-cut ethical decision at a given hour on a given afternoon. I had been duly trained in that splendid tradition of good scholarship and careful thinking which allows at least a couple thousand years to work through any problem. . . .

Daniel Callahan. "Bioethics as a Discipline." Abridged from *Hastings Center Studies*, Volume 1, 1973, pp. 66–73. Reprinted by permission.

When we ask what the place of bioethics might be, we of course need to know just what the problems are in medicine and biology which raise ethical questions and need ethical answers. I will not retail the whole catalogue of issues here; suffice it to say that they begin with "A" (abortion and amniocentesis) and run all the way to "Z" (the moral significance of zygotes). One evident and first task for the ethicist is simply that of trying to point out and define which problems raise moral issues. A second and no less evident task is providing some systematic means of thinking about, and thinking through, the moral issues which have been discerned. A third, and by far the most difficult, task is that of helping scientists and physicians to make the right decisions; and that requires a willingness to accept the realities of most medical and much scientific life, that is, that at some discrete point in time all the talk has to end and a choice must be made, a choice which had best be right rather than wrong. . . .

I used above the phrase "the realities of life." Another one of these realities is that the ethical issues of medicine and biology rarely present themselves in a way nicely designed to fit the kinds of categories and processes of thought which philosophers and theologians traditionally feel secure about. They almost always start off on the wrong foot by coming encumbered with the technical jargon of some other discipline. And only in text books is one likely to encounter cases which present a clear occasion, say, for deciding on the validity of a deontological or utilitarian ethical solution. The issues come, that is, in a mossy, jumbled form, cutting through many disciplines, gumming up all our clean theoretical engines, festooned with odd streamers and complicated knots.

The fact that this is the case immediately invites the temptation of what can be called "disciplinary reductionism." By that I mean a penchant for distilling out of an essentially complex ethical problem one transcendent issue which is promptly labeled *the* issue. Not coincidentally, this issue usually turns out to be a classic, familiar argument in philosophy or theology. By means of this kind of reductionism, the philosopher or theologian is thus enabled to do what he has been trained to do, deal with those classic disputes in a language and a way he is comfortable with—in a way which allows him to feel he is being a good "professional." The results of this tendency are doleful. It is one reason why most biologists and physicians find the contributions of the professional ethicist of only slight value. Their problems, very real to them in their language and their frame of reference, are promptly made unreal by being transmuted into someone else's language and reference system, in the process usually stripping the original case of all the complex facticity with which it actually presented itself. The whole business becomes positively pitiable when the philosopher or theologian, rebuffed or ignored because of his reductionism, can only respond by charging that his critics are obviously "not serious" about ethics, not interested in "real" ethical thinking.

I stress the problem of "disciplinary reductionism" out of a conviction that if a discipline of bioethics is to be created, it must be created in a way which does not allow this form of evading responsibility, of blaming the students for the faults of the teacher, of changing the nature of the problems to suit the methodologies of professional ethicists.

Toward this end, no subject would seem to me more worthy of investigation than what I will call the "ordinary language of moral thinking and discourse." Most people do not talk about their ethical problems in the language of philosophers. And I have yet to meet one professional ethicist who, when dealing with his own personal moral dilemmas, talks the language of his professional writings; he talks like everyone else, and presumably he is thinking through his own problems in banal everyday language like everyone else. Now of course it might be said that this misses the whole point of a serious professional discipline. Is it not like claiming that there must be nothing to theoretical physics simply because the physicist does not talk about the furniture in his house in terms of molecules and electrons? But the analogy does not work, for it is of the essence of moral decision-making to be couched in ordinary language and dealt with by ordinary, non-professional modes of thinking. The reason for this is apparent. An ethical decision will not be satisfactory to the person whose decision it is unless it is compatible with the way in which the person ordinarily thinks about himself and what he takes his life to be. . . .

In trying to create the discipline of bioethics, the underlying question raised by the foregoing remarks bears on what it should mean to be "rigorous" and "serious" about bioethics. . . . it is common enough for ethicists to gather among themselves after some frustrating interdisciplinary session to mutter about the denseness and inanity of their scientific and medical colleagues.

There are two options open here. One is to continue the muttering, being quite certain that the muttering is being reciprocated back in the scientific lab. That is, one can stick to traditional notions of philosophical and theological rigor, in which case one will rarely if ever encounter it in the interdisciplinary work of bioethics. Or, more wisely, the thought may occur that it is definitions of "rigor" which need adaptation. Not the adaptation of expediency or passivity in the face of careless thinking, but rather a perception that the kind of rigor required for bioethics may be of a different sort than that normally required for the traditional philosophical or scientific disciplines.

This is to say no more than that the methodological rigor should be appropriate to the subject matter. I spoke above of three tasks for the bioethicist: definition of issues, methodological strategies, and procedures for decision-making. Each of these tasks requires a different kind of rigor. The first requires what I will paradoxically call the rigor of an unfettered imagination, an ability to see in, through and under the surface appearance of things, to envision alternatives, to get under the skin of people's ethical agonies or ethical insensitivities, to look at things from many perspectives simultaneously.

A different kind of rigor is needed for the development of methodological strategies. Here the traditional methodologies of philosophy and theology are indispensable; there are standards of rigor which can and should come into play, bearing on logic, consistency, careful analysis of terms, and the like. Yet at the same time they have to be adapted to the subject matter at hand, and that subject matter is not normally, in concrete ethical cases of medicine and biology, one which can be stuffed into a too-rigidly structured methodological mold.

I am not about to attempt here a full discourse on what should be the proper and specific methodology of bioethics. Some sketchy, general comments will have to do, mainly in the way of assertions. Traditionally, the methodology of ethics has concerned itself with ethical thinking; how to think straight about ethical problems. However, I believe that the province of the bioethicist can legitimately encompass a concern with three areas of ethical activity: thinking, feeling (attitudes), and behavior. The case for including feelings and behavior along with thinking rests on the assumptions (1) that in life both feelings and behavior shape thinking, often helping to explain why defective arguments are nonetheless, for all that, persuasive and pervasive; and (2) that it is legitimate for an ethicist to worry about what people do and not just what they think and say; a passion for the good is not inappropriate for ethicists.

If ethics was nothing other than seeing to it that no logical fallacies were committed in the process of ethical argumentation, it would hardly be worthy of anyone's attention. It is the premises of ethical arguments, the visions behind ethical systems, the feelings which fuel ethical (or non-ethical) behavior, which make the real difference for human life. Verbal formulations and arguments are only the tip of the iceberg. An ethicist can restrict himself to that tip; he will be on safe enough professional grounds if he does so. But I see no reason why he can't dare more than that, out of a recognition that the source and importance of his field lie not in the academy but in private and public human life, where what people think, feel, and do make all the difference there is. . . .

I will only offer one negative and one positive criterion for ethical methodology. The wrong methodology will be used if it is not a methodology which has been specifically developed for ethical problems of medicine and biology. This does not mean it cannot or should not bear many of the traits of general philosophical or theological methodology. But if it bears only those traits one can be assured that it will not deal adequately with specific issues which arise in the life sciences. My positive criterion for a good methodology is this: it must display the fact that bioethics is an interdisciplinary field in which the purely "ethical" dimensions neither can nor should be factored out without remainder from the legal, political, psychological and social dimensions. The critical question, for example, of who should make the ethical decisions in medicine and biology is falsified at the outset if too sharp a distinction is drawn between what, ethically, needs to be decided and who, politically, should be allowed to decide. It is surely important to ethical theory to make this kind of distinction; unfortunately, if pressed too doggedly it may well falsify the reality of the way decisions are and will continue to be made.

The problem of decision-making, which I include as the third task of the bioethicist, cannot be divorced from the methodological question. Actually it makes me realize that I have a second positive criterion to offer as a test of a good bioethical methodology. The methodology ought to be such that it enables those who employ it to reach reasonably specific, clear decisions in those in-stances which require them—in the case of what is to be done about Mrs. Jones by four o'clock tomorrow afternoon, after which she will either live or die depending upon the decision made. I have already suggested that philosophers are not very good at that sort of thing, and that their weakness in this respect is likely to be altogether vexing to the physician who neither has the right atmosphere nor the time to think through everything the philosopher usually argues *needs* to be thought through.

In proposing that a good methodology should make it possible to reach specific conclusions at specific times, I am proposing a utopian goal. The only kinds of ethical systems I know of which make that possible are those of an essentially deductive kind, with well-established primary and secondary princi-ples and a long history of highly refined casuistical thinking. The Roman Catholic scholastic tradition and the Jewish *responsa* tradition are cases in point. Unfortu-nately, systems of that kind presuppose a whole variety of cultural conditions and shared world-views which simply do not exist in society at large. In their absence, it has become absolutely urgent that the search for a philosophically viable normative ethic, which can presuppose some commonly shared principles, go forward with all haste. Short of finding that, I do not see how ethical methodologies can be developed which will include methods for reaching quick and viable solutions in specific cases. Instead, we are likely to get only what we now have, a lot of very broad and general thinking, full of vagrant insights, but on the whole of limited use to the practicing physician and scientist.

Much of what I have been saying presupposes that a distinction can be drawn between "ethics" understood broadly and ethics understood narrowly. In its narrow sense, to do "ethics" is to be good at doing what well-trained philoso-phers and theologians do: analyze concepts, clarify principles, see logical en-tailments, spot underlying assumptions, and build theoretical systems. There are better and worse ways of doing this kind of thing and that is why philosophers and theologians can spend much of their time arguing with each other. But even the better ways will, I think, not be good enough for the demands of bioethics. That requires understanding "ethics" in a very broad, well-nigh unmanageable sense of the term.

My contention is that the discipline of bioethics should be so designed, and its practitioners so trained, that it will directly—at whatever cost to disciplinary elegance—serve those physicians and biologists whose position demands that they make the practical decisions. This requires, ideally, a number of ingredients as part of the training—which can only be life-long—of the bioethicist: sociologi-cal understanding of the medical and biological communities; psychological understanding of the kinds of needs felt by researchers and clinicians, patients and physicians, and the varieties of pressures to which they are subject; historical understanding of the sources of regnant value theories and common practices; requisite scientific training; awareness of and facility with the usual methods of ethical analysis as understood in the philosophical and theological communi-ties—and no less a full awareness of the limitations of those methods when applied to actual cases; and, finally, personal exposure to the kinds of ethical problems which arise in medicine and biology. . . .

One important test of the acceptance of bioethics as a discipline will be the extent to which it is called upon by scientists and physicians. This means that it should be developed inductively, working at least initially from the kinds of problems scientists and physicians believe they face and need assistance on. As often as not, they will be wrong about the real nature of the issues with which they have to wrestle. But no less often the person trained in philosophy and theology will be equally wrong in his understanding of the real issues. Only a continuing, probably tension-ridden dialectic will suffice to bridge the gap, a dialectic which can only be kept alive by a continued exposure to specific cases in all their human dimensions. Many of them will be very unpleasant cases, the kind which make one long for the security of writing elegant articles for professional journals on such manageable issues as recent distinctions between "rules" and "maxims."

Medical Ethics
Some Uses, Abuses, and Limitations

K. Danner Clouser

In 1969, Dr. K. Danner Clouser, a Harvard-trained philosopher, was invited to join the faculty of the newly established College of Medicine of Pennsylvania State University, Hershey, where a pioneering Department of Medical Humanities had been created.

"Medical Ethics: Some Uses, Abuses, and Limitations" was written to counter early criticisms of the presence of professional ethicists in medicine. He attempts to specify the work of the ethicist as "structuring" the disputed issues by detailing the relevant principles and implications, analyzing the pivotal concepts, and focusing on the relevant facts. He points out the limitations of ethics in analyzing issues and refutes the view that medical ethics is a reform movement or an effort to inspire moral behavior.

N ew thrusts seem inevitably slated for backlash. New drugs, new procedures, new interpretations, new movements sooner or later experience re-think. Zeal is replaced by temperance, and blind commitment by cautious evaluation. Perhaps we too easily go overboard; perhaps the Hegelian Dialectic has fashioned our Being to its pendular patterns.

Medical ethics is no exception. One could always count on a midpoint backlash. On a one-year commission it would happen during June; in a week's conference it happens on Wednesday, and in a one-day consultation, it happens around noon. Suspecting that we are in the fifth year of a decade, I am in a stocktaking frame of mind. I have neither inclination nor talent to tackle the recent history, purpose, and track-record of medical ethics, but in a much more limited way I might initiate some reflection on medical ethics—at least enough to defuse some fears, articulate some nagging doubts, and generally to assess the possibilities and limitations. This is probably not an important enterprise, but, like spring housecleaning, it should be done every now and then just to remind us what is really underneath it all.

When backlash strikes, it is on several levels, emotional and conceptual: haughty attitudes are despaired of; intrusions into medicine by outsiders become annoying; and the difficult language and conceptual gymnastics of ethicists are seen as purposeful obfuscation.

K. Danner Clouser. "Medical Ethics: Some Uses, Abuses, and Limitations." Reprinted from *The New England Journal of Medicine*, Volume 293, 1978, pp. 384–387. Reprinted by permission of *The New England Journal of Medicine*. Copyright © 1978, Massachusetts Medical Society.

In case your own gentle spirits would preclude having angry or questioning thoughts—hear what some others are saying:

A recent letter to the *New England Journal of Medicine* began: "I am increasingly disturbed by the creeping encroachment of people and agencies concerned about medical ethics . . . as they affect medical practice and scientific investigation, and wonder whether the time has not come for medical practitioners and biomedical scientists to assert their views more strongly. . . ."[1] A physician writing in a recent issue of the *Hastings Center Report* says: "I must say that, from the view of the practicing physician, most of the conversations I have had with ethicists have tended to anger me, producing a deep feeling of frustration."[2]

Last year Daniel Greenberg wrote a two-page comment in the *New England Journal of Medicine* entitled "Ethics and Nonsense." Its first paragraph read this way: "At the risk of appearing both dense and perverse, I timorously suggest that perhaps the most inflated non-issue currently absorbing time and energy in the health community and its governmental command posts is that loose amalgamation of anxieties and passions that comes under the banner of medical ethics."[3]

These quotations give voice and authority to the uneasy qualms we all have concerning medical ethics—ethicists, doctors, and consumers alike.

I have no illusions about dealing satisfactorily with all the doubts and dilemmas that exist. More realistically, my aim is to make some basic points in a relatively organized way. My own ethical position would argue that there is a rational foundation for morality. Though that is not at issue here, it may help the reader to put what follows into perspective.

I will first describe two roles of medical ethics. This will be followed by a description of two essential limitations. I will conclude with a series of complaints and responses.

Medical Ethics

Two Roles

To begin with, medical ethics is no big deal. The issues that it raises may be fascinating and important, but it is not as though medical ethics were a recent invention for discovering these intriguing issues or a special method for dealing with them. Medical ethics is simply ethics applied to a particular area of our lives—roughly the area touched by medicine. And being the same old ethics that has been around for a long time, medical ethics has no special principles or methods or rules. It is the "old ethics" trying to find its way around in new, very puzzling circumstances.

To consider the first role, the most obvious task being done by medical ethics is that of sensitizing. Everyone is getting in on this development, calling attention to myriad details of the biomedical world that have ethical implications. It is a consciousness-raising enterprise, alerting us to everything from grossest injustice to subtlest nuance. The majority of literature that has been labeled "medical ethics" does just that. It tends to be short on argument and long on description, anecdotes, and implications. Exposes of human experimentation, of lying to patients, or of refusing to grant patient requests would be examples.

The one thing to notice is that in this identifying of various phenomena as immoral—that is, as cases of needless suffering, or of injustice, or of deceit, or whatever—we are not calling on some special sense of morality, but only on the principles or moral rules that we ordinarily acknowledge in everyday life.

Furthermore, the reasoning about the medical-ethical issues proceeds much as is already familiar to you in everyday circumstances. What do you do? Suppose you genuinely wonder if a particular action is moral. If the action occurs in a context laden with many variables, pressures and causal chains, you try to sort out all the strands of argument, and all the contingent conditions, ". . . if I do this, he will do that . . . on the other hand, if the conditions of the County Home were better I would choose differently . . . unless, of course, the neighbor were to decide to. . . ." You figure out the implications of the action with the best probabilities you can—who will be hurt, how badly, which moral rules will be broken, and who will benefit. And ultimately you try to balance all this out, to determine the best action or the least immoral action you can do in the circumstances.

That is just what the professional ethicist does. This is the second item I would isolate in describing what medical ethics is up to. I would call this "structuring" the issues. The morally relevant strands of a complex situation are teased out.

Several things are involved in this structuring. One is spelling out the variety of conflicting ethical principles that are usually involved in any given situation. For example, in experimentation on human beings many have felt an over-riding obligation to help mankind through their discoveries, but this impulse is in sharp conflict with our moral obligations not to deceive subjects. Then, one must question the validity of each principle or see if there is a higher principle that might resolve the conflict.

Another aspect of this structuring is to isolate pivotal concepts that need clarification, definition, or defense. For example, is abortion killing the fetus or simply removing the pregnancy? Is not-treating the same as killing? What results from interpreting it one way or the other? What arguments are there for interpreting one way or the other? What constitutes being a person? Fetuses, the severely retarded, the senile—are they persons, and do they have certain rights? If yes, then such and such follows; if no, then something else follows. And so on. These are the strands of argument an ethicist must spell out, or "structure."

"Structuring" the issues is an analytic dissection. It is a road map of the issue, showing routes, relations, functions, shortcuts, and central and peripheral locations. It shows where various arguments and actions lead, what facts would be relevant, what concepts are crucial, and what moral principles are at issue and probably in conflict. This discovery and delineation of the issues is perhaps the central contribution of medical ethics.

Notice that structuring in itself does not necessarily mean making a decision on what to do in the situation. It simply lays out the issues, bringing the hidden problems and principles to the surface. This process may involve helping us to dig down through layers of culturation, habit, and verbal debris, to rediscover with clarity our moral purpose and rationale. Notice also that what the professional ethicist does is not different in kind from what we all do in deliberating about a moral issue. This point is important. It is counter to the nature of morality that it be an esoteric body of knowledge that only a few specialists can really comprehend. The medical ethicist cannot be appealing to special theories and remote lines of reasoning and simply delivering his conclusions to us, which we must accept because he is the expert. (It is that kind of reliance on "experts" that got us into trouble in the first place!) Rational people must be able to see, follow, and judge the points made. Morality, to do its job of harmonizing our lives together, must be generally understood by all.

Two Limitations

Without a doubt we are all constantly being guided by moral considerations. We should not allow our conceptual struggle over the very difficult cases to hide the fact that moral deliberations give clear and unambiguous direction in most of our daily dealings.

Nevertheless, a serious limitation of ethics of which we should be aware is that ethics is a fairly blunt instrument; it does not cut finely. It can be precise and rigorous, but it does not determine one and only one action that receives the moral seal of approval. Certain alternatives may be ruled out, but a range of possible actions may remain as morally acceptable. So the field really is not narrowed down much by moral criteria, and frequently the decision is ultimately made on the basis of some belief, predilection, or matter of taste. These often pose as moral determinants, but they are not. In a given situation there may be many possible actions that do not break any moral rule, and hence all would be morally acceptable. But more frequently, I suppose, all the possible actions infringe on one moral rule or another, in which case it is a matter of choosing what one regards as the lesser evil. But equally moral persons can disagree on that. It must be admitted that it is on this level that many a so-called "ethical" debate focuses, whereas what is really the case is that the alternatives are equally moral, and that in truth they are debating either their personal preferences or matters of empirical fact, such as which way will put more people at risk, or which way will lessen the amount of suffering, or whatever.

As one example of this limitation, consider a situation in which the gene pool becomes more polluted and the incidence of genetic disease rises dramatically. One person might choose to deny the right of certain people to have children because of the great increase in the risk of inflicting suffering on the children who will be born. Another person might put great value on the right to have children, arguing that that right outweighs any of the pain and suffering that would result. Equally rational moral persons might disagree on this point.

They are really disagreeing about the relative importance of the moral rules to be broken. One thinks rights are more important than high risk of suffering; the other thinks the "mere" right to procreate is no big deal but rather that elimination of suffering is more critical.

Also consider a debate over voluntary euthanasia. One person argues that the right to self-determination is basic to all our rights. Another argues that in view of the inevitable misuse of euthanasia to do in people who do not really want to die, or doing in oneself for insufficient reasons (say, sheer depression), the possibility of injustice outweighs the right to be helped to die. These are equally moral alternatives, both endorsed by the rather blunt instrument of ethics. The issue must be decided on other than ethical grounds, and usually consists in convincing one's opponent that weighing this right or that result will in the long run have more desirable consequences. But determining what consequences will result or how desirable they will be is often an empirical matter and in the absence of the relevant facts, it becomes guesswork. That an argument is empirical, not moral, makes it no less important, but it does tell us that moral criteria are no longer relevant to the argument. Medical ethics, in structuring the issue, should be giving us the topography of the argument, so we can go looking in the right places for the right things at the right point in the argument.

I have just discussed one limitation of medical ethics—that it does not cut very finely. The other limitation I will mention is that many of its key notions really must be referred to expertise outside of ethics (though I am reluctant to stress this kind of conceptual territoriality). Many of the pivotal notions on which ethical issues turn are themselves outside the domain of ethics. Some, such as "normal," "rational," "sick," "person," "competent," and "voluntary," need considerable conceptual analysis by a variety of specialties, whereas others are more empirical, such as which procedure involves what risks, the effects of certain drugs on judgment, the physiologic reactions of certain people to certain kinds of information, and so on. Sometimes the issue calls for both conceptual analysis and empirical study. For example, in wondering if mongoloid children have happy lives, we must get clear about what is meant by "satisfying" or "happy" or "meaningful" life, and then whether in fact they have it.

This limitation shows the critical importance of joint effort in these matters. Every one is needed, and each must listen to the other.

Unease and Abuses

With the very general description of medical ethics and its limitations behind us, we turn to a list of complaints. My purpose is to articulate some of the spoken and unspoken uneasiness with medical ethics, and to respond to them.

To begin with, there is the unease medical people very understandably might have with ethicists prowling around their domain. (One can see how medical ethicists might be seen as the invading barbarian tribes from the north, intruding on an old and venerable civilization populated and regulated by distinguished, knowledgeable physicians.) I see this unease taking several different forms. One is a fear of getting dogmatic pronouncements. Another is suspicion that the ethicist will spot only the superficial and obvious dimensions of the problem, missing all the nuances and subtleties that constitute its really important aspects. And the third is that the physician is half fearful of being denounced by this underinformed, zealous outsider.

One answer to this question is to recall my insistence on the complexity of the issues, the need for judgment from a variety of experts and the necessity for the reasoning to be transparent to all. This is not to say that someone might not draw quick conclusions and shoot from the hip. But he would be totally misguided if he did. If the ethicist is doing his job properly, he is analyzing, clarifying, developing lines of reasoning, and trying it out on those who must work with these problems to see if he has misunderstood, overlooked important points or stated it too obtusely to be understood.

However, there is a more important distinction that it would be relevant to insist on here: the distinction between reformers and ethicists. Those fearful of ethicists are usually confusing them with reformers. They are not at all the same. Reformers are those who are primarily agents of change. If they see something they regard as clearly immoral, they zealously set about calling attention to it and trying to correct it. They are seldom ethicists as such. They are usually doctors, administrators, consumers, lawyers, and others.

Ethicists, on the other hand, tend to be interested only in the difficult, problematic cases in which what is right or wrong is by no means easy to see. Their interest is in picking through the thicket, trying this or that principle, following out this or that line of reasoning, exploring various concepts, interpretations, definitions, and perspectives. They grapple with an issue trying to help the medical world to see its way clear. It is not in their nature to issue oversimplified pronouncements. Indeed, I worry far more about their generating such a clutter of analyses and alternatives that a decision can never be made!

Another criticism one hears likens the medical ethicist to a medical specialist, and then complains that the ethicist is not much good on a seven-minute consultation because he does not deliver "the solution"! The ethicist might be able to structure the issues for you and perhaps rule out the obviously immoral, but, as we saw earlier, there are still a lot of decisions to be made, and they in turn have to do with how a variety of variables are interpreted and values weighted. The ethicist can help you uncover all the ingredients and sketch out a variety of alternatives and their justifications, but ultimately it is up to you to decide. That is why he must make his thinking clear for you to follow and understand, and why it is more of an educational matter than a consultation— more of a process than a pronouncement.

Ethicists have been heard to complain that whereas most specialist groups are fussy about credentials, everyone thinks he is an expert on ethics. Thus, a conference on medical ethics will have geneticists, surgeons, and internists freely speaking up, but an ethicist would not dare speak up at a medical conference. This is as it should be. Morality is in fact something that we all participate in:

it affects all of us, and it guides our actions. It is something we all must understand. It cannot be esoteric knowledge. And given my description of medical ethics, it needs a great deal of information on facts, concepts, and their implications from the medical sciences. So they very properly participate. There are, of course, areas of ethics in which anyone but professional ethicists might fear to tread—matters concerning theories and foundations of ethics. And like any professional group they have their own vocabulary, strategies, methods and maneuvers, but, nevertheless, when they are dealing in applied ethics of a particular realm, they must work for the participation, understanding and concurrence of the practitioners of that realm.

Turning a medical ethicist into a reformer and specialty consultant is not the only injustice that can be done him. Some try to saddle him with the task of inspiring others to be moral, as though it were his job either to motivate people to be moral or to invent a theory of ethics contrived somehow to stimulate people to be moral. This effort, of course, is a perversion. He is more an analyst than a preacher, more a diagnostician than a therapist, more a scholar than an essayist. The ethicist can only assume that you want to do the moral thing but that you are just not sure in a complicated situation what that would be. It is not his job as ethicist to make you want to be moral.

Some criticize medical ethics for dealing only with the so-called glamorous issues—abortion, euthanasia, human experimentation, genetic engineering, psychosurgery, and so on. Rather, say these critics, they should be helping with the day-to-day issues of medicine, those daily dealings between doctor and doctor, doctor and patient, doctor and staff, etc. In part I agree with this criticism, but at the same time I would issue a warning. This area of concern seems particularly susceptible to the limitation of ethics that I earlier emphasized—namely, that ethics does not cut finely. And pushing it to do so leads to confusion and contrivance. For example, suppose the issue is whether a doctor should come without question whenever and wherever a patient needs him, or perhaps whether doctors may refuse to work more than 60 hours a week. We can squeeze ethical principles and theories of obligations to derive every subtle drop of implication, but my bet is that on most of these issues it would be no help. What we need instead are simply rational social arrangements that will settle these issues by common agreement. Ethics, of course, would give us broad guidelines (e.g., we cannot have deceit, broken promises, or loss of confidentiality), and ethics would generally suggest a fair procedure for reaching such agreement. But for the most part we must work out these arrangements among ourselves by tradeoffs, compromises, convincing arguments, or whatever, so that the interests of all of us will be served so far as possible.

Another misuse of medical ethics is to expect it to be everything that is nonmedical. This is to burden it with expectations it could not possibly fulfill. It would make it such a potpourri of methods, aims and subject matter as to be worthless. A physician's article on the nature of medical ethics lists a number of areas with which he thinks ethicists should deal—among them are interchange with the dying patient and his family, definition of death, premedical and medical-

school curriculum, problems in the clinical training of physicians, public education concerning diseases, and rising costs of hospital care.[2] A program like that
could turn fine minds to jello and return medical ethics to the stone age.

The last criticism I will mention we usually hear stated this way: it is just
a matter of his values against mine; when it comes to these matters anyone's
opinion is just as good as anyone else's.

It of course borders on madness even to raise this issue. It applies not just
to medical ethics, but to all ethics, and indeed to anything concerning values.
Furthermore, volumes could be written in response. However, I will meekly go
to the other extreme, using the occasion summarily to make two points.

The first is that we generally quit the discussion of values long before we
have exhausted meaningful argument. We are too quick to say, "You have your
values and I have mine." Further discussion can elicit much more agreement
either by pursuing the consistency of the value in question with other values
that you hold or in "unpacking" the meaning and empirical criteria underlying
the value in question. Persistent pursuit of each other's values with "why" questions will elicit a lot of hidden assumptions and reasoning, and consequently
more agreement than we would initially expect. In short, I think values can be
meaningfully argued—at least up to a point.

Secondly, ethics very roughly is concerned with the rules or principles that
would harmonize the aims and desires of all men, by allowing those of each
man to be realized so far as it would be compatible with a similar realization of
everyone else's. Ethics is concerned in the sense that it tries to discover, examine,
justify and apply such rules and principles. There are better ways and worse
ways to accomplish this harmonizing task. Hence, there are better reasons for
some moves than for others, and there are ways of showing that they are
better. It is not just one groundless opinion against another's groundless opinion.
Argument, facts, and good reasons are very much to the point. The object of
ethics is a harmonious and just society, and that is a matter for careful reasoning;
one opinion is simply not as useful to that end as any other opinion.

These last two points are declarations and not arguments. But declarations,
being less tedious than arguments, provide a smoother exit from an overly long
editorial comment.

References

1. Hepner GW: Ethics of human experimentation. N Engl J Med 292:321–322,
   1975
2. Moore C: This is medical ethics? Hastings Cent Rep 4:1–3, 1974
3. Greenberg DS: Ethics and nonsense. N Engl J Med 290:977–978, 1974

How Medicine Saved the Life of Ethics

Stephen Toulmin

Stephen Toulmin was a well-established philosopher whose work *Reason in Ethics* (Cambridge University Press, 1950) had long been appreciated, when he took leave from the University of Chicago to work as philosophy consultant to the National Commission for the Protection of Human Subjects of Biomedical and Behavioral Research (1974–1978). He currently serves as director of the Center for Multiethnic and Transnational Studies at the University of Southern California.

"How Medicine Saved the Life of Ethics" was inspired by Toulmin's service with the National Commission. The article, although published somewhat later than the others in this section, had a broad influence on the emerging field of bioethics. Its main ideas are more fully developed in Toulmin's later book, co-authored with Albert Jonsen, *The Abuse of Casuistry: A History of Moral Reasoning* (Berkeley: University of California, 1988).

D uring the first 60 years or so of the twentieth century, two things character-ized the discussion of ethical issues in the United States, and to some extent other English-speaking countries also. On the one hand, the theoretical analyses of moral philosophers concentrated on questions of so-called meta-ethics. Most professional philosophers assumed that their proper business was not to take sides on substantive ethical questions but rather to consider in a more formal way what *kinds* of issues and judgments are properly classified as moral in the first place. On the other hand, in less academic circles, ethical debates repeatedly ran into stalemate. A hard-line group of dogmatists, who appealed either to a code of universal rules or to the authority of a religious system or teacher, confronted a rival group of relativists and subjectivists, who found in the anthropological and psychological diversity of human attitudes evidence to justify a corresponding diversity in moral convictions and feelings.

For those who sought some "rational" way of settling ethical disagreements, there developed a period of frustration and perplexity. Faced with the spectacle of rival camps taking up sharply opposed ethical positions (e.g., toward premarital sex or anti-Semitism), they turned in vain to the philosophers for guidance. Hoping for intelligent and perceptive comments on the actual substance of such issues, they were offered only analytical classifications, which sought to locate the realm of moral issues, not to decide them . . .

How did the fresh attention that philosophers began paying to the ethics of medicine, beginning around 1960, move the ethical debate beyond this stand-off? It did so in four different ways. In place of the earlier concern with attitudes, feelings, and wishes, it substituted a new preoccupation with situations, needs, and interests; it required writers on applied ethics to go beyond the discussion of general principles and rules to a more scrupulous analysis of the particular kinds of "cases" in which they find their application; it redirected that analysis to the professional enterprises within which so many human tasks and duties typically arise; and, finally, it pointed philosophers back to the ideas of "equity," "reason-ableness," and "human relationships," which played central roles in the *Ethics* of Aristotle but subsequently dropped out of sight [1 esp. 5.10.1136b30–1137b32]. Here, these four points may be considered in turn. . . .

The new attention to applied ethics (particularly medical ethics) has done much to dispel the miasma of subjectivity that was cast around ethics as a result of its association with anthropology and psychology. At least within broad limits, an ethics of "needs" and "interests" is objective and generalizable in a way that an ethics of "wishes" and "attitudes" cannot be. Stated crudely, the question of whether one person's actions put another person's health at risk is normally a question of ascertainable fact, to which there is a straightforward "yes" or "no" answer, not a question of fashion, custom, or taste, about which (as the saying goes) "there is no arguing." This being so, the objections to that person's actions can be presented and discussed in "objective" terms. So, proper attention to the example of medicine has helped to pave the way for a reintroduction of "objec-tive" standards of good and harm and for a return to methods of practical reasoning about moral issues that are not available to either the dogmatists or the relativists.

The Importance of Cases

One writer who was already contributing to the renewed discussion of applied ethics as early as the 1950s was Joseph Fletcher of the University of Virginia, who has recently been the object of harsh criticism from more dogmatic thinkers for introducing the phrase "situation ethics."[1] . . .

. . . In retrospect, Joseph Fletcher's introduction of the phrase "situation ethics" can be viewed as one further chapter in a history of "the ethics of *cases*," as contrasted with "the ethics of *rules and principles*"; this is another area in which the ethics of medicine has recently given philosophers some useful pointers for the analysis of moral issues.

Let me here mention one of these, which comes out of my own personal experience. From 1975 to 1978 I worked as a consultant and staff member with the National Commission for the Protection of Human Subjects of Biomedical

---

[1]Just how much of a pioneer Joseph Fletcher was in opening up the modern discussion of the ethics of medicine is clear from the early publication date (1954) of his first publications on this subject [2–4].

and Behavioral Research, based in Washington, D.C.; I was struck by the extent to which the commissioners were able to reach agreement in making recommendations about ethical issues of great complexity and delicacy.[2] If the earlier theorists had been right, and ethical considerations really depended on variable cultural attitudes or labile personal feelings, one would have expected 11 people of such different backgrounds as the members of the commission to be far more divided over such moral questions than they ever proved to be in actual fact. Even on such thorny subjects as research involving prisoners, mental patients, and human fetuses, it did not take the commissioners long to identify the crucial issues that they needed to address, and, after patient analysis of these issues, any residual differences of opinion were rarely more than marginal, with different commissioners inclined to be somewhat more conservative, or somewhat more liberal, in their recommendations. Never, as I recall, did their deliberations end in deadlock, with supporters of rival principles locking horns and refusing to budge. The problems that had to be argued through at length arose, not on the level of the principles themselves, but at the point of applying them: when difficult moral balances had to be struck between, for example, the general claims of medical discovery and its future beneficiaries and the present welfare or autonomy of individual research subjects.

How was the Commission's consensus possible? It rested precisely on this last feature of their agenda: namely, its close concentration on specific types of problematic cases. Faced with "hard cases," they inquired what particular conflicts of claim or interest were exemplified in them, and they usually ended by balancing off those claims in very similar ways. Only when the individual members of the Commission went on to explain their own particular "reasons" for supporting the general consensus did they begin to go seriously different ways. For, then, commissioners from different backgrounds and faiths "justified" their votes by appealing to general views and abstract principles which differed far more deeply than their opinions about particular substantive questions. Instead of "deducing" their opinions about particular cases from general principles that could lend strength and conviction to those specific opinions, they showed a far greater certitude about particular cases than they ever achieved about general matters.

This outcome of the Commission's work should not come as any great surprise to physicians who have reflected deeply about the nature of clinical judgment in medicine. In traditional case morality, as in medical practice, the first indispensable step is to assemble a rich enough "case history." Until that has been done, the wise physician will suspend judgment. If he is too quick to

---

[2]The work of the national commission generated a whole series of government publications— mainly reports and recommendations on the ethical aspects of research involving research subjects from specially "vulnerable" groups having diminished autonomy, such as young children and prisoners. . . As a member of the commission, A. R. Jonsen was also struck by the casuistical character of its work, and this led to the research project of which this paper is one product.

let theoretical considerations influence his clinical analysis, they may prejudice the collection of a full and accurate case record and so distract him from what later turn out to have been crucial clues. Nor would this outcome have been any surprise to Aristotle, either. Ethics and clinical medicine are both prime examples of the concrete fields of thought and reasoning in which (as he insisted) the theoretical rigor of geometrical argument is unattainable: fields in which we should above all strive to be *reasonable* rather than insisting on a kind of *exactness* that "the nature of the case" does not allow [1, 1.3.1094b12–27]. . . .

By taking one step further, indeed, we may view the problems of clinical medicine and the problems of applied ethics as two varieties of a common species. Defined in purely general terms, such ethical categories as "cruelty" and "kindness," "laziness" and "conscientiousness," have a certain abstract, truistical quality: before they can acquire any specific relevance, we have to identify some *actual* person, or piece of conduct, as "kind" or "cruel," "conscientious" or "lazy," and there is often disagreement even about that preliminary step. Similarly, in medicine: if described in general terms alone, diseases too are "abstract entities," and they acquire a practical relevance only for those who have learned the diagnostic art of identifying real-life cases as being cases of one disease rather than another.

In its form (if not entirely in its point) the *art* of practical judgment in ethics thus resembles the art of clinical diagnosis and prescription. In both fields, theoretical generalities are helpful to us only up to a point, and their actual application to particular cases demands, also, a human capacity to recognize the slight but significant features that mark off, say, a "case" of minor muscular strain from a life-threatening disease or a "case" of decent reticence from one of cowardly silence. Once brought to the bedside, so to say, applied ethics and clinical medicine use just the same Aristotelean kinds of "practical reasoning," and a correct choice of therapeutic procedure in medicine is the *right* treatment to pursue, not just as a matter of medical technique but for ethical reasons also.

In the last decades of the nineteenth century, F. H. Bradley of Oxford University expounded an ethical position that placed "duties" in the center of the philosophical picture, and the recent concern of moral philosophers with applied ethics (most specifically, medical ethics) has given them a new insight into his arguments also. It was a mistake (Bradley argued) to discuss moral obligations purely in universalistic terms, as though nobody was subject to moral claims unless they applied to everybody—unless we could, according to the Kantian formula, "will them to become universal laws." On the contrary, different people are subject to different moral claims, depending on where they "stand" toward the other people with whom they have to deal, for example, their families, colleagues, and fellow citizens [5]. . . .

As the modern discussion of medical ethics has taught us, professional affiliations and concerns play a significant part in shaping a physician's obligations and commitments, and this insight has stimulated detailed discussions both about professionalism in general and, more specifically, about the relevance of "the

physician/patient relationship" to the medical practitioner's duties and obligations.[3] . . .

In recent years, as a result, moral philosophers have begun to look specifically
and in greater detail at the situations within which ethical problems typically
arise and to pay closer attention to the human relationships that are embodied
in those situations. In ethics, as elsewhere, the tradition of radical individualism
for too long encouraged people to overlook the "mediating structures" and
"intermediate institutions" (family, profession, voluntary associations, etc.) which
stand between the individual agent and the larger scale context of his actions.
So, in political theory, the obligation of the individual toward the state was
seen as the only problem worth focusing on; meanwhile, in moral theory, the
differences of status (or station) which in practice expose us to different sets of
obligations (or duties) were ignored in favor of a theory of justice (or rights)
that deliberately concealed these differences behind a "veil of ignorance."[4]

On this alternative view, the only just—even, properly speaking, the only
moral—obligations are those that apply to us all equally, regardless of our
standing. By undertaking the tasks of a profession, an agent will no doubt accept
certain special duties, but so it will be for us all. The obligation to perform
those duties is "just" or "moral" only because it exemplifies more general and
universalizable obligations of trust, which require us to do what we have undertaken to do. So, any exclusive emphasis on the universal aspects of morality can
end by distracting attention from just those things which the student of applied
ethics finds most absorbing—namely, the specific tasks and obligations that any
profession lays on its practitioners.

Most recently, Alasdair MacIntyre has pursued these considerations further
in his new book, *After Virtue*.[9] MacIntyre argues that the public discussion of
ethical issues has fallen into a kind of Babel, which largely springs from our
losing any sense of the ways in which *community* creates obligations for us. One
thing that can help restore that lost sense of community is the recognition that,
at the present time, our professional commitments have taken on many of the
roles that our communal commitments used to play. Even people who find
moral philosophy generally unintelligible usually acknowledge and respect the
specific ethical demands associated with their own professions or jobs, and this
offers us some kind of a foundation on which to begin reconstructing our view
of ethics. For it reminds us that we are in no position to fashion individual
lives for ourselves, purely *as individuals*. Rather, we find ourselves born into

---

[3]See Bledstein's discussion [6, p. 107] of the nineteenth-century confusion between codes of
ethics and codes of etiquette within such professional societies as the American Medical
Association.

[4]I borrow this phrase a trifle unfairly from John Rawls [7], but I have argued at greater length
in [8] that *any* unbalanced emphasis on "universality" divorced from "equity" is a recipe for
the ethics of relations between strangers and leaves untouched those important issues that
arise between people who are linked by more complex relationships.

communities in which the available ways of acting are largely laid out in advance: in which human activity takes on different *Lebensformen*, or "forms of life" (of which the professions are one special case), and our obligations are shaped by the requirements of those forms.

In this respect, the lives and obligations of professionals are no different from those of their lay brethren. Professional obligations arise out of the enterprises of the professions in just the same kinds of way that other general moral obligations arise out of our shared forms of life; if we are at odds about the *theory* of ethics, that is because we have misunderstood the basis which ethics has in our actual *practice*. Once again, in other words, it was medicine—as the first profession to which philosophers paid close attention during the new phase of "applied ethics" that opened during the 1960s—that set the example which was required in order to revive some important, and neglected, lines of argument within moral philosophy itself.

Equity and Intimacy

Two final themes have also attracted special attention as a result of the new interaction between medicine and philosophy. Both themes were presented in clear enough terms by Aristotle in the *Nicomachean Ethics*. But, as so often happens, the full force of Aristotle's concepts and arguments was overlooked by subsequent generations of philosophers, who came to ethics with very different preoccupations. Aristotle's own Greek terms for these notions are *epieikeia* and *philia*, which are commonly translated as "reasonableness" and "friendship," but I shall argue here that they correspond more closely to the modern terms, "equity" and "personal relationship" [1].

Modern readers sometimes have difficulty with the style of Aristotle's *Ethics* and lose patience with the book, because they suspect the author of evading philosophical questions that they have their own reasons for regarding as central. Suppose, for instance, that we go to Aristotle's text in the hope of finding some account of the things that mark off "right" from "wrong": if we attempt to press this question, Aristotle will always slip out of our grasp. What makes one course of action better than another? We can answer that question, he replies, only if we first consider what kind of a person the agent is and what relationships he stands in toward the other people who are involved in his actions; he sets about explaining why the kinds of relationship, and the kinds of conduct, that are possible as between "large-spirited human beings" who share the same social standing are simply not possible as between, say, master and servant, or parent and child [1].

The bond of *philia* between free and equal friends is of one kind, that between father and son of another kind, that between master and slave of a third, and there is no common scale in which we can measure the corresponding kinds of conduct. By emphasizing this point, Aristotle draws attention to an important point about the manner in which "actions" are classified, even before we say anything ethical about them. Within two different relationships the very same deeds, or the very same words, may—from the ethical point of view—

represent quite different *acts* or *actions*. Words that would be a perfectly proper command from an officer to an enlisted man, or a straightforward order from a master to a servant, might be a humiliation if uttered by a father to a son, or an insult if exchanged between friends. A judge may likewise have a positive duty to say, from the bench, things that he would never dream of saying in a situation where he was no longer acting *ex officio*, while a physician may have occasion, and even be obliged, to do things to a patient in the course of a medical consultation that he would never be permitted to do in any other context.

. . . For surely, the very deed or utterance by Dr. A toward Mrs. B which would be a routine inquiry or examination within a strictly professional "physician-patient relationship"—for example, during a gynecological consultation—might be grounds for a claim of assault if performed outside that protected context. The *philia* (or relationship) between them will be quite different in the two situations, and, on this account, the "circumstances" do indeed "alter cases" in ways that are directly reflected in the demands of professional ethics.

With this as background, we can turn to Aristotle's ideas about *epieikeia* ("reasonableness" or "equity"). As to this notion, Aristotle pioneered the general doctrine that principles never settle ethical issues by themselves: that is, that we can grasp the moral force of principles only by studying the ways in which they are applied to, and within, particular situations. The need for such a practical approach is most obvious, in judicial practice, in the exercise of "equitable jurisdiction," where the courts are required to decide cases by appeal, not to specific, well-defined laws or statutes, but to general considerations of fairness, of "maxims of equity." In these situations, the courts do not have the benefit of carefully drawn rules, which have been formulated with the specific aim that they should be precise and self-explanatory: rather, they are guided by rough proverbial mottoes—phrases about "clean hands" and the like. The questions at issue in such cases are, in other words, very broad questions—for example, about what would be *just* or *reasonable* as between two or more individuals when all the available facts about their respective situations have been taken into account [10–12].

In ethics and law alike, the two ideas of *philia* ("friendship" or "relationship") and *epieikeia* (or "equity") are closely connected. The expectations that we place on people's lines of conduct will differ markedly depending on who is affected and what relationships the parties stand in toward one another. Far from regarding it as "fair" or "just" to deal with everybody in a precisely *equal* fashion, as the "veil of ignorance" might suggest, we consider it perfectly *equitable*, or *reasonable*, to show some degree of partiality, or favor, in dealing with close friends and relatives whose special needs and concerns we understand. What father, for instance, does not have an eye to his children's individual personalities and tastes? And, apart from downright "favoritism," who would regard such differences of treatment as unjust? Nor, surely, can it be morally offensive to discriminate, within reason, between close friends and distant acquaintances, colleagues and business rivals, neighbors and strangers? We are who we are: we stand in the human relationships we do, and our specific moral duties and obligations can be discussed in practice *only* at the point at which these questions of personal standing and relationship have been recognized and taken into the account.

Conclusion

From the mid-nineteenth century on, then, British and American moral philosophers treated ethics as a field for general theoretical inquiries and paid little attention to issues of application or particular types of cases. The philosopher who did most to inaugurate this new phase was Henry Sidgwick, and, from an autobiographical note, we know that he was reacting against the work of his contemporary, William Whewell [13, 14]. Whewell had written a textbook for use by undergraduates at Cambridge University that resembled in many respects a traditional manual of casuistics, containing separate sections on the ethics of promises or contracts, family and community, benevolence, and so on [15]. For his part, Sidgwick found Whewell's discussion too messy: there must be some way of introducing into the subject the kinds of rigor, order, and certainty associated with, for example, mathematical reasoning. So, ignoring all of Aristotle's cautions about the differences between the practical modes of reasoning appropriate to ethics and the formal modes appropriate to mathematics, he set out to expound the theoretical principles (or "methods") of ethics in a systematic form.

By the early twentieth century, the new program for moral philosophy had been narrowed down still further, so initiating the era of "metaethics." The philosopher's task was no longer to organize our moral beliefs into comprehensive systems: that would have meant *taking sides* over substantive issues. Rather, it was his duty to stand back from the fray and hold the ring while partisans of different views argued out their differences in accordance with the general rules for the conduct of "rational debate," or the expression of "moral attitudes," as defined in *metaethical* terms. And this was still the general state of affairs in Anglo-American moral philosophy in the late 1950s and the early 1960s, when public attention began to turn to questions of medical ethics. By this time, the central concerns of the philosophers had become so abstract and general—above all, so definitional or analytical—that they had, in effect, lost all touch with the concrete and particular issues that arise in actual practice, whether in medicine or elsewhere.

Once this demand for intelligent discussion of the ethical problems of medical practice and research obliged them to pay fresh attention to applied ethics, however, philosophers found their subject "coming alive again" under their hands. But, now it was no longer a field for academic, theoretical, even mandarin investigation alone. Instead, it had to be debated in practical, concrete, even political terms, and before long moral philosophers (or, as they barbarously began to be called, "ethicists"⁵) found that they were as liable as the economists

---

⁵Once again, the *Oxford English Dictionary* has a point to make. It includes the word "ethicist" but leaves it without the dignity of a definition, beyond the bare ethnology, "ethics + ist."

to be called on to write "op ed" pieces for the *New York Times*, or to testify before congressional committees.

Have philosophers wholly risen to this new occasion? Have they done enough to modify their previous methods of analysis to meet these new practical needs? About those questions there can still be several opinions. Certainly, it would be foolhardy to claim that the discussion of "bioethics" has reached a definitive form, or to rule out the possibility that novel methods will earn a place in the field in the years ahead. At this very moment, indeed, the style of current discussion appears to be shifting away from attempts to relate problematic cases to general theories—whether those of Kant, Rawls, or the utilitarians—to a more direct analysis of the practical cases themselves, using methods more like those of traditional "case morality." . . .

Whatever the future may bring, however, these 20 years of interaction with medicine, law, and the other professions have had spectacular and irreversible effects on the methods and content of philosophical ethics. By reintroducing into ethical debate the vexed topics raised by *particular cases*, they have obliged philosophers to address once again the Aristotelean problems of *practical reasoning*, which had been on the sidelines for too long. In this sense, we may indeed say that, during the last 20 years, medicine has "saved the life of ethics," and that it has given back to ethics a seriousness and human relevance which it had seemed—at least, in the writings of the interwar years—to have lost for good.

References

1. Aristotle. *Nicomachean Ethics.*
2. Fletcher, J. *Morals and Medicine.* Princeton, N. J.: Princeton Univ. Press, 1954.
3. Fletcher, J. *Situation Ethics.* Philadelphia: Westminster, 1966.
4. Fletcher, J. *Humanhood.* Buffalo, N.Y.: Prometheus, 1979.
5. Bradley, F. *Ethical Studies.* London, 1876.
6. Bledstein, B. *The Culture of Professionalism.* New York: Norton, 1976.
7. Rawls, J. *A Theory of Justice.* Cambridge, Mass.: Harvard Univ. Press, 1971.
8. Toulmin, S. The tyranny of principles. *Hastings Cent. Rep.* 11:6, 1981.
9. MacIntyre, A. *After Virtue.* South Bend, Ind.: Notre Dame Univ. Press, 1981.
10. Davis, K. *Discretionary Justice.* Urbana: Univ. Illinois Press, 1969.
11. Newman, R. *Equity and Law.* Dobbs Ferry, N. Y.: Oceana, 1961.
12. Hamburger, M. *Morals and Law: The Growth of Aristotle's Legal Theory.* New Haven, Conn.: Yale Univ. Press, 1951.
13. Sidgwick, H. *The Methods of Ethics,* Introduction to 6th ed. London and New York: Macmillan, 1901.
14. Schneewind, J. *Sidgwick's Ethics and Victorian Moral Philosophy.* Oxford and New York: Oxford Univ. Press, 1977.
15. Whewell, W. *The Elements of Morality,* 4th ed. Cambridge: Bell, 1864.

Questions for Discussion
Part I, Section 4

1. Do you agree or disagree with Callahan's position that bioethicists must adapt their standards of rigor in order to deal effectively with the problems they encounter in medicine?
2. Clouser maintains that bioethics is not properly understood as a reform movement or effort to inspire moral behavior. Do you agree or disagree with Clouser's position?
3. According to Clouser, what are the limits of the professional ethicist's role in health care?
4. How does Toulmin describe the role of the ethicist in the world of medicine? How has this role changed since the 1960s and 1970s?

PART II

The Methods of Bioethics

Introduction to the Methods of Bioethics

Nancy S. Jecker

Once bioethics became established as a formal field of scholarly inquiry, bioethicists were initially concerned to address the immediate problems facing practitioners in the clinical setting. While clinical ethics remains at the heart of bioethics, the field has recently broadened to include new areas such as conceptual analyses of bioethical principles; empirical assessments of the beliefs and attitudes health care workers hold; ethical critiques of health policies; and interdisciplinary analyses from fields such as anthropology, literature, and history. In addition, bioethicists have turned a critical eye on the very tools and methods of ethical analysis that they themselves use. It is this latter debate about the methods of bioethical analysis that will be the focus of Part II. This introductory section will familiarize the reader with the development of central principles of bioethics. It will then offer a thumbnail sketch of different positions regarding the role of bioethical principles in ethical analysis.

Principles of Bioethics

The origins of ethics in medicine go back well before the twentieth century to a school of thought associated with the fourth century B.C. physician Hippocrates. The Hippocratic tradition places emphasis on the health professional's special knowledge, training, and experience, which are to be used to direct the course of treatment. According to this approach, the doctor gives orders, and the good patient follows those orders, knowing that a person with superior knowledge and skill is working to promote the patient's best interests. Specifically, the Hippocratic tradition holds that the principle health professionals should heed is to "Follow that method of treatment which, according to my ability and judgment, I consider for the benefit of my patients, and abstain from whatever is deleterious and mischievous" (Hippocrates, trans. Jones, 1923).

In the language of contemporary bioethics, "employing the method that benefits" is expressed in terms of the principle of beneficence. This principle calls upon health professionals to promote the patient's good. It requires that any action a health professional undertakes be in the best interest of the patient. Similarly, "abstaining from whatever is deleterious and mischievous" is expressed in contemporary terms as a principle of nonmaleficence. This principle requires health care workers to avoid any action that would harm the patient. Taken together, the requirements of beneficence and nonmaleficence are often understood in modern times to be maximizing principles: not simply do good and avoid harm, but create the *greatest* good and the *least* amount of harm.

The Hippocratic tradition expressed in the principles of beneficence and nonmaleficence dominated bioethics during the early days of the field and continues to exert a powerful influence. However, beginning in the 1960s, the foundations of Hippocratic ethics came under a cross fire of criticism from a variety of sources. Not only patients, but health professionals, attorneys, academic philosophers, medical sociologists, and others began to call into question physicians' authority to make medical decisions on the patient's behalf. These challenges had many sources. In general, the 1960s was a time of rebellion against formal authorities. The civil rights movement, the anti-Vietnam war movement, and the beginnings of the feminist movement of the 1970s and 1980s caused large numbers of people to question paternalism in many spheres of life. The autonomy of the physician to determine what constitutes harm and benefit was likewise called into question. Critics of Hippocratic ethics noted that nothing in the Hippocratic oath empowers the patient to give or withhold informed consent to treatment.

Coupled with suspicion of authority was patient experience with new technologies. Assisted ventilation and other life-extending technologies did not always have happy endings. Even when interventions such as kidney dialysis and cardiopulmonary resuscitation provided dramatic short-term benefits, long-term outcomes for patients were often poorly understood. Thus both patients and health professionals began to feel less comfortable than they previously had with letting physicians decide whether or not to use medical treatments.

The public was also becoming better educated and informed about their own health and about health care treatments; as a result they were more reluctant than they had been in the past simply to accept the advice of health care experts. For example, patients were more likely to request a second opinion and to expect treatment options to be fully explained to them.

The courts also began to develop an enforceable requirement of informed consent for medical treatment as well as for human subject participation in medical experimentation. By 1972, three important appellate decisions (*Canterbury v. Spence, Cobbs v. Grant,* and *Wilkinson v. Vesey*) had debated the standards of informed consent. Whereas previous judicial decisions had required physicians to disclose to patients only information that it was customary to disclose, *Canterbury, Cobbs,* and *Wilkinson* established that physicians must "divulge any fact that is material to a reasonable person's decision" (Faden, Beauchamp, 1986, p. 32). In their history of informed consent, Ruth Faden and Tom Beauchamp argue that it was primarily courts and the legal profession—rather than physicians—that spearheaded the interest in informed consent that occurred during the 1960s and 1970s. Indeed, some physicians regarded the requirements of full disclosure and informed consent as incompatible with good patient care (Ingelfinger, 1972).

It was partly in response to these developments that the principle of patient autonomy began to play a more prominent role in bioethical analyses. Autonomy comes from the Greek words *autos,* meaning self, and *nomos* meaning rule. It was originally used to refer to political self-rule in ancient Greek city states. In health care, the principle of autonomy states that one ought to respect a competent patient's autonomous choices. In other words, people are entitled to be self-ruling and self-governing when they are able. Thus, a health professional should not stand in the way of what a competent patient wishes to do, even if what a patient wishes is harmful to the patient or entails foregoing a medical benefit, that is, even if respecting patient autonomy violates ethical principles of nonmaleficence or beneficence.

According to this approach, the relationship between patients and health care providers is somewhat analogous to a contract model that operates in other areas, such as law or business. Like an attorney or accountant, a health professional provides his or her client with all information necessary for the patient to make an informed choice about treatment. In its most extreme form, sometimes called the "scientific," "engineering," or "informative" model, the responsibility of the health professional is simply to guarantee that the patient has full information, rather than to do or recommend what the health professional believes to be in the best interest of the patient (Emanuel and Emanuel, 1992). Informed consent to treatment then becomes the crucial test of ethical health care. Thus, when autonomy conflicts with other bioethical principles, it takes precedence.

In summary, during the 1960s and early 1970s the physician's role changed dramatically. In the words of sociologist Eliot Friedson, the physician became "more or less a servitor, someone that the patient calls when he thinks he needs it" (Friedson, 1975, p. 42). Increasingly, doctors, like other professionals, were seen as "on tap" and their services were considered to be at the disposal of their clients (Carr-Saunders, 1955, p. 287).

Most agree that an emphasis on autonomy was a much needed corrective. However this approach is not without problems. One concern is that the patient's autonomy and decision-making skills may be routinely compromised by illness. Hence, patients may generally not be capable of making autonomous decisions about their care. According to Edmund Pellegrino and David Thomasma,

> The patient autonomy model does not give sufficient attention to the impact of disease on the patient's capacities for autonomy . . . Ill persons often become so anxious, guilty, angry, fearful, or hostile that they make judgments they would not make in calmer times . . . These primary characteristics of illness alter personal wholeness to a profound degree. They also change some of our assumptions about the operation of personal autonomy in the one who is ill (Pellegrino and Thomasma, 1988, pp. 14–15).

According to these authors, patient autonomy is properly understood as the goal of treatment, rather than as a starting assumption. Howard Brody (1992) voices a similar concern, noting that the greatest barrier to patient autonomy is often the patient's illness, not the physician. The physician, Brody claims, "should work actively with the patient to identify and remove those barriers and not be content with providing information and then standing back to allow the patient to choose" (Brody, 1992, p. 51).

A different objection is that in the quest to respect the autonomy of patients, the health practitioner's own autonomy may be compromised. For example, doing what the patient wishes may run contrary to the health professional's own personal or professional values.

A further objection to autonomy as a dominant ethic for health care is that abiding by patients' wishes may require health professionals to abdicate their responsibility to promote the public's health and welfare. For instance, in modern times vaccination can reduce the risk to others of contracting certain infectious diseases. But a patient may not be especially concerned about potential harms to others, or may believe that the threat of others' contracting a disease is already minimal because enough other people are vaccinated. In such a situation, society may mandate overriding patient autonomy by adopting mandatory immunization programs.

Another charge raised against the autonomy model has been that it falsely pictures the individual as an independent and self-sufficient decision maker. In fact, individuals exist within a network of personal and social relationships. These relationships partly define who the self is and thereby enable autonomy to function meaningfully. Thus, Nancy Rhoden has argued that

> The family is the context within which a person first develops her powers of autonomous choice, and the values she brings to these choices spring from, and are intertwined with, the family's values. A parent may understand a child's values because she helped to form them, a child may grasp a parent's values because the parent imparted them to her, and a couple may have developed and refined their views in tandem (Rhoden, 1988, pp. 438–439).

According to Rhoden, persons cannot be self-governing and self-reliant in isolation from others as the autonomy model suggests.

Finally, the principle of autonomy can be challenged on the ground that it cannot stand alone because it provides no incentive for cost containment or a fair distribution of scarce health care resources. The imperative is instead to do whatever an autonomous patient wishes, even if the patient wishes that "everything possible" be done. For this reason, the principle of autonomy does not always work well at the macro level, because resources can run out long before an autonomous patient's desire for them does.

In light of such objections to an autonomy-based ethic, a principle of social justice has been presented as an alternative guiding principle for health care. Generally speaking, social justice requires distributing scarce resources so that burdens and benefits are borne fairly by different groups in society. Social justice does not always call for serving the immediate good of the patient (as beneficence does) nor does it always coincide with the patient's autonomous choices about medical care (as autonomy does). Rather, a social justice perspective underscores that health professionals have responsibilities to the society as well as to individual patients.

Under the general heading of social justice a variety of substantive ethical principles have been put forward to govern the allocation of scarce resources. These principles require, for example, that the distribution of scarce goods conforms to ethical criteria of equality, need, ability, effort, social utility, or supply and demand. Among these, the standard of need is commonly defended as a just basis for distributing health care resources. A need-based standard attempts to evaluate patients' needs for treatment on the basis of the quality and likelihood of medical benefit that they can derive from treatment, and it awards treatment first to those who stand to benefit most.

Although a social justice orientation is well-suited to ethical debates about health care policy, its application to the clinical setting and to the doctor-patient relationship has met with some resistance. This is owing in part to the fact that such an orientation goes against the grain of health professionals' training and skills, which are primarily patient-centered. As the physician Marcia Angell has argued, "As individual physicians, we must do the very best we can for each patient. The patient rightly expects his physician to act single-mindedly in his best interests. If very expensive care is indicated, then the physician should do his utmost to obtain it for the patient" (Angell, 1985, p. 1206). Norman Levinsky has voiced a similar position, insisting that the doctor cannot serve two masters— the patient and society. Instead, Levinsky compares the health professional who cares for a patient with the lawyer who defends a client against a criminal charge:

> The attorney is obligated to use all ethical means to defend the client, regardless of the cost of prolonged legal proceedings or even of the possibility that a guilty person may be acquitted through skillful advocacy. Similarly, in the practice of medicine, physicians are obligated to do all that they can for their patients without regard to any costs to society. (Levinsky, 1984, pp. 1573–4).

A further objection mounted against a social-justice perspective in health care has been that the substantive criteria of justice put forward to guide the allocation of health care resources are very difficult to apply in practice. For example, a needs-based standard for distributing health care assumes that the meaning of *need* is relatively fixed. Yet *need* is a slippery term; what a patient "needs" can sometimes be changed to suit the circumstances at hand. For example, in Britan general practitioners have sometimes defined need for kidney dialysis narrowly to exclude older patients who, despite advanced age, could benefit from dialysis. As a result, older patients may not seek this treatment because they assume that they do not "need" it (Aaron, Schwartz, 1984). In the United States, the opposite tack has sometimes been taken: physicians may recommend dialysis or other life-saving interventions as medically necessary even when patients have an exceedingly low chance of successful outcome (Schneiderman, Jecker, Jonsen, 1990).

Models of Ethical Reasoning

The ethical principles of beneficence, nonmaleficence, autonomy, and social justice reviewed above are often considered to be the most central ethical principles in health care. In light of this, one might wonder how, more specifically, these four principles illuminate practical ethical problems. Without providing a complete answer to this question, it will be instructive to consider the trajectories of two quite different responses. I refer to these as different methodological approaches or models, although it would be misleading to think of either as constituting a fully developed framework. It would also be inaccurate to assume that bioethicists themselves always subscribe to a particular methodological approach. To the contrary, many do not consciously deploy any method; others deploy a variety of different methods. As the selections in other parts of this book attest, a single author sometimes uses a variety of methods of analyses in the same article as a way of building the strongest possible case for a particular position.

There is typically no explicit mention of methodology in bioethical literature dealing with practical ethical issues. Nor should this come as a surprise. In many fields where scholars engage in so-called applied studies, methodological debates do not take center stage. The value of becoming more self-conscious about the methods used to debate practical ethical issues, however, is that it places us in a better position to evaluate critically the assumptions that lie behind these methods. Sometimes these assumptions influence the outcome of ethical analysis in important respects.

Turning to the methodological approaches themselves, it is possible to distinguish at least two distinct models. The first regards answers to practical ethical problems as deductively derived from philosophical principles and theories of ethics. According to this approach, ethics is sciencelike in the sense that it offers a decision procedure for making particular ethical judgments. The first step in applying this decision procedure is to identify what the preferred philosophical theory of ethics is. This will presumably be the theory among those available that offers the greatest number of advantages and the fewest disadvantages. An ethical *theory* refers to a set of normative ethical principles. Typically, the principles that comprise a theory are *general* rather than referring to particular individuals; *universal* (that is, they apply to all persons); and internally consistent. From this general theory, one deduces a relevant ethical principle or principles. Next, from these principles one deduces a more specific ethical rule. Finally, the rule is applied to the case at hand to determine an answer to the ethical problem that the case presents. For example, "Equality and Its Implications" (Singer, 1980), which is included in Part II of this anthology, argues that utilitarianism is the preferred philosophical theory of ethics.

According to this model, practical dilemmas are resolved in a *deductive* fashion. What distinguishes deductive reasoning is that it is *demonstrative* or *certain*. In other words, the premises *force* the conclusion, on pain of inconsistency. Thus, the deductive model of ethical analysis is a decision procedure in the strict sense: a theory *logically entails* certain principles/rules, which in turn *logically require* a particular judgment about a case. The deductive method of analysis is summarized as follows.

Deductive Method

1. Identify a preferred philosophical theory of ethics
2. Deduce the relevant ethical principle
3. Deduce the relevant ethical rule
4. Apply the rule to the case at hand

For example, consider a practical ethical problem: a physician wants to know whether or not to tell a particular patient the truth about the patient's medical condition. According to the deductive method of ethical reasoning, one should proceed along the following lines. First, one embraces a general *ethical theory*, say, Kantian ethics. Rather than presenting a set of ethical principles to which our conduct must conform, Kantian ethics is sometimes interpreted as offering a test or procedure that possible ethical principles must pass in order to be considered genuine and binding (Herman, 1993). The name Kant gives to this test is the *categorical imperative*. In one formulation, the categorical imperative instructs us to act only on those principles that we can at the same time will to become a universal law. So understood, Kantian ethics provides a way of determining for ourselves which principles and rules we are ethically required to submit to, among the many possible principles and rules presented to us. The selection from Fred Feldman (Feldman, 1978) included in this anthology summarizes the approach of Kantian ethics.

One of the well-known and widely debated *ethical principles* that Kantian ethics sanctions is veracity. According to Kantian ethics, the categorical imperative shows us that veracity represents an *exceptionless* duty. Therefore, lying, which Kant defined as "an intentional untruthful declaration to another person," (Kant, 1979, p. 286), is universally prohibited, regardless of the consequences. Indeed, Kant goes so far as to say that if a would-be murderer knocks on your door and inquires whether your friend, who is pursued by the would-be murderer, had taken refuge in your house, you are forbidden to lie in order to save the friend's life. He adds: "After you had honestly answered the murderer's question as to whether the intended victim is at home, it may be that he has slipped out so that he does not come in the way of the murderer, and thus that the murder may not be committed" (Kant, 1979, p. 287).

However this may be, the principle of veracity is relevant to the ethical dilemma that the physician faces because the principle of veracity, in turn, entails a specific *professional rule*: doctors should always tell the truth to their patients. This rule implies a *specific judgment*: the physician should tell the patient the truth regarding the patient's medical condition. In this example, the justification for a particular *judgment* about truth telling is a professional *rule*; the rule is itself justified by showing that it follows from a more general *principle*; the principle is in turn justified by showing that it is part of a system of ethical principles—a *theory*, such as Kantian ethics.

Notice that the deductive method identifies the premises of ethical reasoning to be ethical theories. Hence, engaging in ethical argument requires mastery of those theories, together with rules of logical inference. These are the heart and soul of ethical understanding.

A quite different method of ethical analysis is the inductive method. This method proposes to begin ethical analysis with actual observations of the details of a particular case: the persons, circumstances, and relationships involved in the dilemma. It holds that experience and observation, rather than philosophical principles and theories, provide the premises of ethical argument. The papers in Part II, Section 3 show the relevance of quantitative and qualitative methods of empirical observation to the identification and analysis of ethical issues. According to the inductive conception, one should begin by giving ethical attention to concrete particulars. This is the first step because without the ability to respond to the particular features of a case, one cannot begin to decipher what more general principles and obligations are operative. Next, one determines what ethical principles are suitable to the case at hand. Finally, without ever resorting to a philosophical theory, one attempts to balance general principles and obligations with particular facts and insights. This may require, for example, using imagination to place oneself in the midst of the moral situation in order to discern the limits of general principles and obligations. Rather than remaining a detached observer, a person engaged in ethical analysis attempts to comprehend various perspectives or imagine what might be done in analogous situations.

In contrast to the deductive method, the inductive method treats uncertainty and residual tension in ethical judgments as unavoidable. The move from particular to general and back to particular is not accomplished by logical inference but by practical judgment. In inductive reasoning, premises lend *support* to a conclusion without logically guaranteeing it. In other words, an inductive argument intends to make a certain conclusion more probable but does not make it logically necessary. The inductive approach also assumes that general guides are not universally applicable, and so asks reasoners to supplement general normative principles with a clear understanding of their uses and limitations. According to the inductive model, the heart of ethical understanding is not mastery of philosophical theories, but moral experience and judgment. The inductive method of ethical analysis is summarized below.

Inductive Method

1. Pay attention to concrete particulars
2. Find operative ethical principles and obligations
3. Balance concrete particulars and general principles

In rare cases, a fourth step may be required in order to achieve the balance called for in the third. This occurs primarily in situations where the validity of a particular principle or obligation is persuasively challenged. Such a challenge may spring from a recognition that certain assumptions animate the principle or obligation and are no longer considered tenable. For example, the ethical commentaries on marriage that medieval casuists wrote were eventually challenged on the grounds that they were based on outmoded beliefs about sexuality and about equality between the sexes. When a general principle or obligation invoked in ethical analysis is called into question, a fourth step requires us to reevaluate the general claim directly. Thus, we might

4. Reject or modify a general ethical principle after identifying untenable assumptions underlying it.

The papers by Jonsen (1986) and Hunter (1991) are included in Part II to illustrate two different versions of the inductive method of analysis.

To return to the example of truth-telling we considered before, let us see how an inductive model might approach the same problem. In presenting an inductive analysis of truth-telling in the physician-patient relationship, I will borrow from a 1903 essay by the physician Richard Cabot (reprinted in Reiser et al. 1990). As we shall see, Cabot's approach to the problem of truth-telling is quite different from Kant's. Cabot first directs attention to the concrete particulars of the case. He describes the following situation.

A patient has gastric cancer. He is told that he has neuralgia (pain which extends along the course of 1 or more nerves) of the stomach, and feels greatly relieved by the reassurance . . . Meanwhile the truth is told to the patient's wife, and she makes whatever preparations are necessary for the inevitable end.

Cabot proceeds to ask,

Now what harm can be done by such a lie as this? The sufferer is protected from those anticipations and forebodings which are often the worst portion of misery, and yet his wife, knowing the truth and thoroughly approving of the deception, is able to see to it that her husband's financial affairs are straightened out and to prepare, as well as may be, for his death. Surely this seems a humane and sensible way to ease the patient's hard path.

To address this question, Cabot recalls an analogous case:

I was talking not long ago on this subject with a girl of 22. "Oh, of course *I* never believe what doctors say," was her comment, "for I've helped 'em lie too often and helped fix up the letters that were written so that no one should suspect the truth."

On the basis of this analogous case, Cabot identifies an operative principle. He states, "We have added to the lot of one person the sufferings which we spare another. We rob Peter to pay Paul." In other words, the patient himself may be saved some suffering through deception, but those who participate in deception (e.g., his wife) will not trust physicians in the future should they become ill. Cabot concludes by melding general insights and obligations with concrete features of the situation:

Many may be worse off for it [i.e., deception], and some must be. The patient himself is very possibly saved some suffering. But consider a minute. His wife has now acquired, if she did not have it already, a knowledge of the circumstances under which doctors think it merciful and useful to lie. She will be sick herself someday, and when the doctors tell her that she is not seriously ill, is she likely to believe them?

Like Kant, Cabot concludes that truth-telling is required. The doctor should tell the truth.

In response to Cabot's analysis, a feminist critique might cast doubt on central assumptions underlying the ethical principles that Cabot invokes. Or a feminist critique of Cabot's analysis also might argue for supplementing these principles with other general requirements, such as protecting from harm the various interpersonal relationships affected by the case. For a discussion of feminist approaches see "Feminist and Medical Ethics" (Sherwin, 1989), which is included in Part II of this book. If Cabot's reasoning is challenged on feminist or other grounds, it will be necessary to move the discussion of truth-telling to the fourth level of analysis mentioned above. Thus, it might be argued that the assumption underlying Cabot's analysis is that the general obligation of nonmaleficence applies to individual persons. Yet an alternative interpretation might regard the scope of this obligation as including avoiding harm to relationships between persons. If this proposal was accepted, then the requirement to tell the truth would be suitably modified. In the case under discussion, the physician may still be required to disclose to the patient his medical diagnosis but may be required not to disclose to the patient that his wife knew this diagnosis all along and said nothing. Arguably, the latter disclosure would harm the relationship between the patient and his wife by causing the patient to feel angry at and betrayed by his wife.

Let us close this discussion of inductive methods by considering how well such an approach can accommodate multiple disciplinary perspectives. A multidisciplinary inductive model might incorporate under general principles not only principles drawn from philosophical theories but general lessons drawn from multiple disciplines and sources. These sources may include *life experience*, that is, practical experience where one sees first-hand how ethical problems and resolutions play out in the course of people's lives. The discipline of history is also relevant as most ethical problems have long-standing and rich histories; even if a particular case is novel it may bear important similarities to cases that have occurred in the past. Literature is another possible source of general ethical insight. As Martha Nussbaum has shown, the genre of the novel can be an especially powerful tool for eliciting ethical imagination because it shows characters and situations up close (Nussbaum, 1990). Finally, other cultures can provide a valuable perspective from which to identify and assess basic ethical presuppositions that we bring to the ethical analysis of cases. However, as the articles by Fox and Swazey (1984) and Dula (1992) caution, the assumptions of a dominant culture can function to silence the ethical perspectives of other cultural groups in the society (see Part II, Section 4 of this anthology, where these articles appear). Or, as Arras points out in his article "Getting Down to Cases" (in Part

II of this anthology), the values of a single culture may yield conflicting moral conclusions.

To summarize, deductive and inductive methods present very different strategies for the resolution of practical ethical problems. Deductive analyses claim to provide a decision procedure whose premises are philosophical theories and principles of ethics and whose conclusions are specific answers to concrete moral dilemmas. Inductive methods, by contrast, begin by paying careful attention to concrete particulars of the case at hand. They may find operative general insights from philosophical theories and principles or from other sources and disciplines. Whereas deductive reasoning is demonstrative and certain, inductive reasoning lends support to a particular conclusion without establishing it as logically necessary. Admittedly, this description oversimplifies the complexities of each approach. Yet it does serve to highlight that very different epistemological assumptions underlie different forms of bioethical analysis.

Combining Deductive and Inductive Methods

As noted already, bioethicists engaged in practical ethical analysis frequently use both deductive and inductive forms of reasoning. Although this may appear to reveal an underlying confusion or inconsistency, it may instead reflect a considered commitment to using multiple methods of analysis. To the extent that no single method of ethical analysis enjoys an exclusive authoritative status, employing multiple methods arguably affords the most comprehensive analysis of an issue.

Some bioethicists argue that the practice of combining deductive and inductive methods itself constitutes a third model of ethical reasoning. Thus Beauchamp and Childress use the term *coherentism* to refer to ethical analysis that "is neither top-down nor bottom up; it moves in both directions" (Beauchamp and Childress, 1994, p. 20). A general strategy of this sort has also been suggested by the philosopher John Rawls who argues that the goal of ethical reasoning is for a person to achieve a coherent set of moral beliefs. This occurs only when the considered judgments that a person makes about practical issues are consistent with the more general moral principles or theories the person espouses. Rawls refers to the achievement of a coherent set of moral beliefs as *reflective equilibrium* (Rawls, 1971). Bioethicists such as John Arras (see Arras's paper "Getting Down to Cases," [1991], reprinted in Part II) endorse reflective equilibrium as an alternative to strict deductive or inductive methods.

However, it is important to bear in mind that an approach to ethical reasoning is truly eclectic only if the process of achieving reflective equilibrium allows for the possibility of modifying both specific and general moral judgments. For example, someone committed to truth-telling who endorses a general prohibition against lying may nonetheless think that lying is acceptable in a particular case. To resolve this conflict the general prohibition against lying may be modified in order to recognize justified exceptions of the sort that the case represents. Alternatively, once the judgment about the case is seen as conflicting with a general prohibition the person holds, the judgment about the case may be sacrificed to achieve consistency with the general principle of truth-telling. An eclectic position cannot be committed in advance to holding on to either particular general judgments, but instead considers each as subject to revision.

One objection to which an eclectic strategy falls prey is that it does not provide clear guidance about the crucial process of balancing specific and general moral judgments. For example, Beauchamp and Childress defend a role for ethical principles in the selection included in Part II, Section 1, but they do not offer specific guidance about how to decide whether to sacrifice a concrete moral judgment or a general moral principle in particular cases. In the absence of such instruction, one concern is that moral reasoners will make arbitrary decisions based on their prereflective leanings toward a deductive or inductive model. This is among the objections that Clouser and Gert raise in "A Critique of Principlism," which can be found in Part II, Section 1. If either a deductive or an inductive method is generally relied on when an "eclectic" method is used, then an eclectic form of moral reasoning does not represent a separate model of ethical analysis, but instead involves movement back and forth between deductive and inductive methodologies.

Rawls himself may accept this conclusion because, unlike Beauchamp and Childress, Rawls does not indicate that the technique of arriving at reflective equilibrium represents an alternative to deductive and inductive models. Rather, Rawls describes reflective equilibrium as a process that applies specifically to our sense of justice. He uses the technique for the limited purpose of setting out and defending a coherent account of the principles governing our sense of justice.

Conclusion

Perhaps the true measure of the various methods described here will be their usefulness in facilitating rigorous ethical argument and analysis. Part I of this book has already illustrated historically important examples of both inductive and deductive approaches. For example, Duff and Campbell began their essay, "Moral and Ethical Problems in the Special-Care Nursery" (included in Part I, Section 3, of this book), by inductively citing specific empirical data; they proceeded to raise and attempt to answer more general ethical questions. In Part III of this book, deductive and inductive methods will be further illustrated as we consider contemporary bioethical issues that arise in clinical practice.

References

Aaron, Henry J., Schwartz, William B. *The Painful Prescription*. Washington, DC: Brookings Institution, 1984.

Angell, Marcia. "Cost containment and the physician." *New England Journal of Medicine* 254, 1985: 1203–1207.

Beauchamp, Tom, Childress, James. *Principles of Biomedical Ethics*, 4th Ed. New York: Oxford University Press, 1994.

Brody, Howard. *The Healer's Power.* New Haven, CT: Yale University Press, 1992.

Cabot, Richard C. "The use of truth and falsehood in medicine: an experimental study" *American Medicine* 5, 1990: 344–349, reprinted in Stanley Joel Reiser, Arthur J. Dyck, William J. Curran (eds.), *Ethics in Medicine: Historical and Contemporary Concerns* (Cambridge, MA: MIT Press, 1977): 213–219.

Carr-Saunders, A.M. "Metropolitan conditions and traditional professional relationships." In R.M. Fisher, ed., *The Metropolis in Modern Life.* New York: Russell and Russell, 1955.

Emanuel, Ezekiel J., Emanuel, Linda L. "Four models of the physician-patient relationship." *Journal of the American Medical Association* 267, 1992: 2221–2226.

Faden, Ruth R., Beauchamp, Tom L. *A History and Theory of Informed Consent.* New York: Oxford University Press, 1986.

Friedson, Eliot. *Doctoring Together: A Study of Professional Social Control.* New York: Elsevier, 1975.

Herman, Barbara. *The Practice of Moral Judgment.* Cambridge, MA: Harvard University Press, 1993.

Hippocrates. "Oath." In W.H.S. Jones, *The Loeb Classical Library* (Cambridge, MA: Harvard University Press, 1923) vol. 1, pp. 164–165.

Ingelfinger, Franz J. "Informed (but uneducated) consent." *New England Journal of Medicine* 287, 1972: 465–466.

Kant, Immanuel. "On a supposed right to life from altruistic motives." Reprinted in Sissela Bok, *Lying: Moral Choices in Public and Private Life* (New York: Vintage Books, 1979): 285–290.

Levinsky, Norman. "The doctor's master." *New England Journal of Medicine* 311, 1984: 1573–1575.

Nussbaum, Martha C. "Finely aware and richly responsible." In Nussbaum, *Love's Knowledge: Essay on Philosophy and Literature* (New York, Oxford University Press, 1990).

Pellegrino, Edmund D., and Thomasma, David C. *For the Patient's Good: The Restoration of Beneficence in Health Care.* New York: Oxford University Press, 1988.

Rawls, John. *A Theory of Justice.* Cambridge, MA: Harvard University Press, 1971.

Rhoden, Nancy. "Litigating life and death." *Harvard Law Review* 102, 1988: 375–446.

Schneiderman, Lawrence J., Jecker, Nancy S., Jonsen, Albert R. "Medical futility: its meaning and ethical implications." *Annals of Internal Medicine* 112, 1990:949–954.

DEDUCTIVE APPROACHES

ETHICAL THEORIES AND PRINCIPLES

ࠨ

Equality and Its Implications

Peter Singer

Peter Singer studied moral and social philosophy at Oxford University during the 1970s under the direction of philosopher R.M. Hare. Singer is currently professor of philosophy and director of the Centre of Human Bioethics at Monash University in Australia. In this essay, excerpted from the book *Practical Ethics*, Singer espouses a principle requiring the equal consideration of each person's interests. He specifically rejects the possibility of taking into account any facts about persons other than their interests. One implication of this idea—which Singer does not address—is that it provides no ethical justification for showing partiality toward persons with whom we stand in special relationships (e.g., friends, parents, siblings).

The principle that all humans are equal is now part of the prevailing political and ethical orthodoxy. But what, exactly, does it mean and why do we accept it? . . .

John Rawls has suggested, in his influential book *A Theory of Justice*, that equality can be founded on the natural characteristics of human beings, provided we select what he calls a "range property." Suppose we draw a circle on a piece of paper. Then all points within the circle—this is the "range"—have the property of being within the circle, and they have this property equally. Some points may be closer to the centre and others nearer the edge, but all are, equally, points inside the circle. Similarly, Rawls suggests, the property of "moral personality" is a property which virtually all humans possess, and all humans who possess

Peter Singer. "Equality and Its Implications." Abridged from *Practical Ethics*, 1980, pp. 14–23. Reprinted by permission of Cambridge University Press.

this property possess it equally. By "moral personality" Rawls does not mean "morally good personality"; he is using "moral" in contrast to "amoral." A moral person, Rawls says, must have a sense of justice. More broadly, one might say that to be a moral person is to be the kind of person to whom one can make moral appeals, with some prospect that the appeal will be heeded. . . .

There are problems with using moral personality as the basis of equality. One objection is that moral personality is, unlike being inside a circle, a matter of degree. Some people are highly sensitive to issues of justice and ethics generally; others, for a variety of reasons, have only a very limited awareness of such principles. The suggestion that being a moral person is the minimum necessary for coming within the scope of the principle of equality still leaves it open just where this minimal line is to be drawn. Nor is it intuitively obvious why, if moral personality is so important, we should not have grades of moral status, with rights and duties corresponding to the degree of refinement of one's sense of justice.

Still more serious is the objection that it is not true that all humans are moral persons, even in the most minimal sense. Infants and small children, along with some mentally defective humans, lack the required sense of justice. Shall we then say that all humans are equal, except for very young or mentally defective ones? This is certainly not what we ordinarily understand by the principle of equality. If this revised principle implies that we may disregard the interests of very young or mentally defective humans in ways that would be wrong if they were older or more intelligent, we would need far stronger arguments to induce us to accept it. (Rawls deals with infants and children by including *potential* moral persons along with actual ones within the scope of the principle of equality. But this is an *ad hoc* device, confessedly designed to square his theory with our ordinary moral intuitions, rather than something for which independent arguments can be produced. Moreover although Rawls admits that those with irreparable mental defects "may present a difficulty" he offers no suggestions towards the solution of this difficulty.)

So the possession of "moral personality" does not provide a satisfactory basis for the principle that all humans are equal. I doubt that any natural characteristic, whether a "range property" or not, can fulfill this function, for I doubt that there is any morally significant property which all humans possess equally.

There is another possible line of defence for the belief that there is a factual basis for a principle of equality. . . . We can admit that humans differ as individuals, and yet insist that there are no morally significant differences . . . . Knowing that someone is black or white, female or male, does not enable us to draw conclusions about her or his intelligence, sense of justice, depth of feelings, or anything else that would entitle us to treat her or him as less than equal. . . .

The fact that humans differ as individuals, not as races or sexes, is important . . . yet it provides neither a satisfactory principle of equality, nor an adequate defence against a more sophisticated opponent of equality. . . .

. . . the claim to equality does not rest on intelligence, moral personality, rationality or similar matters of fact. There is no logically compelling reason for assuming that a difference in ability between two people justifies any difference in the amount of consideration we give to their interests. Equality is a basic ethical principle, not an assertion of fact . . .

. . . when I make an ethical judgment I must go beyond a personal or sectional point of view and take into account the interests of all those affected. This means that we weigh up interests, considered simply as interests and not as my interests, or the interests of Australians, or of whites. This provides us with a basic principle of equality: the principle of equal consideration of interests.

The essence of the principle of equal consideration of interests is that we give equal weight in our moral deliberations to the like interests of all those affected by our actions. This means that if only X and Y would be affected by a possible act, and if X stands to lose more than Y stands to gain, it is better not to do the act. We cannot, if we accept the principle of equal consideration of interests, say that doing the act is better, despite the facts described, because we are more concerned about Y than we are about X. What the principle really amounts to is: an interest is an interest, whoever's interest it may be.

We can make this more concrete by considering a particular interest, say the interest we have in the relief of pain. Then the principle says that the ultimate moral reason for relieving pain is simply the undesirability of pain as such, and not the undesirability of X's pain, which might be different from the undesirability of Y's pain. Of course, X's pain might be more undesirable than Y's pain because it is more painful, and then the principle of equal consideration would give greater weight to the relief of X's pain. Again, even where the pains are equal, other factors might be relevant, especially if others are affected. If there has been an earthquake we might give priority to the relief of a doctor's pain so she can treat other victims. But the doctor's pain itself counts only once, and with no added weighting. The principle of equal consideration of interests acts like a pair of scales, weighing interests impartially. True scales favour the side where the interest is stronger or where several interests combine to outweigh a smaller number of similar interests; but they take no account of whose interests they are weighing. . . .

The principle of equal consideration of interests prohibits making our readiness to consider the interests of others depend on their abilities or other characteristics, apart from the characteristic of having interests. It is true that we cannot know where equal consideration of interests will lead us until we know what interests people have, and this may vary according to their abilities or other characteristics. Consideration of the interests of mathematically gifted children may lead us to teach them advanced mathematics at an early age, which for different children might be entirely pointless or positively harmful. But the basic element, the taking into account of the person's interests, whatever they may be, must apply to everyone, irrespective of race, sex or scores on an intelligence test. . . .

Equal consideration of interests is a minimal principle of equality in the sense that it does not dictate equal treatment. Take a relatively straightforward example of an interest, the interest in having physical pain relieved. Imagine that after an earthquake I come across two victims, one with a crushed leg, in agony, and one with a gashed thigh, in slight pain. I have only two shots of morphine left. Equal treatment would suggest that I give one to each injured person, but one shot would not do much to relieve the pain of the person with the crushed leg. She would still be in much more pain than the other victim, and even after I have given her one shot, giving her the second shot would bring greater relief than giving a shot to the person in slight pain. Hence equal consideration of interests in this situation leads to what some may consider an inegalitarian result: two shots of morphine for one person, and none for the other.

There is a still more controversial inegalitarian implication of the principle of equal consideration of interests. In the case above, although equal consideration of interests leads to unequal treatment, this unequal treatment is an attempt to produce a more egalitarian result. By giving the double dose to the more seriously injured person, we bring about a situation in which there is less difference in the degree of suffering felt by the two victims than there would be if we gave one dose to each. Instead of ending up with one person in considerable pain and one in no pain, we end up with two people in slight pain. This is in line with the principle of declining marginal utility, a principle well-known to economists, which states that for a given individual, a set amount of something is more useful when the individual has little of it than when he has a lot. If I am struggling to survive on 200 grammes of rice a day, and you provide me with an extra fifty grammes per day, you have improved my position significantly; but if I already have a kilo of rice per day, I probably couldn't care less about the extra fifty grammes. When marginal utility is taken into account the principle of equal consideration of interests inclines us towards an equal distribution of income, and to that extent the egalitarian will endorse its conclusions. What is likely to trouble the egalitarian about the principle of equal consideration of interests is that there are circumstances in which the principle of declining marginal utility does not hold or is overridden by countervailing factors.

We can vary the example of the earthquake victims to illustrate this. Let us say, again, that there are two victims, one more severely injured than the other, but this time we shall say that the more severely injured victim, A, has lost a leg and is in danger of losing a toe from her remaining leg; while the less severely injured victim, B, has an injury to her leg, but the limb can be saved. We have medical supplies for only one person. If we use them on the more severely injured victim the most we can do is save her toe, whereas if we use them on the less severely injured victim we can save her leg. In other words, we assume that the situation is: without medical treatment, A loses a leg and a toe, while B loses only a leg; if we give the treatment to A, A loses a leg and B loses a leg; if we give the treatment to B, A loses a leg and a toe, while B loses nothing.

Assuming that it is worse to lose a leg than it is to lose a toe (even when that toe is on one's sole remaining foot) the principle of declining marginal utility does not hold in this situation. We will do more to further the interests, impartially considered, of those affected by our actions if we use our limited resources on the less seriously injured victim than on the more seriously injured one. Therefore this is what the principle of equal consideration of interests leads us to do. . . .

Kantian Ethics

Fred Feldman

Fred Feldman received his formal training in philosophy at Brown University during the late 1960s. He is a faculty member of the Department of Philosophy at the University of Massachusetts, Amherst. This essay, which is taken from a larger work entitled *Introductory Ethics*, analyzes Kant's formulation of the categorical imperative. According to Feldman, Kantian philosophy regards the requirements of morality as derived from the requirements of rationality, such that the person who wills an immoral act wills inconsistently. This approach holds that the universality of moral imperatives is as self-evident as the universality of reason itself.

Sometimes our moral thinking takes a decidedly nonutilitarian turn. That is, we often seem to appeal to a principle that is inconsistent with the whole utilitarian standpoint. One case in which this occurs clearly enough is the familiar tax-cheat case. A person decides to cheat on his income tax, rationalizing his misbehavior as follows: "The government will not be injured by the absence of my tax money. After all, compared with the enormous total they take in my share is really a negligible sum. On the other hand, I will be happier if I have the use of the money. Hence, no one will be injured by my cheating, and one person will be better off. Thus, it is better for me to cheat than it is for me to pay."

In response to this sort of reasoning, we may be inclined to say something like this: "Perhaps you are right in thinking that you will be better off if you cheat. And perhaps you are right in thinking that the government won't even know the difference. Nevertheless, your act would be wrong. For if everyone were to cheat on his income taxes, the government would soon go broke. Surely you can see that you wouldn't want others to act in the way you propose to act. So you shouldn't act in that way." While it may not be clear that this sort of response would be decisive, it should be clear that this is an example of a sort of response that is often given.

There are several things to notice about this response. For one, it is not based on the view that the example of the tax cheat will provoke everyone else to cheat too. If that were the point of the response, then the response might be explained on the basis of utilitarian considerations. We could understand the responder to be saying that the tax cheater has miscalculated his utilities. Whereas

Feldman, Fred. "Kantian Ethics." *Introductory Ethics*, © 1978, pp. 97–99, 101–117. Adapted by permission of Prentice Hall, Upper Saddle River, New Jersey.

he thinks his act of cheating has high utility, in fact it has low utility because it will eventually result in the collapse of the government. It is important to recognize that the response presented above is not based upon any such utilitarian considerations. This can be seen by reflecting on the fact that the point could just as easily have been made in this way. "Of course, very few other people will know about your cheating, and so your behavior will not constitute an example to others. Thus, it will not provoke others to cheat. Nevertheless, your act is wrong. For if everyone were to cheat as you propose to do, then the government would collapse. Since you wouldn't want others to behave in the way you propose to behave, you should not behave in that way. It would be wrong to cheat."

Another thing to notice about the response in this case is that the responder has not simply said, "What you propose to do would be cheating; hence, it is wrong." The principle in question is not simply the principle that cheating is wrong. Rather, the responder has appealed to a much more general principle, which seems to be something like this: If you wouldn't want everyone else to act in a certain way, then you shouldn't act in that way yourself.

This sort of general principle is in fact used quite widely in our moral reasoning. . . [It is] used against the person who refrains from giving to charity; the person who evades the draft in time of national emergency; the person who tells a lie in order to get out of a bad spot; and even the person who walks across a patch of newly seeded grass. In all such cases, we feel that the person acts wrongly not because his actions will have bad results, but because he wouldn't want others to behave in the way he behaves.

A highly refined version of this nonutilitarian principle is the heart of the moral theory of Immanuel Kant.[1] In his *Groundwork of the Metaphysic of Morals*,[2] Kant presents, develops, and defends the thesis that something like this principle is the "supreme principle of morality.". . .

Kant formulates his main principle in a variety of different ways.

> I ought never to act except in such a way that my maxim should become a universal law.[3]
>
> Act only on that maxim through which you can at the same time will that it should become a universal law.[4]
>
> Act as if the maxim of your action were to become through your will a universal law of nature.[5]
>
> We must be able to will that a maxim of our action should become a universal law—this is the general canon for all moral judgment of action.[6]

Before we can evaluate this principle, which Kant calls the *categorical imperative*, we have to devote some attention to figuring out what it is supposed to mean. To do this, we must answer a variety of questions. What is a maxim? What is meant by "universal law"? What does Kant mean by "will"? Let us consider these questions in turn.

Maxims

. . . Kant defines *maxim* as "a subjective principle of volition. . . .[7]

Kant apparently believes that when a person engages in genuine action, he always acts on some sort of general principle. The general principle will explain what the person takes himself to be doing and the circumstances in which he takes himself to be doing it. For example, if I need money, and can get some only by borrowing it, even though I know I won't be able to repay it, I might proceed to borrow some from a friend My maxim in performing this act might be, "Whenever I need money and can get it by borrowing it, then I will borrow it, even if I know I won't be able to repay it."

Notice that this maxim is *general*. If I adopt it, I commit myself to behaving in the described way *whenever* I need money and the other conditions are satisfied. In this respect, the maxim serves to formulate a general principle of action rather than just some narrow reason applicable in just one case.[8] So a maxim must describe some general sort of situation, and then propose some form of action for the situation. To adopt a maxim is to commit yourself to acting in the described way whenever the situation in question arises. . . .

It would be implausible to maintain that before we act, we always consciously formulate the maxim of our action. Most of the time we simply go ahead and perform the action without giving any conscious thought to what we're doing, or what our situation is. We're usually too intent on getting the job done. Nevertheless, if we are asked after the fact, we often recognize that we actually were acting on a general policy, or maxim. . . .

For our purposes, it will be useful to introduce a concept that Kant does not employ. This is the concept of the *generalized form* of a maxim. Suppose I decide to go to sleep one night and my maxim in performing this act is this:

M: Whenever I am tired, I shall sleep.

My maxim is stated in such a way as to contain explicit references to me. It contains two occurrences of the word "I." The generalized form of my maxim is the principle we would get if we were to revise my maxim so as to make it applicable to everyone. Thus, the generalized form of my maxim is this:

GM: Whenever anyone is tired, he will sleep.

In general, then, we can represent the form of a maxim in this way:

M: Whenever I am———, I shall———.

Actual maxims have descriptions of situations in the first blank and descriptions of actions in the second blank. The generalized form of a maxim can be represented in this way:

GM: Whenever anyone is———, she will———.

So much, then, for maxims. Let us turn to our second question, "What is meant by universal law?"

When, in the formulation of the categorical imperative, Kant speaks of "universal law,". . . sometimes he seems to be thinking of a *universal law of nature*. . . .

A *law of nature* is a fully general statement that describes not only how things are, but how things always *must* be. Consider this example: If the temperature of a gas in an enclosed container is increased, then the pressure will increase too. This statement accurately describes the behavior of gases in enclosed containers. Beyond this, however, it describes behavior that is, in a certain sense, necessary. The pressure not only *does* increase, but it *must* increase if the volume remains the same and the temperature is increased. This "must" expresses not logical or moral necessity, but "physical necessity." Thus, a law of nature is a fully general statement that expresses a physical necessity. . . .

Willing

. . . The Kantian concept of willing is a bit more complicated. . .

Some states of affairs are impossible. They simply cannot occur. For example, consider the state of affairs of your jumping up and down while remaining perfectly motionless. It simply cannot be done. Yet a sufficiently foolish or irrational person might will that such a state of affairs occur. That would be as absurd as commanding someone else to jump up and down while remaining motionless. Kant would say of a person who has willed in this way that his will has "contradicted itself." We can also put the point by saying that the person has willed inconsistently.

Inconsistency in willing can arise in another, somewhat less obvious way. Suppose a person has already willed that he remain motionless. He does not change this volition, but persists in willing that he remain motionless. At the same time, however, he begins to will that he jump up and down. Although each volition is self-consistent, it is inconsistent to will both of them at the same time. This is a second way in which inconsistency in willing can arise.

It may be the case that there are certain things that everyone must always will. For example, we may have to will that we avoid intense pain. Anyone who wills something that is inconsistent with something everyone must will, thereby wills inconsistently.

Some of Kant's examples suggest that he held that inconsistency in willing can arise in a third way. . . . Suppose a person wills to be in Boston on Monday and also wills to be in San Francisco on Tuesday. Suppose, furthermore, that because of certain foul-ups at the airport it will be impossible for her to get from Boston to San Francisco on Tuesday. In this case, Kant would perhaps say that the person has willed inconsistently.

In general, we can say that a person wills inconsistently if he wills that p be the case and he wills that q be the case and it is impossible for p and q to be the case together.

With all this as background, we may be in a position to interpret the first version of Kant's categorical imperative. Our interpretation is this:

> CI_1: An act is morally right if and only if the agent of the act can consistently will that the generalized form of the maxim of the act be a law of nature.

We can simplify our formulation slightly by introducing a widely used technical term. We can say that a maxim is *universalizable* if and only if the agent who acts upon it can consistently will that its generalized form be a law of nature. Making use of this new term, we can restate our first version of the categorical imperative as follows:

CI_1': An act is morally right if and only if its maxim is universalizable.

As formulated here, the categorical imperative is a statement of necessary and sufficient conditions for the moral rightness of actions. Some commentators have claimed that Kant did not intend his principle to be understood in this way. They have suggested that Kant meant it to be understood merely as a necessary but not sufficient condition for morally right action. Thus, they would prefer to formulate the imperative in some way such as this:

CI_1'': An act is morally right only if its maxim is universalizable.

Understood in this way, the categorical imperative points out one thing to avoid in action. That is, it tells us to avoid actions whose maxims cannot be universalized. But it does not tell us the distinguishing feature of the actions we should perform. Thus, it does not provide us with a criterion of morally right action. Since Kant explicitly affirms that his principle is "the supreme principle of morality," it is reasonable to suppose that he intended it to be taken as a statement of necessary and sufficient conditions for morally right action. In any case, we will take the first version of the categorical imperative to be CI_1, rather than CI_1''. . . .

In a very famous passage in Chapter II of the *Groundwork*, Kant presents four illustrations of the application of the categorical imperative.[9] In each case, in Kant's opinion, the act is morally wrong and the maxim is not universalizable. Thus, Kant holds that his theory implies that each of these acts is wrong. If Kant is right about this, then he has given us four positive instances of his theory. That is, he has given us four cases in which his theory yields correct results. . . .

Kant distinguishes between "duties to self" and "duties to others." He also distinguishes between "perfect" and "imperfect" duties. This gives him four categories of duty: "perfect to self," "perfect to others," "imperfect to self," and "imperfect to others." Kant gives one example of each type of duty. By "perfect duty," Kant says he means a duty "which admits of no exception in the interests of inclination."[10] Kant seems to have in mind something like this: If a person has a perfect duty to perform a certain kind of action, then he must *always* do that kind of action when the opportunity arises. For example, Kant apparently holds that we must always perform the (negative) action of refraining from committing suicide. This would be a perfect duty. On the other hand, if a person has an imperfect duty to do a kind of action, then he must at least *sometimes* perform an action of that kind when the opportunity arises. For example, Kant maintains that we have an imperfect duty to help others in distress. We should devote at least some of our time to charitable activities, but we are under no obligation to give all of our time to such work. . . .

Kant's first example illustrates the application of CI_1 to a case of perfect duty to oneself—the alleged duty to refrain from committing suicide. Kant describes the miserable state of the person contemplating suicide, and tries to show that his categorical imperative entails that the person should not take his own life. In order to simplify our discussion, let us use the abbreviation "a_1," to refer to the act of suicide the man would commit, if he were to commit suicide. According to Kant, every act must have a maxim. Kant tells us the maxim of a_1: "From self-love I make it my principle to shorten my life if its continuance threatens more evil than it promises pleasure."[11] Let us simplify and clarify this maxim, understanding it as follows:

> M (a_1): When continuing to live will bring me more pain than pleasure, I shall commit suicide out of self-love.

The generalized form of this maxim is as follows:

> GM(a_1): Whenever continuing to live will bring anyone more pain than pleasure, he will commit suicide out of self-love.

Since Kant believes that suicide is wrong, he attempts to show that his moral principle, the categorical imperative, entails that a_1 is wrong. To do this, of course, he needs to show that the agent of a_1 cannot consistently will that GM (a_1) be a law of nature. Kant tries to show this in the following passage:

> . . . a system of nature by whose law the very same feeling whose function is to stimulate the furtherance of life should actually destroy life would contradict itself and consequently could not subsist as a system of nature. Hence this maxim cannot possibly hold as a universal law of nature and is therefore entirely opposed to the supreme principle of all duty.[12]

The general outline of Kant's argument is clear enough:

Suicide Example

1. GM (a_1) cannot be a law of nature.
2. If GM (a_1) cannot be a law of nature, then the agent of a_1 cannot consistently will that GM (a_1) be a law of nature.
3. a_1 is morally right if and only if the agent of a_1 can consistently will that GM (a_1) be a law of nature.
4. Therefore, a_1 is not morally right. . . .

Let us turn now to the second illustration. Suppose I find myself hard-pressed financially and I decide that the only way in which I can get some money is by borrowing it from a friend. I realize that I will have to promise to repay the money, even though I won't in fact be able to do so. For I foresee that my financial situation will be even worse later on than it is at present. If I perform this action, a_2, of borrowing money on a false promise, I will perform it on this maxim:

$M(a_2)$: When I need money and can get some by borrowing it on a false promise, then I shall borrow the money and promise to repay, even though I know that I won't be able to repay.

The generalized form of my maxim is this:

$GM(a_2)$: Whenever anyone needs money and can get some by borrowing it on a false promise, then he will borrow the money and promise to repay, even though he knows that he won't be able to repay.

Kant's view is that I cannot consistently will that $GM(a_2)$ be a law of nature. This view emerges clearly in the following passage:

> . . . I can by no means will a universal law of lying; for by such a law there could properly be no promises at all, since it would be futile to profess will for future action to others who would not believe my profession or who, if they did so overhastily, would pay me back in like coin; and consequently my maxim, as soon as it was made a universal law, would be bound to annul itself.[13]

It is important to be clear about what Kant is saying here. He is not arguing against lying on the grounds that if I lie, others will soon lose confidence in me and eventually won't believe my promises. Nor is he arguing against lying on the grounds that my lie will contribute to a general practice of lying, which in turn will lead to a breakdown of trust and the destruction of the practice of promising. These considerations are basically utilitarian. Kant's point is more subtle. He is saying that there is something covertly self-contradictory about the state of affairs in which, as a law of nature, everyone makes a false promise when in need of a loan. Perhaps Kant's point is this: Such a state of affairs is self-contradictory because, on the one hand, in such a state of affairs everyone in need would borrow money on a false promise, and yet, on the other hand, in that state of affairs no one could borrow money on a false promise—for if promises were always violated, who would be silly enough to loan any money?

Since the state of affairs in which everyone in need borrows money on a false promise is covertly self-contradictory, it is irrational to will it to occur. No one can consistently will that this state of affairs should occur. But for me to will that $GM(a_2)$ be a law of nature is just for me to will that this impossible state of affairs occur. Hence, I cannot consistently will that the generalized form of my maxim be a law of nature. According to CI_1, my act is not right unless I can consistently will that the generalized form of its maxim be a law of nature. Hence, according to CI_1, my act of borrowing the money on the false promise is not morally right.

We can restate the essentials of this argument much more succinctly:

Lying-Promise Example

1. $GM(a_2)$ cannot be a law of nature.
2. If $GM(a_2)$ cannot be a law of nature, then I cannot consistently will that $GM(a_2)$ be a law of nature.

3. a_2 is morally right if and only if I can consistently will that $GM(a_2)$ be a
   law of nature.
4. Therefore, a_2 is not morally right. . . .

Let us turn, then, to the third example. Kant now illustrates the application
of the categorical imperative to a case of imperfect duty to oneself. The action
in question is the "neglect of natural talents." Kant apparently holds that it is
wrong for a person to let all of his natural talents go to waste. Of course, if a
person has several natural talents, he is not required to develop all of them.
Perhaps Kant considers this to be an imperfect duty partly because a person has
the freedom to select which talents he will develop and which he will allow to
rust.

Kant imagines the case of someone who is comfortable as he is and who,
out of laziness, contemplates performing the act, a_3, of letting all his talents
rust. His maxim in doing this would be:

$M(a_3)$: When I am comfortable as I am, I shall let my talents rust.

When generalized, the maxim becomes:

$GM(a_3)$: Whenever anyone is comfortable as he is, he will let his talents rust.

Kant admits that $GM(a_3)$ could be a law of nature. Thus, his argument in this
case differs from the arguments he produced in the first two cases. Kant proceeds
to outline the reasoning by which the agent would come to see that it would
be wrong to perform a_3:

> He then sees that a system of nature could indeed always subsist under such a
> universal law, although (like the South Sea Islanders) every man should let his talents
> rust and should be bent on devoting his life solely to idleness, indulgence, procreation,
> and, in a word, to enjoyment. Only he cannot possibly *will* that this should become
> a universal law of nature or should be implanted in us as such a law by a natural
> instinct. For as a rational being he necessarily wills that all his powers should be
> developed, since they serve him, and are given him, for all sorts of possible ends.[14]

Once again, Kant's argument seems to be based on a rather dubious appeal
to natural purposes. Allegedly, nature implanted our talents in us for all sorts
of purposes. Hence, we necessarily will to develop them. If we also will to let
them rust, we are willing both to develop them (as we must) and to refrain
from developing them. Anyone who wills both of these things obviously wills
inconsistently. Hence, the agent cannot consistently will that his talents rust.
This, together with the categorical imperative, implies that it would be wrong
to perform the act, a_3, of letting one's talents rust.

The argument can be put as follows:

Rusting-Talents Example

1. Everyone necessarily wills that all his talents be developed.
2. If everyone necessarily wills that all his talents be developed, then the
   agent of a_3 cannot consistently will that $GM(a_3)$ be a law of nature.

3. a₃ is morally right if and only if the agent of a₃ can consistently will that GM(a₃) be a law of nature.
4. Therefore a₃ is not morally right. . . .

In Kant's fourth illustration the categorical imperative is applied to an imperfect duty to others—the duty to help others who are in distress. Kant describes a man who is flourishing and who contemplates performing the act, a₄, of giving nothing to charity. His maxim is not stated by Kant in this passage, but it can probably be formulated as follows:

M(a₄): When I'm flourishing and others are in distress, I shall give nothing to charity.

When generalized, this maxim becomes:

GM(a₄): Whenever anyone is flourishing and others are in distress, he will give nothing to charity.

As in the other example of imperfect duty, Kant acknowledges that GM (a₄) could be a law of nature. Yet he claims once again that the agent cannot consistently will that it be a law of nature. He explains this by arguing as follows:

For a will which decided in this way would be in conflict with itself, since many a situation might arise in which the man needed love and sympathy from others, and in which, by such a law of nature sprung from his own will, he would rob himself of all hope of the help he wants for himself.[15]

Kant's point here seems to be this: The day may come when the agent is no longer flourishing. He may need charity from others. If that day does come, then he will find that he wills that others give him such aid. However, in willing that GM(a₄) be a law of nature, he has already willed that no one should give charitable aid to anyone. Hence, on that dark day, his will will contradict itself. Thus, he cannot consistently will that GM(a₄) be a law of nature. This being so, the categorical imperative entails that a₄ is not right. . . .

References

1. Immanuel Kant (1724–1804) is one of the greatest Continental philosophers. He produced quite a few philosophical works of major importance. The *Critique of Pure Reason* (1781) is perhaps his most famous work.
2. Kant's *Grundlegungzur Metaphysik der Sitten* (1785) has been translated into English many times. All references here are to Immanuel Kant, *Groundwork of the Metaphysic of Morals*, translated and analysed by H. J. Paton (New York: Harper & Row, 1964).
3. Kant, *Groundwork*, p. 70.
4. *Ibid.*, p. 88.
5. *Ibid.*, p. 89.
6. *Ibid.*, p. 91.
7. *Ibid.*, p. 69n.
8. In some unusual cases, it may accidentally happen that the situation to which

the maxim applies can occur only once, as, for example, in the case of successful suicide. Nevertheless, the maxim is general in form.

9. *Ibid.*, pp. 89–91.
10. *Ibid.*, p. 89n.
11. *Ibid.*, p. 89.
12. *Ibid.*
13. *Ibid.*, p. 71.
14. *Ibid.*
15. *Ibid.*, p. 91.

From *Principles of Biomedical Ethics*

Tom L. Beauchamp and James F. Childress

Philosopher Tom Beauchamp was a member of the Kennedy Institute of Ethics at Georgetown University when the first edition of *Principles of Biomedical Ethics* appeared in 1977. He continues to serve in this capacity, and as a professor in the Department of Philosophy at Georgetown. James Childress is professor of religious studies at the University of Virginia, Charlottesville. Now in its fourth edition, the excerpt from *Principles of Bioethics* reprinted below espouses a "common-morality theory," which takes its basic premises from the shared morality of society's members. Elsewhere in the book, Beauchamp and Childress set forth the principles of autonomy, beneficence, nonmaleficence, and justice as the central ethical considerations that constitute a common-morality theory in health care.

Principle-Based, Common-Morality Theories

. . . A common-morality theory takes its basic premises directly from the morality shared in common by the members of a society—that is, unphilosophical common sense and tradition. Such a theory need not be principle-based, but we treat these two types of theories together in order to develop the tradition of ethics in which our account should be situated. This [discussion], then, is best understood overall as a statement of the type of ethical theory that we accept and utilize. . . .

Principle-based theories share with utilitarian and Kantian theories an emphasis on principles of *obligation*, but these theories share little else. Two main differences distinguish them. First, utilitarianism and Kantianism are *monistic* theories. One supreme, absolute principle supports all other action-guides in the system. Common-morality theories, as we here stipulatively define them, are *pluralistic*. Two or more nonabsolute (prima facie) principles form the general level of normative statement. Second, common-morality ethics relies heavily on ordinary shared moral beliefs for its content, rather than relying on pure reason, natural law, a special moral sense, and the like. The principles embedded in these shared moral beliefs are also usually accepted by rival ethical theories. Although not the most general principles in many normative theories, the principles are nonetheless accepted in most types of ethical theory. . . .

Any theory that eventuates in moral judgments that cannot be brought into reflective equilibrium with pretheoretical commonsense judgments will be considered seriously flawed. However, this is not to maintain *either* that . . . a common-morality theory is merely a systematizing of commonsense judgments

Tom L. Beauchamp and James F. Childress. Abridged from *Principles of Biomedical Ethics*, 1994, pp. 100–106. Reprinted by permission of Oxford University Press.

or that all *customary moralities* qualify as part of the *common morality*. An important function of the standards in the common morality (from which the principles we defend and their correlative rights are developed) is to provide a basis for the evaluation and criticism of actions in countries and communities whose customary moral viewpoints fail to acknowledge basic principles. A customary morality, then, is not synonymous with the common morality. The latter is a pretheoretic moral point of view that transcends merely local customs and attitudes. Analogous to beliefs in the universality of basic human rights, the principles of the common morality are universal standards.

Our method . . . is to unite principle-based, common-morality ethics with the coherence model of justification. . . . This strategy allows us to rely on the authority of the indispensable principles in the common morality, while incorporating tools to refine and correct its weaknesses and unclarities and to allow for additional specification. Because our strategy accepts the goal of reflective equilibrium and, in part, *constructs* principles and rules from considered judgments in the common morality, while also *specifying* principles and rules, we will not end with the identical content with which we began. . . .

The Common Morality as Primary Source

As a rough generalization, what Henry Sidgwick called the commonsense morality (morality's core principles and assorted rules of veracity, fidelity, and the like) is the source of the initial moral content for this type of theory. Ethical theory augments this sparse content by a method (1) to clarify and interpret the content, (2) to make the various strands coherent, and (3) to further specify and balance the requirements of norms. . . .

Consider why the common morality should play an essential role in ethical theory. If we could be confident that some abstract moral theory was a better source for codes and policies than the common morality, we could work constructively on practical and policy questions by progressive specification of the norms in that theory. But fully analyzed norms in ethical theories are invariably more contestable than the norms in the common morality. We cannot reasonably expect that a contested moral theory will be better for practical decisionmaking and policy development than the morality that serves as our common denominator. Far more social consensus exists about principles and rules drawn from the common morality (for example, our four principles) than about theories. This is not surprising, given the central social role of the common morality and the fact that its principles are, at least in schematic form, usually embraced in some form by all major theories. Theories are rivals over matters of justification, rationality, and method, but they often converge on mid-level principles. . . .

Common-morality ethics does not preclude the possibility of reform, which often occurs through interpretation, specification, and balancing. . . . Interpretation and innovation are almost always carried out by appeal to justifications *within* rather than *beyond* norms already shared in the community. For example, if our policies on AIDS are so uncompassionate that we need to alter our conception of how therapeutic drugs are brought to the market, purchased, and distributed, this reevaluation will invoke available conceptions of compassion, fair funding, and distribution, rather than totally new principles of justice. Moreover, social agreements, traditions, and norms are inherently indeterminate, thereby failing to anticipate adequately the full range of moral problems and solutions. Interpretation and specification of norms, reconstruction of traditional beliefs, balancing different values, and negotiation are essential. This approach to construction in theory invites evolutionary change while insisting that the common morality provides the starting point and the constraining framework.

Two Examples of Principle-Based Theories

Commonsense convictions played only a minor role in ethical theory prior to the eighteenth century, when philosophers such as Francis Hutcheson, Jean-Jacques Rousseau, and Joseph Butler argued that a native moral sense or an intuitive conscience possessed by all persons is far more important in the moral life than the more complicated systems of philosophers. Their moral psychology did not survive, but their commonsense emphasis did, and Hume, Kant, Hegel, and other leading moral theorists were deeply affected by it. Two twentieth-century writers in ethical theory will serve here to illustrate how a principle-based, common-morality theory is still alive and well.

Frankena's theory. An elegant and simple example of a common-morality theory that resembles ours is William Frankena's version of Hume's postulate that the two major "principles of morals" are beneficence and justice. Frankena appeals to what Bishop Butler called "the moral institution of life," together with what Frankena calls "the moral point of view," meaning a dispassionate attitude of sympathy in which moral decisions are reached by appeal to principled good reasons. For Frankena, the principle of beneficence . . . resembles, but is not identical to, the utilitarian demand that we maximize good over evil, whereas the principle of justice (primarily an egalitarian principle) guides "our distribution of good and evil" independently of judgments about maximizing and balancing good outcomes. Frankena's theory comprises these two general principles, together with an argument that they capture the essence of the moral point of view.

Ross's theory. A second example is the ethics of W. D. Ross, who has had a particularly imposing influence on twentieth-century ethical theory, and more influence on the present authors than any recent writer in ethical theory. He is best known for his intuitionism and his scholarship on Aristotle, but we will largely ignore these dimensions of his work. Ross's starting point is Aristotelian. The moral convictions of thoughtful persons are "the data of ethics just as sense-perceptions are the data of a natural science. Just as some of the latter have to be rejected as illusory, so have some of the former." The "plain" person is, for Ross, the beginning rather than the end of the matter. Using this data base of ordinary standards, Ross thinks *acts* are properly categorized as right and wrong, whereas *motivation* and character are good and bad. This allows him to say that a right act can be done from a bad motive and that a good motive may eventuate in a wrong act.

Ross defends several basic and irreducible moral principles that express prima facie obligations. For example, promises create obligations of fidelity, wrongful actions and debts create obligations of reparation, and the generous services or gifts of others create obligations of gratitude. In addition to fidelity, reparation, and gratitude, Ross lists obligations of self-improvement, justice, beneficence, and nonmaleficence. He holds that the principle of nonmaleficence (noninfliction of harm) takes precedence over the principle of beneficence (production of benefit) when the two come into conflict, but he assigns no priorities among the other principles. This list of obligations is not grounded in any overarching principle.

In a noteworthy methodological statement, Ross maintains that principles are "recognized by intuitive induction as being implied in the judgments already passed on particular acts." His studies of Greek philosophy also led him to distinguish knowledge from opinion. We know principles in the same way the plain person knows the main lines of moral obligation. Here we have *knowledge*, not *opinion*. However, when two or more obligations conflict and balancing, overriding, and judgment are necessary, Ross says we must examine the situation carefully until we form a "considered opinion (it is never more)" that one obligation is more incumbent in the circumstances than any other. These judgments are about the *weight* of principles. They are not judgments that straightforwardly *apply* principles.

The Centrality of Principles and Rules

We can now develop the perspectives and assumptions that make [our theory] a form of common-morality ethics.

The source of the principles.   To say that principles have their origins in the common morality is not to suggest that the final form in which they greet a reader of this book is identical to their appearance in the common morality. Conceptual clarification and methods to introduce coherence are needed to give shape and substance to our moral commitments, much as grammarians, lexicographers, and stylists investigate the nature of our commitments in using words, punctuation, forms of citation, and the like. If unacceptable content is discovered in formulations of principles (for example, if a vigorous strong paternalism in clinical medicine is uncovered) or if incoherence is located, an attempt is made to find acceptable content and achieve coherence. This is work *in* ethical theory, even if its product should not be spoken of as *an* ethical theory. The objective is to give each principle a precise, plausible, thorough, and independent statement, without presupposing that our familiar ways of formulating principles are necessarily the best or the most coherent ways. After the principles are so formulated, they will still have to be further interpreted, specified, and balanced to produce an ethics for biomedicine. This is the heart of our strategy.

The prima facie and specifiable nature of the principles. Like Ross, we construe principles as prima facie binding. Some theories recognize rules, but treat them as expendable rules of thumb that summarize past experience by expressing better and worse ways to handle recurrent problems. Other theories contain absolute principles. Still other theories give a hierarchical (or lexical) ordering to moral norms. We reject all three interpretations as inadequate to capture the nature of moral norms and moral reasoning. Rules of thumb permit too much discretion, as if principles or rules were not binding; absolute principles and rules disallow all discretion for moral agents and also encounter unresolvable moral conflicts; and a hierarchy of rules and principles suffers from damaging counterexamples whose force depends on our reservoir of considered judgments. (Unlike Ross, we assign no form of priority weighing or hierarchical ranking to our principles.)

By contrast, we treat principles as both prima facie binding and subject to revision. So understood, a prima facie principle is a normative guideline stating conditions of the permissibility, obligatoriness, rightness, or wrongness of actions that fall within the scope of the principle. The latitude to balance principles in cases of conflict leaves room for compromise, mediation, and negotiation. The account is thereby rescued from the charge that principles cannot be compromised and so become tyrannical. In stubborn cases of conflict there may be no single right action, because two or more morally acceptable actions are unavoidably in conflict and yet have equal weight in the circumstances. Here we can give good but not decisive reasons for more than one action.

For instance, although murder is absolutely prohibited because of the normative content in the word *murder,* it is not plausible to hold that killing is absolutely prohibited. Killing persons is *prima facie* wrong, but killing to prevent a person's further extreme pain or suffering is not wrong in every circumstance. Killing may be the only way to meet some obligations, even though it is prima facie wrong. However, when a prima facie obligation is outweighed or overridden, it does not simply disappear or evaporate. It leaves what Nozick calls "moral traces," which should be reflected in the agent's attitudes and actions.

A disadvantage of this account, some say, is that it moves relentlessly to the paradoxical conclusion that, as Hume put it, "the principles upon which men reason in morals are always the same; though the conclusions which they draw are often very different." True, a relativity of judgment is inevitable, but a relativity of the principles embedded in the common morality is not. When people reach different conclusions, their moral judgments are still subject to justification by good reasons. They are not purely arbitrary or subjective judgments. A judgment can be proposed for consideration on any basis a person chooses—random selection, emotional reaction, mystical intuition, etc.—but to propose is not to justify, and one part of justification is to test judgments and norms by their coherence with the other norms in the moral life.

We conclude that although flexibility and diversity in judgment are inelimi-nable, judgment generally should be constrained by the demands of moral justification, which typically involves appeal to principles. Our presentation of principles—together with arguments to show the coherence of these principles with other aspects of the moral life, such as the moral emotions, virtues, and rights [will] *constitutes* [our] theory. This web of norms and arguments *is* the theory. There is no single unifying principle or concept, no description of the highest good, and the like.

A Critique of Principlism

K. Danner Clouser and Bernard Gert

Danner Clouser was one of the first American philosophers to join the faculty at a major medical school. He is currently professor of humanities at the Pennsylvania State University College of Medicine. Bernard Gert is professor of intellectual and moral philosophy at Dartmouth College. This essay rejects the use of principles to replace both moral theory and particular moral rules, arguing that such an approach lacks logical consistency and fails to provide a workable method of resolving practical ethical problems.

I. Introduction and Overview

Throughout the land, arising from the throngs of converts to bioethics awareness, there can be heard a mantra ". . . beneficence . . . autonomy . . . justice . . ." It is this ritual incantation in the face of biomedical dilemmas that beckons our inquiry.

In the last twenty years the field of biomedical ethics has expanded in an unprecedented way. The numbers of persons involved, its acceptance as an important field, the myriad university courses, the ubiquitous workshops and conferences, and the plethora of articles, books, and journals have exceeded all expectations. In response to this enormous demand for training in ethics, there have appeared countless books, workshops, and courses that package the theories and methods of ethics, making them readily available to more people in a shorter time.

The major strategy in the most influential of these responses is the deployment of "principles" of biomedical ethics. Conceptually, as diagrammed for example by Beauchamp and Childress (1983), the principles are located just below theories and just above rules. The general notion is that principles follow from moral theories and, in turn, generate particular rules that are then used to make moral judgments. Brandishing these several principles, adherents to the "principle approach" go forth to confront the quandaries of biomedical ethics.

We believe that the "principles of biomedical ethics" approach (hereinafter referred to as "principlism") is mistaken and misleading. Principlism is mistaken about the nature of morality and is misleading as to the foundations of ethics. It misconceives both theory and practice. By no means do we wish to impugn

K. Dan Clouser and Bernard Gert. "A Critique of Principlism." Abridged from *The Journal of Medicine and Philosophy*, Volume 15,1990, pp. 219–236. Reprinted by permission of Kluwer Academic Publishers.

the many significant moral insights of the proponents of principlism. Our quarrel is not so much with the content of the various "principles" as it is with the use of "principles" at all. We consider this to be crucial and not just a matter of philosophical style. Our focus is on [one] philosophical point: the conceptual or systematic status of "principles" as used in principlism.

Our bottom line, starkly put, is that "principle," as conceived by the proponents of principlism, is a misnomer and that "principles" so conceived cannot function as they are in fact claimed to be functioning by those who purport to employ them. At best, "principles" operate primarily as checklists naming issues worth remembering when considering a biomedical moral issue. At worst "principles" obscure and confuse moral reasoning by their failure to be guidelines and by their eclectic and unsystematic use of moral theory. . . .

A. Our General Claim

Our general contention is that the so-called "principles" function neither as adequate surrogates for moral theories nor as directives or guides for determining the morally correct action. Rather they are primarily chapter headings for a discussion of some concepts which are often only superficially related to each other. When, for example, we are told that a particular case calls for the application of the principle of beneficence, this can mean that the case involves either (1) the utilitarian ideal of promoting some good, or (2) the moral ideal of preventing some harm or removing some harm, or (3) some duty which is morally required. This use of "principles" bears no similarity to principles that "summarize" theories, e.g., as used by Rawls and Mill. Rawls's principle of justice and Mill's principle of utility or principle of liberty are directives toward a moral resolution of particular cases. The principles of Rawls and Mill are effective summaries of their theories; they are shorthand for the theories that generated them. However, this is not the case with principlism, because principlism often has two, three, or even four competing "principles" involved in a given case, for example, principles of autonomy, justice, beneficence, and nonmaleficence. This is tantamount to using two, three, or four conflicting moral theories to decide a case. Indeed some of the "principles"—for example, the "principle" of justice—contain within themselves several competing theories. . . .

Why do we make so much of the fact that in principlism the "principles" provide no systematic guidance? After all, the proponents of principlism would simply say, "Principles are complicated directives. When we say 'apply the principle of beneficence,' we mean consider those points that we discuss in our chapter on the principle of beneficence." In other words, they would say that "the principle of beneficence" is shorthand for their discussion of beneficence. But in that case there is really nothing to be "applied." In effect the agent is being told "think about beneficence and here's thirty pages of distinctions and deliberations to get you started," and that is very different from being told, e.g., "Do that act which will create the greatest good for the greatest number." At best the agent may be reflecting on the relevance of beneficence to the current problem, but he is only deceiving himself if he believes that he has some useful guideline to apply.

There are two problems with an agent's being deceived about whether or not he has a principle that can be applied. One is that the principles are assumed to be firmly established and justified. A person feels secure in applying or in presuming to apply them. The other problem is that an agent will not be aware of the real grounds for his moral decision. If the principle is not a clear, direct imperative at all, but simply a collection of suggestions and observations, occasionally conflicting, then he will not know what is really guiding his action nor what facts to regard as relevant nor how to justify his action. The language of principlism suggests that he has applied a principle which is morally well-established and hence *prima facie* correct. But a closer look at the situation shows that in fact he has looked at and weighed many diverse moral considerations, which are superficially interrelated and herded under a chapter heading named for the "principle" in question.

The agent meanwhile may have "applied" other competing "principles" as well, e.g., autonomy and justice, to the same case. This actually amounts simply to thinking about the case from diverse and conflicting points of view. By "applying" the "principles" of autonomy, beneficence, and justice, the agent is unwittingly using several diverse and conflicting accounts rather than simply applying a well-developed unified theory. It is risky to be doing the former while believing one is doing the latter. . . .

B. Our Thesis Illustrated

It is necessary to see some real examples of principlism. . . .

. . . what is surely the most popular of all biomedical ethics textbooks [is]Beauchamp and Childress's *Principles of Biomedical Ethics* (1983). The authors enunciate four basic principles, each of which illustrates the problems that we have been delineating. Consider their principle of beneficence. For Beauchamp and Childress beneficence is a duty "to help others further their important and legitimate interests" (1983, p. 149); it is morally required (p. 148). The "principle" explicitly prescribes at least two very different kinds of action: (1) to prevent and remove harm, and (2) to confer benefits. These are both included in the general duty of beneficence. Additionally, there seem to be other subprinciples buried in the general "principle." Some are genuine duties to help, which accrue by virtue of special relationships and roles, whereas others are triggered by needs and one's ability to meet those needs, though without clear limitations on the scope of such obligations. All these are included in "*the* principle of beneficence." Clearly, this "principle" is simply a chapter heading under which many superficially related topics are discussed; it is primarily a label for a general concern with consequences. . . .

The Beauchamp and Childress "principle of justice" manifests our point even more than their other "principles." There is not even a glimmer of a usable guide to action. There is a discussion of the concept of justice and about various well-known and conflicting accounts of justice, yet there is no specific action-guide stated. Nevertheless, they refer to a principle of justice as though it is something we ought to apply to moral situations. It is clearly not a guide to action, but rather a checklist of considerations that should be kept in mind when reflecting on moral problems. Not being the kind of classical principle that summarizes a theory and yields specific action-guides, it is deceptive in purporting to have conceptual status and systematic validity. Their "principle" is neither derived from a theory nor does it provide a usable guide to action. . . .

III. Principlism: Systematic Considerations
Relativism: The Anthology Syndrome

Beauchamp and Childress accompany their account of moral reasoning with [the following] diagram:

4. *Ethical Theories*
↑
3. *Principles*
↑
2. *Rules*
↑
1. *Particular Judgments and Actions*

"According to this diagram, judgments about what ought to be done in particular situations are justified by moral rules, which in turn are justified by principles, which ultimately are justified by ethical theories" (p. 5). Admitting that their diagram "may be oversimplified," they nevertheless claim that "its design indicates that in moral reasoning we appeal to different reasons of varying degrees of abstraction and systematization" (p. 5).

The authors give no argument for this account of moral reasoning. We suspect that they give no argument because none exists to support the role of principles in the hierarchy they propose. We believe that giving principles a significant role in moral reasoning is not only mistaken, but it also has unfortunate practical and theoretical consequences.

We had earlier seen a kind of relativism embodied by their "principles." Each principle seemed to have a life and logic of its own, as well as a number of internal conflicts. This relativism seems to be endorsed by their diagram having *theories* at the top of the hierarchy rather than a single unified ethical theory. This same kind of ethical relativism is endorsed by almost all anthologies in medical ethics, as well as in all other areas of applied and professional ethics. These anthologies (as well as most courses) almost invariably start by providing brief summaries of some standard ethical theories, e.g., utilitarianism, Kantianism, and contractualism. Next, the inadequacies of each of these theories are pointed out. There is no attempt to repair or remedy these defects, nor to present readers with a theory that they can actually use in solving the problems that are presented in the main body of the book (or course). Rather, the theories are either completely ignored and each problem is dealt with on an *ad hoc* basis, or the student is told to apply whatever inadequate theory he thinks is most useful in dealing with the problem at hand. Often he is told to apply several different, inadequate theories to a given problem, using whatever part of each theory seems most appropriate. This is an extraordinary way to proceed. It is difficult to imagine any respectable discipline proceeding in a similar fashion. Having acknowledged that all of the standard theories are inadequate, one is then told to apply them anyway, and even to apply competing theories, without any attempt to show how the theories can be reconciled.

In effect, the "anthology" approach is that of principlism. The proponents of principlism claim to derive principles from several different theories, none of which they judge to be adequate, and then they urge the student or health care professional to apply one or more of these competing principles to a given case. There is no attempt to show how or even whether these different principles can be reconciled. There is no attempt to show that the different theories, from which the principles are presumably derived, can be reconciled, or that any one of the theories can be revised so as to remove its defects and inadequacies.

References

Beauchamp, T.L., and Childress, J.F.: 1983, *Principles of Biomedical Ethics*, second edition, Oxford University Press, New York.

Feminism and Moral Theory

Virginia Held

Virginia Held received her Ph.D. from Columbia University in the late 1960s and is currently on the faculty of Hunter College of the City University of New York. She argues here that women's moral experience has generally been discounted in the construction of ethical theories and principles. To remedy this omission, Held analyzes the experience of women who engage in mothering. She concludes that the practice of mothering has important perspectives to contribute to ethics; these perspectives emphasize an ethic of caring, place a premium on sensitivity to the particularity of context, and are suspicious of general, impartial rules.

The tasks of moral inquiry and moral practice are such that different moral approaches may be appropriate for different domains of human activity. I have argued in a recent book that we need a division of moral labor.[1] In *Rights and Goods*, I suggest that we ought to try to develop moral inquiries that will be as satisfactory as possible for the actual contexts in which we live and in which our experience is located. Such a division of moral labor can be expected to yield different moral theories for different contexts of human activity, at least for the foreseeable future. In my view, the moral approaches most suitable for the courtroom are not those most suitable for political bargaining; the moral approaches suitable for economic activity are not those suitable for relations within the family, and so on. The task of achieving a unified moral field theory covering all domains is one we may do well to postpone, while we do our best to devise and to "test" various moral theories in actual contexts and in light of our actual moral experience.

What are the implications of such a view for women? Traditionally, the experience of women has been located to a large extent in the context of the family. In recent centuries, the family has been thought of as a "private" domain distinct not only from that of the "public" domain of the polis, but also from the domain of production and of the marketplace. Women (and men) certainly need to develop moral inquiries appropriate to the context of mothering and of family relations, rather than accepting the application to this context of theories developed for the marketplace or the polis. We can certainly show that the moral guidelines appropriate to mothering are different from those that

---

Virginia Held. "Feminism and Moral Theory." Abridged from *Women and Moral Theory*, 1987, pp. 112–127. Reprinted by permission of Rowman and Littlefield.

152

now seem suitable for various other domains of activity as presently constituted. But we need to do more as well: we need to consider whether distinctively feminist moral theories, suitable for the contexts in which the experience of women has or will continue to be located, are better moral theories than those already available, and better for other domains as well.

The Experience of Women

We need a theory about how to count the experience of women. It is not obvious that it should count equally in the construction or validation of moral theory. To merely survey the moral views of women will not necessarily lead to better moral theories. In the Greek thought that developed into the Western philosophical tradition,[2] reason was associated with the public domain from which women were largely excluded. If the development of adequate moral theory is best based on experience in the public domain, the experience of women so far is less relevant. But that the public domain is the appropriate locus for the development of moral theory is among the tacit assumptions of existing moral theory being effectively challenged by feminist scholars. We cannot escape the need for theory in confronting these issues.

We need to take a stand on what moral experience is. As I see it, moral experience is "the experience of consciously choosing, of voluntarily accepting or rejecting, of willingly approving or disapproving, of living with these choices, and above all of acting and of living with these actions and their outcomes. . . . Action is as much a part of experience as is perception."[3] Then we need to take a stand on whether the moral experience of women is as valid a source or test of moral theory as is the experience of men, or on whether it is more valid.

Certainly, engaging in the process of moral inquiry is as open to women as it is to men, although the domains in which the process has occurred has been open to men and women in different ways. Women have had fewer occasions to experience for themselves the moral problems of governing, leading, exercising power over others (except children), and engaging in physically violent conflict. Men, on the other hand, have had fewer occasions to experience the moral problems of family life and the relations between adults and children. Although vast amounts of moral experience are open to all human beings who make the effort to become conscientious moral inquirers, the contexts in which experience is obtained may make a difference. It is essential that we avoid taking a given moral theory, such as a Kantian one, and deciding that those who fail to develop toward it are deficient, for this procedure imposes a theory on experience, rather than letting experience determine the fate of theories, moral and otherwise.

We can assert that as long as women and men experience different problems, moral theory ought to reflect the experience of women as fully as it reflects the experience of men. The insights and judgments and decisions of women as they engage in the process of moral inquiry should be presumed to be as valid as those of men. In the development of moral theory, men ought to have no privileged position to have their experience count for more. If anything, their privileged position in society should make their experience more suspect rather than more worthy of being counted, for they have good reasons to rationalize their privileged positions by moral arguments that will obscure or purport to justify these privileges.[4] . . .

Mothering and Markets

When we bring women's experience fully into the domain of moral consciousness, we can see how questionable it is to imagine contractual relationships as central or fundamental to society and morality. . . .

The most central and fundamental social relationship seems to be that between mother or mothering person and child. It is this relationship that creates and recreates society. It is the activity of mothering which transforms biological entities into human social beings. Mothers and mothering persons produce children and empower them with language and symbolic representations. Mothers and mothering persons thus produce and create human culture.

Despite its implausibility, the assumption is often made that human mothering is like the mothering of other animals rather than being distinctively human. In accordance with the traditional distinction between the family and the polis, and the assumption that what occurs in the public sphere of the polis is distinctively human, it is assumed that what human mothers do within the family belongs to the "natural" rather than to the "distinctively human" domain. Or, if it is recognized that the activities of human mothers do not resemble the activities of the mothers of other mammals, it is assumed that, at least, the difference is far narrower than the difference between what animals do and what humans who take part in government and industry and art do. But, in fact, mothering is among the most human of human activities.

Consider the reality. A human birth is thoroughly different from the birth of other animals, because a human mother can choose not to give birth. However extreme the alternative, even when abortion is not a possibility, a woman can choose suicide early enough in her pregnancy to consciously prevent the birth. A human mother comprehends that she brings about the birth of another human being. A human mother is then responsible, at least in an existentialist sense, for the creation of a new human life. The event is essentially different from what is possible for other animals.

Human mothering is utterly different from the mothering of animals without language. The human mother or nurturing person constructs with and for the child a human social reality. The child's understanding of language and of symbols, and of all that they create and make real, occurs in interactions between child and caretakers. Nothing seems more distinctively human than this. In comparison, government can be thought to resemble the governing of ant colonies, industrial production to be similar to the building of beaver dams, a market exchange to be like the relation between a large fish that protects and a small fish that grooms, and the conquest by force of arms that characterizes so much of human history to be like the aggression of packs of animals. But the imparting of language and the creation within and for each individual of a human social reality, and often a new human social reality, seems utterly human.

An argument is often made that art and industry and government create new human reality, while mothering merely "reproduces" human beings, their cultures, and social structures. But consider a more accurate view: in bringing up children, those who mother create new human *persons*. They change persons, the culture, and the social structures that depend on them, by creating the kinds of persons who can continue to transform themselves and their surroundings. Creating new and better persons is surely as "creative" as creating new and better objects or institutions. It is not only bodies that do not spring into being unaided and fully formed; neither do imaginations, personalities, and minds.

Perhaps morality should make room first for the human experience reflected in the social bond between mothering person and child, and for the human projects of nurturing and of growth apparent for both persons in the relationship. In comparison, the transactions of the marketplace seem peripheral; the authority of weapons and the laws they uphold, beside the point. . . .

Between the Self and the Universal

Perhaps the most important legacy of the new insights will be the recognition that more attention must be paid to the domain *between* the self—the ego, the self-interested individual—on the one hand, and the universal—everyone, others in general—on the other hand. . . .

. . . Moral theory has neglected the intermediate region of family relations and relations of friendship, and has neglected the sympathy and concern people actually feel for particular others. . . .

Standard moral philosophy has construed personal relationships as aspects of the self-interested feelings of individuals, as when a person might favor those he loves over those distant because it satisfies his own desires to do so. Or it has let those close others stand in for the universal "other," as when an analysis might be offered of how the conflict between self and others is to be resolved in something like "enlightened self-interest" or "acting out of respect for the moral law," and seeing this as what should guide us in our relations with those close, particular others with whom we interact. . . .

. . . What feminist moral theory will emphasize, in contrast, will be the domain of particular others in relations with one another. . . .

Moral theories must pay attention to the neglected realm of particular others in actual contexts. In doing so, problems of egoism vs. the universal moral point of view appear very different, and may recede to the region of background insolubility or relative unimportance. The important problems may then be seen to be how we ought to guide or maintain or reshape the relationships, both close and more distant, that we have or might have with actual human beings.

Particular others can, I think, be actual starving children in Africa with whom one feels empathy or even the anticipated children of future generations, not just those we are close to in any traditional context of family, neighbors, or friends. But particular others are still not "all rational beings" or "the greatest number.". . .

In recognizing the component of feeling and relatedness between self and particular others, motivation is addressed as an inherent part of moral inquiry. Caring between parent and child is a good example.[5] . . . When the relationship between "mother" and child is as it should be, the caretaker does not care for the child (nor the child for the caretaker) because of universal moral rules. The love and concern one feels for the child already motivate much of what one does. This is not to say that morality is irrelevant. One must still decide what one ought to do. But the process of addressing the moral questions in mothering and of trying to arrive at answers one can find acceptable involves motivated acting, not just thinking. . . .

Principles and Particulars

When we take the context of mothering as central, rather than peripheral, for moral theory, we run the risk of excessively discounting other contexts. It is a commendable risk, given the enormously more prevalent one of excessively discounting mothering. But I think that the attack on principles has sometimes been carried too far by critics of traditional moral theory. . . .

We should not forget that an absence of principles can be an invitation to capriciousness. Caring may be a weak defense against arbitrary decisions, and the person cared for may find the relation more satisfactory if both persons, but especially the person caring, are guided, to some extent, by principles concerning obligations and rights. To argue that no two cases are ever alike is to invite moral chaos. Furthermore, for one person to be in a position of caretaker means that that person has the power to withhold care, to leave the other without it. The person cared for is usually in a position of vulnerability. The moral significance of this needs to be addressed along with other aspects of the caring relationship. Principles may remind a giver of care to avoid being capricious or domineering. While most of the moral problems involved in mothering contexts may deal with issues above and beyond the moral minimums that can be covered by principles concerning rights and obligations, that does not mean that these minimums can be dispensed with. . . .

That aspect of the attack on principles which seems entirely correct is the view that not all ethical problems can be solved by appeal to one or a very few simple principles. It is often argued that all more particular moral rules or principles can be derived from such underlying ones as the Categorical Imperative or the Principle of Utility, and that these can be applied to all moral problems. The call for an ethic of care may be a call, which I share, for a more pluralistic view of ethics, recognizing that we need a division of moral labor employing different moral approaches for different domains, at least for the time being.[6] Satisfactory intermediate principles for areas such as those of international affairs, or family relations, cannot be derived from simple universal principles, but must be arrived at in conjunction with experience within the domains in question.

Attention to particular others will always require that we respect the particularity of the context, and arrive at solutions to moral problems that will not give moral principles more weight than their due. But their due may remain considerable. And we will need principles concerning relationships, not only concerning the actions of individuals, as we will need evaluations of kinds of relationships, not only of the character traits of individuals.

Notes

1. See Virginia Held, *Rights and Goods: Justifying Social Action* (New York: Free Press, Macmillan, 1984).
2. See Genevieve Lloyd, *The Man of Reason: "Male" and "Female" in Western Philosophy* (Minneapolis: University of Minnesota Press, 1984).
3. Virginia Held, *Rights and Goods*, p. 272. See also V. Held, "The Political 'Testing' of Moral Theories," *Midwest Studies in Philosophy* 7 (1982):343–63.
4. For discussion, see especially Nancy Hartsock, *Money, Sex, and Power* (New York: Longman, 1983), chaps. 10, 11.
5. See, e.g., Nell Noddings, *Caring: A Feminine Approach to Ethics and Moral Education* (Berkeley: University of California Press, 1984) pp. 91–94.
6. Participants in the conference on Women and Moral Theory offered the helpful term "domain relativism" for the version of this view that I defended.

Questions for Discussion
Part II, Section 1

1. Do you think that ethical reasoning can be reduced to a single fundamental principle, such as Singer's principle of equal consideration of interests or the categorical imperative?

2. According to Feldman's interpretation of Kantian ethics, why is it logically inconsistent for a person to will to perform an ethically impermissible action?

3. In what sense, if any, are the four principles of biomedical ethics that Beauchamp and Childress describe "derived" from utilitarian or Kantian ethics?

4. If Clouser's and Gert's objections to principlism are sound, what alternative methods of ethical reasoning remain?

5. Does Held's description of women's experience capture accurately the variety of women's lives?

6. Do utilitarian and Kantian ethics discount the moral experience of women, as Held charges?

INDUCTIVE METHODS

CASUISTRY AND NARRATIVE ETHICS

ॐ

Casuistry and Clinical Ethics

Albert R. Jonsen

Albert Jonsen received his training in religious studies at Yale during the late 1960s. He currently serves as chair of the Department of Medical History and Ethics at the University of Washington School of Medicine. The essay that appears here reviews the method of casuistry and defends its use for contemporary bioethics.

The remoteness of academic ethics from moral problems was dramatically revealed in the 1960s. The war in Southeast Asia and the civil rights activities, which had fired the nation, excited college students. Moral philosophy courses and their teachers were expected to speak to these issues. Yet the finest elaboration of rule utilitarianism or ideal observer theory seemed weak instruments when brought to bear on anxious questions about civil disobedience and draft avoidance. I was a graduate student in ethics during these years; we were struggling to make our ethical theories match the reality of moral perplexities. Our professors were questioning the "relevance" of their theories. They began to write, at first hesitantly then with greater assurance, about conscientious objection and divestment in South African firms. They began to look at cases as seriously as they had looked at theories.

At about the same time, the interest in medical ethics was stimulated by the advent of cardiac transplantation and the rationing of renal dialysis. These interests brought the ethicists closer to the case than had any other issue. As they read about medical care and talked with physicians, they realized that the

Albert Jonsen. "Casuistry and Clinical Ethics." Abridged from *Theoretical Medicine*, Volume 7, 1986, pp. 65–74. Reprinted by permission of Kluwer Academic Publishers.

"case" was the unit of health care and the unwaning center of attention of its providers. They learned that cases were filled with details, obscured by many unknowns, described differently by different observers. They came to recognize stable elements about which generalizations could be competently made and idiosyncratic features that were irreducibly singular. Agents A and B were now this young Dr. Smith and that elderly, very sick Mrs. Jones. Act M became "turning off the respirator," or was it "allowing to die" or was it "killing"?. . .

Those ethicists who did venture into the hospital discovered quickly that their philosophical skills, while certainly useful, needed supplementation. They needed to learn the added skill of *interpreting the case*. Many of these ethicists devised their own approaches to the cases, their methods, systems, paradigms and matrices. Common to all these was the need to comprehend the complexity of detail and the variety of values and principles that seemed embedded in the case. These ethicists often described their work as "helping to clarify thinking" about these difficult cases. But unquestionably, their "clarification" was far different than the programs of clarification proposed by the modern moral philosophers. One of the most distinguished of these, R. M. Hare, has recently expressed this in his book *Moral Thinking*. It is in the modern tradition, concerned with helping us think more clearly about moral issues, but, unlike the preponderant tradition, Hare affirms "we can get a long way by logic alone but, in the selection of principles for use in this world of ours, facts about the world and the people in it are relevant" ([3] p. 5).

A case is filled with facts about the world and the people in it. Ethicists' methods must find a way to take them into account, to think about principles in their presence and to draw conclusions that seem to fit them. This sort of ethicist then becomes a casuist *malgre lui*. Without knowing much about casuistry and casuists, they act as did those shadowy forebearers who counseled kings and conquistadors, bankers and bishops.

The Casuistical Method

What was the casuistical method? Strangely enough, it is difficult to discover. Although they produced a vast literature (600 works, many in multiple editions between 1550 and 1650), casuists rarely exposed their method in explicit terms. Indeed, they may not have thought much about method, as we understand the idea. Yet, several features of their style emerge after much reading of their dusty tomes.

The first feature is surprising: they did not apply principles to cases in any carefully deductive or inferential fashion. True, they universally acknowledged a doctrine of "natural law," but that doctrine, although elaborated in considerable intricacy by the theologians of the era, remained at a high level of abstraction and served more as a source of maxims than a system of premises. . . .

The "system" they were familiar with was not a philosophical structure of linked ideas as in the Cartesian or better, Spinozan fashion—an *ethica modo geometrica demonstrata*—but the system of the ancient discipline of rhetoric. It is hardly known today that rhetoric and moral philosophy were closely associated in the ancient and medieval education. Aristotle's *Rhetoric* (hardly opened by modern philosophers) begins with a synopsis of his *Nicomachean Ethics*, then goes on to set out the sorts of reasoning appropriate to recommendations about "acts to be pursued or avoided, with justification or condemnation of actions performed" [1]. The forms of reasoning, namely examples, the enthymene, maxims, and commonplaces are, for Aristotle, the probabilistic counterparts of formal reasoning based on induction and deductions. Examples are real or fictitious presentations of cases; the enthymeme is a syllogism starting from a general proposition true only for the most part; maxims are familiar, widely accepted, but inconclusive statements about the moral life, such as "know thyself" or "nothing in excess." Certain basic and common understandings about the world and about people give structure to certain forms of argument which the rhetoricans called "topics" or "commonplace." In the most general form, these might be cause and effect, before and after, possible and impossible, greater or less. Cicero, also writing about rhetoric, adds to the Aristotelian framework the element of the particular occasion or the circumstances of the case. These elements came to be summarized as "Who did what? Where? Why? In what manner? With what help?" [2]

These rhetorical categories informed the minds of the casuists. The categories, more than the categories of formal logic, were used to formulate a case and devise a recommendation about "acts to be pursued or avoided, justification or condemnation of acts performed." The broad concepts of moral philosophy, whether Aristotle's virtues, Plato's ideals, Augustine's charity or Aquinas' natural law were an inexhaustible source of examples and maxims. Casuists were not adherents of one or another master or school. All the ancients provided wisdom about the mystery of life. Also, the Church Law, Roman Law and Jurisprudence were dipped into when convenient. . . .

The "new" casuistry must be more than talking about cases. It must be an articulated art, that is, it must be able to discuss the singular and unique in terms that can be generally understood and appreciated. It must have the quality of moral discourse, that is, its judgments about particulars must reflect the features of universality and prescriptivity now commonly appreciated as essential to moral thought [3]. . . .

Modern casuists may avail themselves of certain features of classical casuistry, even without delving into the actual history of that arcane endeavor. . . . However, the features that can be profitably copied are first, reliance on paradigm cases, second, reference to broad consensus, and, finally, acceptance of "probable certitude."

The casuists' thinking moved from the clear and obvious cases toward the more problematic ones. They had a base, the manifest relevance of a strong principle to a certain case, and moved away from that base by the moral judgments, but the questions do not, in themselves, rule out the prudent assertion of "probable certitudes."

Ethicists associated with the provision of medical care can be casuists in ways that their counterparts in other fields do not enjoy. They daily meet cases in urgent need of practical resolution. They are aware that elegant theory and critical questions do not lead to answers for demanding clinical problems. They have at hand a series of paradigm cases which they understand and which can be readily communicated to their listeners. They have an ample body of carefully assessed opinions about these cases that reveal both areas of consensus and points of disagreement. They can assure their hearers, on the grounds of the paradigms, of considered opinions and of reasoning by analogy, that this or that resolution lies within the realm of "probable certitude" [4]. In this way, the spirits of the antique casuists inhabit the corridors of modern hospitals.

References

[1] Aristotle: 1941, *The Rhetoric*, R. McKeon (trans.), Random House, New York.
[2] Cicero: 1949, *De Inventione*, H. M. Hubbell (trans.), Harvard University Press, Cambridge, I, 33–44.
[3] Hare, R. M.: 1981, *Moral Thinking: Its Levels, Method and Point*, Clarendon Press, Oxford, p. 5.
[4] Jonsen, A. R., Siegler, M., Winslade, W.: 1982, *Clinical Ethics*, Macmillan Publishing Co., New York.

From *Doctors' Stories*

Kathryn M. Hunter

Kathryn M. Hunter is on the faculty of Northwestern University School of Medicine and serves as Co-Director of Northwestern's Ethics and Human Value Program. The essay below, excerpted from her 1991 book, *Doctors' Stories*, explores how narrative shapes clinical judgment. Hunter defends a case-based empirical way of making ethical decisions which requires health professionals to become familiar with patients' stories.

Early in his illness, Tolstoy's Ivan Ilych recognizes in his physician the "new method" he has perfected for himself as an examining magistrate. In that office he "acquired a method of eliminating all considerations irrelevant to the legal aspect of the case, and reducing even the most complicated case to a form in which it would be presented on paper only in its externals, completely excluding his personal opinion of the matter, while above all observing every prescribed formality." Now, with his physician, there is

> the sounding and listening, and the questions which called for answers that were foregone conclusions and were evidently unnecessary, and the look of importance which implied that "if only you put yourself in our hands we will arrange everything—we know indubitably how it has to be done, always in the same way for everybody alike." It was all just as it was in the law courts. The doctor put on just the same air towards him as he himself put on towards an accused person.[1]

Although impartiality and restraint in the new bureaucratic administration of power are preferable to bribe-taking and favoritism, we are meant to see the deficits of the "new method" for Ivan Ilych—first as a person who practices it and then, once he is ill, as the victim of such cool professionalism in its medical form. Patients need more than diagnoses, and to supply their need physicians must have richer case narratives than the traditional medical case history.

Narrative shapes clinical judgment. In medical practice, the vast body of knowledge about human biology is applied to the patient analogically through narratives of the experience of comparable instances. The capacity to provide good medical care depends upon both the physician's stock of clinical stories and an understanding of how they are (or are not) relevant to this particular case. Maxims and rules are absorbed during clinical training, just as the principles

Kathryn M. Hunter. Abridged from *Doctors' Stories*. 1991, pp. 148–160. Reprinted by permission of Princeton University Press.

of the biomedical sciences are memorized in the first two years of medical school. But despite the increased specificity of practice-based maxims, their applicability is still often uncertain. As in other case-based inquiry—law, moral theology, criminal detection—judgment in medicine is shaped (and the relativism of the individual interpretation of principle controlled) by comparing the narrated circumstances of the present case with others of more or less the same kind.

The prevalence of narrative in medicine suggests that this case-based, experiential way of knowing is well accepted in clinical practice, even if its implications are seldom acknowledged. Ethical decisions are made in much the same case-based way, and as a consequence, philosophers fresh from the classroom in the early days of the bioethics movement were frustrated at what seemed to be physicians' ignorance or unconsciousness of the overarching principles that guided their ethical decision making. They soon learned the strength of case-based deliberations. Not surprisingly, the recent defense of the philosophical position of casuistry has been undertaken by philosophers working in medicine and influenced by the methods used in the work of their clinical colleagues.[2] Medicine, as Leon Kass has observed, is a fertile ground for understanding "the moral relation between knowledge or expertise and the concerns of life."[3]

The construction of the case history is an integral part of medical thinking, essential to clinical education and to making decisions about the care of an individual patient. But good decisions about patient care beyond the diagnosis call for a richer narrative than the traditional medical case. In an era dominated by chronic disease, a physician's narrative stock should include not only clinical cases, which traditional medical education provides, but also a practical knowledge of human character and life patterns for both the well and the ill. In addition to an encyclopedic, Sherlock Holmesian knowledge of pathological cases, physicians need a literary sense of the lives in which illness and medical care take place. In the past twenty-five years medical thinkers have sought to broaden the practitioner's understanding of the individual case. Whether by increasing the number and kind of "facts" regarded as relevant to the grasp of a case, by organizing what is observed into a more coherent chronicle, or by attending to narrative shape and subtleties of representation, these critics have expanded and enriched the concept of the "case" itself. Taken together, they are working toward reshaping the medical narrative. Their arguments have met with only mixed success at a time when medical practice has been altered by technology and economic constraints. Yet these pressures only make more necessary a richer sense of patients and their life choices. Physicians feel strongly the danger of becoming mere technicians. Whether they treat patients in brief, almost anonymous encounters or take care of the chronically ill, intellectual and moral support for patient care can be found in the "color and life" of enriched case narrative. A larger sense of the patient's story enlivens the everyday practice of medicine and improves the quality of attention given to the person who is ill.

The Shield of Achilles

In the midst of the *Iliad* Homer interrupts the progress of the war to describe the making of a new shield for Achilles. It is a narrative digression that (among other things) is itself about narrative art. Because the besieged Trojans have driven the Greeks back to their ships, Achilles has allowed his friend Patroclus to go into battle disguised in the armor Achilles inherited from his father. Patroclus has been slain by Hector and his body and the armor have been taken captive. Grief-stricken and enraged, Achilles is ready at last to return to battle, and his mother, the nymph Thetis, persuades Hephaistos, "smith of the strong arms," to forge new armor for her son. At this turning point in the war Homer gives us a long digressive account of the wonders of the god's creation. The shield is marvelous. Homer describes it as "fivefold," five layers thick, but it is easy to imagine that the phrase might mean five layers folded like pages, for the whole world is represented there. First is the physical universe:

> earth, heaven, and sea,
> unwearied sun, moon waxing, all the stars
> that heaven bears for garland.
> (XVIII, 557–560, trans. Robert Fitzgerald)

Next are two cities, one at peace, celebrating weddings and adjudicating a blood quarrel; the other at war, besieged like Troy, refusing a treaty, attempting an ambush, breaking into open battle. As Homer describes them, these are not still scenes but moving pictures, full of action. They are eventful slices of narratable life. Only with difficulty can we anchor such descriptions to static representation on the surface of a shield, and as readers immersed in the narrative we do not try. It seems right that this visual representation convey action over time; it is, after all, a god's handiwork.

Cosmology and politics are not the shield's only themes nor, evidently, has Hephaistos begun to fill the available space. He adds a field being plowed, the gathering of a king's wheat, and the preparation by the people of a celebratory feast. Elsewhere, an irrigated vineyard is harvested by singing children; cattle in a pasture are surprised by a pair of lions; shepherds not far away tend their sheep in a quiet valley. Last, there is a dancing floor where young men and women link arms, moving effortlessly in a circle, and all around the shield's rim runs the circle of the mighty ocean stream.

Here in the midst of the *Iliad*'s account of bravery, death, and loss we find a full, richly detailed representation of human life, and, moreover, it is a part of what we might have expected to be a simple piece of military equipment. The digression's unexpected length and its intrusion on the principal action of the epic suggest the importance of the shield and its art. Despite Achille's renown and his connection with the gods, the scenes represent small, ordinary events. They are the life out of which the story of the *Iliad* arises. Their representation of the whole of human experience places war and the epic poem itself in a larger context of human activity, and we are led to feel that this representation is a part of the protection offered to the hero returning to battle.

The shield is an epitome of narrative and its representation of human life. Works of art generally give us intellectual pleasure by representing to us the things that are not. These are not lies, of course, but fiction: true accounts of the way things would be, if only we had experienced them in just this way. In the ninth year of the Trojan War, Hephaistos paints enameled pictures of a besieged, chaotic city and a peaceful, orderly one. We recognize Troy in the one and are reminded, perhaps reassured, that, outside the *Iliad*, the other still exists. Beyond is the countryside at peace where life is marked by (and stories are part of) the regular events of the seasons—plowing, harvest, festival. There nature and art provide all that is narratable: lions rampage; one boy among the happy grape harvesters sings "a summer dirge"; two tumblers handspring across the circle of the "magical" dance.

The representative wholeness of Hephaistos's creation, which might be a metaphor for all art for all of us, seems to have a special relevance for physicians. Literature in particular constitutes a source of knowledge. For those to whom the experiences are familiar, narrative is confirming; for those reading about something new, the view of human possibility is enlarged. This is especially useful for physicians and for medical students. Their education often proceeds as if the practice of medicine were only a science and not also a social enterprise subject to cultural and emotional variants. Illness is assumed to be an inhuman evil, death is wrong, and medicine's task is simply described: to restore the sick to health, preventing or at least forestalling death. There are few sick people and no physicians at all in medical textbooks and none of the human experience that gives illness and the practice of medicine their meaning. "Cure sometimes, relieve often, comfort always." Only the old maxim, more often read than heard these days, exists as a reminder of medicine's role in the face of the entropic reality of human life.

Literature and Medicine

Where does medicine look for an understanding of its activities and its values? What is the source of its ideas about its place in the sum of human activity? In its confidence in its knowledge and the significance of that knowledge, the medical profession emulates early twentieth-century positivist physical scientists rather than the social scientists and the humanists whose work physicians' work more nearly resembles. The human sciences, by contrast, have begun to study themselves obsessively. Anthropology and sociology puzzle over how other human beings can be reliably understood, and historians are absorbed by the impossibility of separating the event from its telling. Social science generally has been gripped by debate over its suspension, like quantum mechanics, between the knower and what is known. Literary scholars approach their texts armed with theories of reading, writing, and knowing, and philosophers debate not only the foundations of knowledge but their very possibility. Medicine, however, has remained turned resolutely outward toward the "real world."

Medicine cannot of itself address questions of its meaning or the meaning of illness. This is not a part of its province as it is currently conceived, but is rather the province of religion, the humanities, and the values-oriented social sciences. Philosophers, historians, and sociologists have studied medicine as they have studied science, and these studies include valuable descriptions of what medicine is and does. Although many literary critics find inadequate the view that literature provides an unmediated record of social reality, it is nevertheless a vivid means of understanding the physician's often quite lonely job, the hard work of nursing the desperately ill, the patient's experience of illness, the process of dying. Fiction, poetry, and drama all offer medicine their visions of human experience. Within its representation of the full range of human possibility, we may see how doctoring, being sick, and learning to heal fit into the whole.

Literature and medicine are distinguished from most other studies of humankind by the particular account they give of individual experience. Just as literary criticism can be abstract, so can medical knowledge, especially in its textbook form; but as medicine, it has meaning only in its applicability to the individual case. The medical case history, like literary narrative, can be about only one set of circumstances at a time. Medicine has its origin—in several senses—in the patient's presentation to medical attention, and it has its end—also in more than one sense—in the treatment of that sick person. Like literature, the medical case history embodies the attention medicine accords the individual. The case history concerns instances that at once test our generalizations about human beings and embody the aggregate of human experience.

Reading about Patients

This particularization of widespread experience is easily seen in contemporary stories about illness. In recent years, the patient's story of "my operation" has gathered force in a flood of books and articles. There are a few traditional plays and stories in which illness plays an essential part—the Book of Job, Sophocles's *Philoctetes* come to mind. But only recently, as we have begun to live long enough to fall victim to chronic disease, have very many stories been written to examine illness as the individual experiences it. Thomas Mann's *The Magic Mountain* is in some ways the model of the genre, yet in that novel the hero is distanced from the narrator and both are distanced from the author; its story becomes a metaphor for a sick society. The contemporary narrative of illness in the United States is instead a midlife version of the growing-up novel. Hero-narrator and author are collapsed into one figure in an autobiographical (or autobiographically fictional) account of an individual's growth in circumstances not of his or her choosing.

The lack of choice compels our attention. As medicine has become central to our understanding of what it means to be human in an unreligious, technocratic time, a voracious public appetite has developed for medical narrative:

fiction, autobiography, reportage, played out in drama. These stories are about the failure of control and the threat of extinction. They enable us to think about the value society places on a human life, about the meaning of pain, the definition of the person, the limits of even an American autonomy, and our attitudes toward authority, choice, chance, and the death of the individual. Much of our public discourse, even before the AIDS epidemic, concerned disease and medical care. Fleshed out with "human interest" detail, case narrative has become the stuff of the well-publicized adventures of transplantation teams. It is a mainstay of television's daily dose of hospital crisis and intrigue. Pathographies of the seriously ill have become a subgenre of contemporary biography.[4] Issues of health-care policy are debated and necessarily have their legal manifestation not in the abstract realm of public policy but as individual cases. Names of individual people come to stand for issues—and now and then for their resolution: Dax Cowart, Karen Ann Quinlan, Baby Jane Doe, Elizabeth Bouvier, Rock Hudson, Baby M., Nancy Cruzan. Medical cases are often the germ of fiction and, especially, drama. Brian Clark's *Whose Life Is It Anyway?*,[5] which stirred public discussion of unwanted life-sustaining medical treatment, was very probably inspired by the 1975 discussion of Cowart's case by Robert White and H. Tristram Engelhardt, Jr., in the *Hastings Center Report*.[6] In 1985 Larry Kramer's *The Normal Heart*[7] and William Hoffman's *As Is*[8] gave their newly alarmed off-Broadway audiences a glimpse of the human and political costs of ignoring AIDS. We look to such accounts of illness to tell us who we are as a society. Their crises concern the exercise of individual rights, the problem of balancing conflicting interests in decision making, and the allocation of resources that our political choices have made scarce. In their imaginative exploration of the ordinary person's opportunity for self-definition and even for heroism, they depict for us a boundary condition of our humanity.

These stories and plays and autobiographies are based on what are, at other times and places, with other narrators, plain, stripped-down medical case histories. They go beyond the conventions of medical storytelling to supply plots and themes missing from medical narrative. Indeed, pathographies, especially first-person narratives of fatal illness, seem to have been written by patients precisely to supply those things that the case history rigorously excludes. Many of them are quite forthright about this motive. They write not simply to supply that lack for us as readers (although, having few other ways to think about the unthinkable, we are morbidly curious about fatal diagnoses) but primarily to repair the loss to themselves. As Eric Cassell has pointed out, suffering is quite distinct from pain and even from dying, and, although the goal of medicine is the relief of suffering, many patients suffer not from their disease but from their medical treatment.[9] Pathographies address and sometimes seek to avenge the damage done by medical care to their bodies, care that took no care of them. They tackle complex questions of human suffering and response to illness, the difficulties and hopes of the doctor-patient relationship, the acceptance or rejection of medical therapy, and the meaning of illness in the life of the person who is ill. In so doing, they bring to bear on the medical "facts" of the case

assumptions broader than rigorously scientific ones about causality and consequence in the course of human illness.

Physicians' familiarity with patients' stories may ultimately enrich their
understanding of medical cases, but pathography cannot substitute for case
narrative. However valuable pathography may be, its focus is on the patient
rather than the disease. The case, by contrast, serves an essential diagnostic
purpose, and for this purpose its narrowness makes sense. It orders the messy
and confusing details of experience and filters out clinical "irrelevancies." It
promotes medicine's focus on—indeed, its obsession with—the particular in the
care of patients, for it serves as a constant reminder that not all cases of the
same kind are actually the same. It clarifies medical intervention by preserving
the physician's awareness of the problematic relation between general laws and
a particular circumstance. It encourages a tolerance of uncertainty by providing
the means of recording and memorializing exceptions to the rule. For all these
reasons, case narrative is central to the epistemology as well as to the practice
of medicine. It is a construct of that epistemology, necessary to rational investigation in a domain where subjective experience (and subjective accounts of that
experience by another person) are the original and grounding data of clinical
care. As patient history, narrative makes possible the communication of one
human being's experience to another and underlines its status as mediated fact:
it is often the best we have to go on. As the account of a patient's course of
illness, the case narrative's representation of change through time is an essential
tool of clinical reasoning, facilitating the comparison and contrast of developing
patterns. Narrative accommodates the uncontrolled, uncontrollable variables of
the individual circumstance, making possible a clinical flexibility that dare not
ossify into inalterable rules. Scientifically it fosters a fidelity to the phenomena
and a recognition that they are the final arbiters of the explanatory power of
the principles themselves. Pedagogically, narrative encourages and improves
clinical judgment by making possible a kind of practical, clinical knowledge that
mediates biological principles and the facts of the particular clinical case.

Nevertheless, in any situation but acute emergency care—and sometimes
even there—the traditional medical case is restrictive, limiting the practice of
medicine and the care of patients to diagnosis and prescription. Just as that
narrative hones clinical judgment, so fiction and pathography enlarge the physician's awareness of the human problems that are the context of disease and injury.
Knowledge of cases sharpens the awareness of clinical possibilities; knowledge of
life stories helps cultivate attention to patients, an interest in their oddities and
their ordinariness—and a tolerance of both. Especially in primary-care practice,
this interest and attention can be vital. John Berger in his portrait of a physician,
A Fortunate Man, describes the daily rounds of a general practitioner in the
north of England. By the standards of a resident in a North American tertiary-
care hospital, the array of illness this village physician sees is grindingly "uninter-
esting."[10] Its only distinction from a general practice anywhere at all lies in the
recent decline in the region's standard of living as industry has departed. What
fascinates the physician (and thus the narrator and his readers) is the role he

plays in his patients' lives: for them he is the "requested clerk of their records."[11] It is a historical, even a literary task. He is not simply a bystander in the unfolding story of their lives. He knows the hard truths. He understands something of what goes wrong in their lives. William Carlos Williams, fascinated by his own quite ordinary patients, admitted, "my 'medicine' was the thing which gained me entrance to these secret gardens of the self."[12] But fewer physicians these days have such a practice, and, although "continuity of care" has been a medical buzzword off and on for more than two decades, few schools set out to prepare their students to understand its pleasures.

Is reading autobiography and fiction necessary to the formation of this narrative sensibility? The wisdom and sensitivity of experienced physicians may have been gathered without benefit of literature through a lifetime of careful attention to patients. But what are young practitioners to do before they have acquired a store of cases on which to found a sustaining overview of life? And what are middle-aged physicians to do when the physical consequences of bad luck and folly and human evil lead them to harden themselves to the life stories of their patients? Physicians turn to professional journals for accounts of difficult or unusual cases and new developments that offer hope of altering the plots in old stories of disease. Likewise, in fiction, autobiography, and drama they can broaden their knowledge of human beings not only beyond the textbooks in human behavior but beyond the ethnic and chronological limits of their own experience. The physician who has read Tolstoy's *The Death of Ivan Ilych*, for instance, has imagined a patient's unwilling slide toward death. He or she is also able to entertain the possibility that the horrors of illness are not entirely physical; an apparently self-possessed, successful, now terminally ill patient may lack the support of family and friends, but in some sense may have before him the discovery of an authentic life. Years of practice may provide wisdom to equal this awareness, but, unrelieved and unassessed, those years may also callous the physician who has "seen it all."

To cultivate practical wisdom in the diagnosis and treatment of patients, physicians are taught to employ a narratively mediated casuistry. The residencies are long apprenticeships that at once foster the accumulation of a large number of cases and guide the new physician in their judicious use. Most physicians, especially those who enter primary-care practice, extend this case-based reasoning beyond diagnosis and treatment to judgment about the people who are ill and how best to provide effective care. To some degree, physicians are prepared for this by attention given during their education to "case management."[13] To increase this preparation, the Association of American Medical Colleges' 1984 report on the general professional education of the physician, *Physicians for the Twenty-First Century* (the GPEP Report) calls for, among other things, more experience in ambulatory care.[14] Such exposure gives students an opportunity to begin to acquire a fuller collection of cases, one that takes into account the vagaries—economic, social, psychological—of the human beings who are ill. For effective and satisfying practice, a collection of life histories is needed. Years of experience taking care of patients may foster the clinical wisdom necessary to handle difficult cases well, but meanwhile for physicians, as for all of us, the vicarious experience offered by narrative increases familiarity with the range of human character and the life outside office and hospital to which medicine aims to restore them.

In particular, literature is a source of knowledge about the operation of values through time. Just as medical narrative is the repository of much of the professional ethos learned by students and residents, so narrative generally— biography, fiction, history—shapes moral sensibility and models clinical distance. Several recent works by physicians make this point. Robert Coles's recent book, *The Call of Stories: Teaching and the Moral Imagination*, extends the argument of his 1979 *New England Journal of Medicine* essay, "Medical Ethics and Living a Life," to argue the centrality of narrative in moral education.[15] In the earlier essay, which addresses the moral life of physicians, he distinguishes ethical reflection from its more academic cousin, ethical analysis, and recommends reading novels about doctors (*Middlemarch, Arrowsmith, Wonderland*) for their account of the peril that lies in wait for the unsuspecting and, particularly, the idealistic practitioner. In *Stories of Sickness*, Howard Brody finds an even more practical role for literature in delineating the responses to illness that govern the lives of patients.[16] With an eye to developing an ethical analysis grounded in the story of the patient's life, he surveys (among other works) *Philoctetes, The Magic Mountain, The Metamorphosis*, and *Cancer Ward* to offer physicians what he sees as the best available knowledge of the experience of illness. Arthur Kleinman samples the life stories of actual patients in *The Illness Narratives*, a framed collection of mostly autobiographical accounts of the experience of chronic disease.[17] They are ordinary, sad, sometimes frustrating, often heroic, always revealing about the role of medicine and health-care practitioners in the lives of the ill. Kleinman argues persuasively that the patient's culture is one the physician must enter carefully, ethnographically, openly.

Narrative, in medicine and out, cultivates the power of observation. No one is able to observe carefully details that are not known to exist or have dropped from memory. Narrative's clinical usefulness is most obvious in constructing the history of the patient's present illness. Into what category does this illness fall, the physician asks, and does it differ in any way from the index case of its kind? What has the patient's life been? How has it contributed to this illness? How will it help or hinder recovery? The conviction that such information is important must be acquired. It is not standard equipment that comes with a medical education. Medical students in the late-twentieth century find in Francis Peabody's 1927 essay, "The Care of the Patient," a still painfully accurate description of information overload and the neglect of the patient. But it is the actual experiences of illness in which they begin to take part that, for them, will illustrate the diagnostic and therapeutic importance of life histories and make Peabody's essay most persuasive. Familiarity with the life stories in fiction and drama fill out the range of human possibility. Many medical students, for example, have not known well a vigorous, healthy old person; outside their families few have known someone alert but steadily failing. Stereotypes abound, and narrative about the lives of the elderly—D. L. Coburn's "The Gin Game," Alice Adam's *Second Chances*—can subject them to scrutiny. William L. Morgan, Jr., has given the pages about Aunt Leonie from Proust's *Swann's Way* to his residents in internal medicine. Near ninety, she takes to her bed and from that vantage rules the family and the neighborhood. When she naps, "three streets away, a tradesman who had to hammer nails into a packing-case would send first to Françoise to make sure that my aunt was not resting."[18] "Is Aunt Leonie ill?" the residents were asked. "What should be the goals of her physician?"

A narrative view of medicine does not neglect the biomedical sciences. Instead, it adds to that scientific view a privileged humility in the care of the patient through its recognition that the larger biological story in which each human being participates moves, with or without medical attention, from birth to death. We may organize our life stories, plot them, change their course, shorten them—but their direction and the fact of their end are givens. For most of us these days disease is a small part of life—and as we move into our seventh decade, a not unexpected part. The perspective offered by this larger pattern of life-narrative can ease the expectation (held as often by physician as patient) that death can be defeated. By locating us all on the common narrative trajectory from birth to death, narrative restores the physician to the proper place in the patient's story. This larger view may offer help to the physician in thinking about and communicating prognostics: the meaning of the illness for the patient may be set by the medical meaning—the diagnosis and the customary course of treatment—but it is not confined to it. Likewise, even in chronic or fatal illnesses, the meaning of the illness is not the meaning of the patient's life. Thus hope need not always be construed as the hope of cure,[19] and therapy may be tailored to the patient's life stage and wishes.[20] Of little use is the enthusiastic athleticism that expects of every patient a no-holds-barred struggle against death or a run for the record books that is often more valuable to clinical pioneers than to their patients. Good physicians offer their patients all that is appropriate, urge them to make use of technological advances that are promising in their case, soothe fears, alleviate pain, persuade. But they do not lose sight of the lives out of which patients' choices come and into which medical therapy must intrude.

Narrative also offers physicians a way of confronting the pain of a patient's illness or loss. A physician who does not ask an elderly patient about her family because the answer may be, "There's no one; my husband died this last year," might justify the reluctance by saying that such a question will "make her sad." But such a physician has either a maimed sense of what causes sadness or a partial, perhaps rigid, sense of life patterns. The real threat is surely that the physician will feel the pain of her sadness. This is at once egocentric and much too self-deprecating: the question does not cause the sadness and may in fact do much to ease its pain. The bereaved are not all sad in the same way. Some are sad for reasons that can be addressed, some feel guilt and anger, which the physician as an arbiter of normality can render less painful. Many are stronger and healthier for having their sadness acknowledged. Physicians who read more than the bodies of their patients and are acquainted with more life stories than the ones in which they are asked to intervene are better prepared to see an individual's life as a moral trajectory and have a firmer grasp of the challenges we face at every stage of life.[21] They see more clearly the mix of pain, pleasure, and loss in most people's lives and know what, if anything, suffering may be good for. An understanding of the human condition gained from literary narrative may make it easier to meet patients' suffering with an educated innocence, an openness of observation that in itself can be some comfort to the patient. "It is difficult/to get the news from poems," William Carlos Williams wrote, "yet men die miserably every day/ for lack/ of what is found there."[22]

By enabling us to envision the whole of life into which our lives somehow must fit, literature, like Achilles' shield, offers us a little shelter from inevitable pain. Although it was forged for his protection, neither the shield nor the representation of life's wholeness emblazoned on it can save the hero from the death he is bound for or restore his friend Patroclus to life. Achilles knows it: his mother has told him that he will not long survive Hector, and it is Hector he means to kill. The gods know it: Hephaistos acknowledges the hero's mortality even as he agrees to set to work on the shield. The shield has a problematic, even paradoxical usefulness. It alters Achilles's fate not one bit. He nevertheless cannot return to battle without it. It will cover him meanwhile, enabling him to fight again, protecting him while he goes on to meet his fate.

Like Achilles, we readers retain our vulnerability. There is no protection from death or from the loss of the people whom we love—even for those of us who become physicians. In a literal sense, the work of art, like Achilles's shield, may be entirely useless. It serves no practical purpose in the world, but it is difficult, sometimes impossible, to return to battle without it. It sets its bearer's action in a context of meaning: violence and death are all around, but although inescapable, they are not all. The work of art shelters us meanwhile from injury and pain. Physicians, whose profession is not a protection from human suffering but a deliberate exposure to it, stand in need of that shield. Literature enables medical students and seasoned clinicians alike to face the onslaught of experience, bearing a knowledge of life that is both painfully particular and clear-sightedly whole. Reminded that the single individual has only a small part in the scheme of things, no matter how heroic, they may better equip themselves with a protecting, protected concern for those who seek their help. Literature's representation of life provides its readers a little space between themselves and the onslaught in which to see clearly both their own deeds and the lives of others.

Notes

1. Leo Tolstoy, "The Death of Ivan Ilych," *The Death of Ivan Ilych and Other Stories*, trans. Aylmer Maude (New York: Signet, 1960), p. 121.
2. Albert R. Jonsen and Stephen Toulmin, *The Abuses of Casuistry* (Berkeley: Univer-

sity of California Press, 1988), was preceded by Toulmin's "The Tyranny of
Principles," *Hastings Center Report* 11 (1981), 30–39, and Jonsen's "Casuistry in
Clinical Ethics," *Theoretical Medicine* 7 (1986), 65–74.

See also Warren Thomas Reich, "Caring for Life in the First of It: Moral
Paradigms for Perinatal and Neonatal Ethics," *Seminars in Perinatology* 11 (1987),
279–87, and Howard Brody, *Stories of Sickness* (New Haven: Yale University Press,
1988). All are on the faculty of a medical school; Brody is also a physician. In a
new preface to his first book, *The Place of Reason in Ethics* [1950] (Chicago:
University of Chicago Press, 1986), Stephen Toulmin describes the influences that
drew him away from analytical philosophy's way of conducting moral philosophy
toward a more historical, contextual proto-casuist method.

3. Leon Kass, *Toward a More Natural Science: Biology and Human Affairs* (New York:
   Free Press, 1985), p. 12.
4. The term "pathography" is Anne Hunsaker Hawkins's; see "Two Pathographies:
   A Study in Illness and Literature," *Journal of Medicine and Philosophy* 9 (1984),
   231–52.
5. Brian Clark, *Whose Life Is It Anyway?* (Derbyshire, Eng.: Amber Lane Press,
   1978).
6. Robert B. White and H. Tristram Engelhardt, Jr., "A Demand to Die," *Hastings
   Center Report* 5 (1975), 9–10.
7. Larry Kramer, *The Normal Heart* (New York: New American Library, 1985).
8. William M. Hoffman, *As Is* (New York: Vintage, 1985).
9. Eric J. Cassell, "The Nature of Suffering and the Goals of Medicine," *New
   England Journal of Medicine* 306 (1982), 639–45.
10. Terry Mizrahi, *Getting Rid of Patients: Contradictions in the Socialization of Physicians*
    (New Brunswick, N.J.: Rutgers University Press, 1986).
11. John Berger, *A Fortunate Man*, with photographs by Jean Mohr (New York:
    Holt, 1967), p. 103.
12. William Carlos Williams, "The Autobiography" (1951), in *The William Carlos
    Williams Reader*, ed. M. L. Rosenthal (New York: New Directions Press, 1966),
    p. 307.
13. A. C. Dornhurst argues for a pragmatic approach to medical education in
    "Information Overload: Why Medical Education Needs a Shake-up," *Lancet* 2
    [8245] (1981), 513–14.
14. Association of American Medical Colleges Project on the General Professional
    Education of the Physician, "Physicians for the Twenty-First Century," *Journal
    of Medical Education* 59 (1984), no. 11, part 2.
15. Robert Coles, *The Call of Stories: Teaching and the Moral Imagination* (Boston:
    Houghton Mifflin, 1989); "Medical Ethics and Living a Life," *New England
    Journal of Medicine* 301 (1979), 444–46.
16. Howard Brody, *Stories of Sickness* (New Haven: Yale University Press, 1988).
17. Arthur Kleinman, *The Illness Narratives: Suffering, Healing, and the Human Condi-
    tion* (New York: Basic Books, 1988).
18. Marcel Proust, *Remembrance of Things Past: Swann's Way*, trans. C. K. Scott
    Moncrief and Terence Kilmartin (New York: Vintage, 1982).
19. Howard Brody, "Hope," *Journal of the American Medical Association* 246 (1981),
    1411–12.
20. See Daniel Callahan, *Setting Limits: Medical Goals in an Aging Society* (New York:

Simon and Schuster, 1987), and Brody, "The Physician-Patient Relationship as a Narrative," in *Stories of Sickness*, pp. 171–81.

21. David Burrell and Stanley Hauerwas, "From System to Story: An Alternative Pattern for Rationality in Ethics," *Knowledge, Value and Belief*, vol. 2: *The Foundations of Ethics and Its Relationship to Science*, ed. H. Tristram Engelhardt, Jr., and Daniel Callahan (Hastings-on-Hudson, N.Y.: The Hastings Center, 1977), pp. 111–52.

22. William Carlos Williams, "Asphodel, That Greeny Flower," in *Reader*, pp. 73–74.

Getting Down to Cases
The Revival of Casuistry in Bioethics

John Arras

A philosopher by training, John Arras is on the faculty of the Division of Legal and Ethical Issues in Health Care at the Montefiore Medical Center, Albert Einstein College of Medicine, New York. This article critically evaluates the method of casuistry espoused by Al Jonsen and others. After identifying important shortcomings, Arras recommends ways of improving casuistic analysis in health care.

The Revival of Casuistry

Developed in the early Middle Ages as a method of bringing abstract and universal ethico-religious precepts to bear on particular moral situations, casuistry has had a checkered history (Jonsen and Toulmin, 1988). In the hands of expert practitioners during its salad days in the 16th and 17th centuries, casuistry generated a rich and morally sensitive literature devoted to numerous real-life ethical problems, such as truth-telling, usury, and the limits of revenge. By the late 17th century, however, casuistical reasoning had degenerated into a notoriously sordid form of logic-chopping in the service of personal expediency. To this day, the very term "casuistry" conjures up pejorative images of disingenuous argument and moral laxity.

In spite of casuistry's tarnished reputation, some philosophers have claimed that casuistry, shorn of its unfortunate excesses, has much to teach us about the resolution of moral problems in medicine. Indeed, through the work of Albert Jonsen (1980, 1986a, 1986b, 1988) and Stephen Toulmin (1981; Jonsen and Toulmin, 1988) this "new casuistry" has emerged as a definite alternative to the hegemony of the so-called "applied ethics" method of moral analysis that has dominated most bioethical scholarship and teaching since the early 1970s (Beauchamp and Childress, 1989). In stark contrast to methods that begin from "on high" with the working out of a moral theory and culminate in the deductivistic application of norms to particular factual situations, this new casuistry works from the "bottom up," emphasizing practical problem-solving by means of nuanced interpretations of individual cases.

John Arras. "Getting Down to Cases: The Revival of Casuistry in Bioethics." Abridged from the *Journal of Medicine and Philosophy*, Volume 16, 1991, pp. 29–51. Reprinted by permission of Kluwer Academic Publishers.

This paper will assess the promise of this reborn casuistry for bioethics education. . . .

Problems with the Casuistical Method

Since the new casuistry attempts to define itself by turning applied ethics on its head, working from cases to principles rather than vice-versa, it should come as no surprise to find that its strengths correlate perfectly with the weaknesses of applied ethics. Thus, whereas applied ethics, and especially deductivism, are often criticized for their remoteness from clinical realities and for their consequent irrelevance (Fox *et al.*, 1984; Noble, 1982) casuistry prides itself on its concreteness and on its ability to render useful advice to caregivers in the medical trenches. Likewise, if the applied ethics model appears rather narrow in its single-minded emphasis on the application of principles and in its corresponding neglect of moral interpretation and practical discernment, the new casuistry can be viewed as a defense of the Aristotelian virtue of *phronesis* (or sound, practical judgment).

Conversely, it should not be surprising to find certain problems with the casuistical method that correspond to strengths of the applied ethics model. I shall devote the second half of this essay to an inventory of some of these problems. It should be stressed, however, that not all of these problems are unique to casuistry, nor does applied ethics fare much better with regard to some of them.

What Is "a Case"?

For all of their emphasis upon the interpretation of particular cases, casuists have not said much, if anything, about how to select problems for moral interpretation. What, in other words, gets placed on the "moral agenda" in the first place, and why? This is a problem because it is quite possible that the current method of selecting agenda items, whatever that may be, systematically ignores genuine issues equally worthy of discussion and debate (O'Neil, 1988).

I think it safe to say that problems currently make it onto the bioethical agenda largely because health practitioners and policy makers put them there. While there is usually nothing problematic in this, and while it always pays to be scrupulously attentive to the expressed concerns of people working in the trenches, practitioners may be bound to conventional ways of thinking and of conceiving problems that tend to filter out other, equally valid experiences and problems. As feminists have recently argued, for example, much of the current bioethics agenda reflects an excessively narrow, professionally driven, and male outlook on the nature of ethics (Carse, 1989). As a result, a whole range of important ethical problems—including the unequal treatment of women in health care settings, sexist occupational roles, personal relationships, and strategies of *avoiding* crisis situations—have been either downplayed or ignored completely (Warren, 1989, pp. 77–82). It is not enough, then, for casuistry to tell us *how* to interpret cases; rather than simply carrying out the agenda dictated by health professionals, all of us (casuists and applied ethicists alike) must begin to think more about the problem of *which* cases ought to be selected for moral scrutiny.

An additional problem, which I can only flag here, concerns not the identification of "a case"—i.e., what gets placed on the public agenda—but rather the specification of "the case"—i.e., what description of a case shall count as an adequate and sufficiently complete account of the issues, the participants and the context. One of the problems with many case presentations, especially in the clinical context, is their relative neglect of alternative perspectives on the case held by other participants. Quite often, we get the attending's (or the house officer's) point of view on what constitutes "the case," while missing out on the perspectives of nurses, social workers and others. Since most cases are complicated and enriched by such alternative medical, psychological and social interpretations, our casuistical analyses will remain incomplete without them. Thus, in addition to being long, the cases that we employ should reflect the usually complementary (but often conflicting) perspectives of all the involved participants.

Is Casuistry Really Theory-Free?

The casuists claim that they make moral progress by moving from one class of cases to another without the benefit of any ethical principles or theoretical apparatus. Solutions generated for obvious or easy categories of cases adumbrate solutions for the more difficult cases. In a manner somewhat reminiscent of pre-Kuhnian philosophers of science clinging to the possibility of "theory free" factual observations, to a belief in a kind of epistemological "immaculate perception," the casuists appear to be claiming that the cases simply speak for themselves.

. . . One problem with this suggestion is that it does not acknowledge or account for the way in which different theoretical preconceptions help determine which cases and problems get selected for study in the first place. Another problem is that it does not explain what allows us to group different cases into distinct categories or to proceed from one category to another. In other words, the casuists' account of case analysis fails to supply us with principles of relevance that explain what binds the cases together and how the meaning of one case points beyond itself toward the resolution of subsequent cases. The casuists obviously cannot do without such principles of relevance; they are a necessary condition of any kind of moral taxonomy. Without principles of relevance, the cases would fly apart in all directions, rendering coherent speech, thought, and action about them impossible.

But if the casuists rise to this challenge and convert their implicit principles of relevance into explicit principles, it is certainly reasonable to expect that these will be heavily "theory laden." Take, for example, the novel suggestion that anencephalic infants should be used as organ donors for children born with fatal heart defects. What is the relevant line of cases in our developed "morisprudence" for analyzing this problem? To the proponents of this suggestion, the brain death debates provide the appropriate context of discussion. According to this line of argument, anencephalic infants most closely resemble the brain dead; and since we already harvest vital organs from the latter category, we have a moral warrant for harvesting organs from anencephalics (Harrison, 1986). But to some of those opposed to any change in the status quo, the most relevant line of cases is provided by the literature on fetal experimentation. Our treatment of the anencephalic newborn should, they claim, reflect our practices regarding nonviable fetuses. If we agree with the judgment of the National Commission that research which would shorten the already doomed child's life should not be permitted, then we should oppose the use of equally doomed anencephalic infants as heart donors (Meilaender, 1986).

How ought the casuist to triangulate the moral problem of the anencephalic newborn as organ donor? What principles of relevance will lead him to opt for one line of cases instead of another? Whatever principles he might eventually articulate, they will undoubtedly have something definite to say about such matters as the concept of death, the moral status of fetuses, the meaning and scope of respect, the nature of personhood, and the relative importance of achieving good consequences in the world versus treating other human beings as ends in themselves. Although one's position on such issues perhaps need not implicate any full-blown ethical theory in the strictest sense of the term, they are sufficiently theory-laden to cast grave doubt on the new casuists' ability to move from case to case without recourse to mediating ethical principles or other theoretical notions.

Although the early work of Jonsen and Toulmin can easily be read as advocating a theory-free methodology comprised of mere "summary principles," their recent work appears to acknowledge the point of the above criticism. Indeed, it would be fair to say that they now seek to articulate a method that is, if not "theory free," then at least "theory modest." Drawing on the approach of the classical casuists, they now concede an indisputably normative role for principles and maxims drawn from a variety of sources, including theology, common law, historical tradition, and ethical theories. Rather than viewing ethical theories as mutually exclusive, reductionistic attempts to provide an apodictic *foundation* for ethical thought, Jonsen and Toulmin now view theories as limited and complementary *perspectives* that might enrich a more pragmatic and pluralistic approach to the ethical life (1988, Chapter 15). They thus appear reconciled to the usefulness, both in research and education, of a severely chastened conception of moral principles and theories.

One lesson of all this for bioethics education is that casuistry, for all its usefulness as a method, is nothing more (and nothing less) than an "engine of thought" that must receive *direction* from values, concepts and theories outside of itself. Given the important role such "external" sources of moral direction must play even in the most case-bound approaches, teachers and students need to be self-conscious about which traditions and theories are in effect driving their casuistical interpretations. This means that they need to devote time and energy to studying and criticizing the values, concepts and rank-orderings implicitly or explicitly conveyed by the various traditions and theories from which they derive their overall direction and tools of moral analysis. In short, it means that adopting the casuistical method will not absolve teachers and students from studying and evaluating either ethical theories or the history of ethics.

Indeterminacy and Consensus

One need not believe in the existence of uniquely correct answers to all moral questions to be concerned about the casuistical method's capacity to yield determinate answers to problematical moral questions. Indeed, anyone familiar with Alastair MacIntyre's (1981) disturbing diagnosis of our contemporary moral culture might well tend to greet the casuists' announcement of moral consensus with a good deal of skepticism. According to MacIntyre, our moral culture is in a grave state of disorder: lacking any comprehensive and coherent understanding of morality and human nature, we subsist on scattered shards and remnants of past moral frameworks. It is no wonder, then, according to MacIntyre, that our moral debates and disagreements are often marked by the clash of incommensurable premises derived from disparate moral cultures. Nor is it any wonder that our debates over highly controversial issues such as abortion and affirmative action take the form of a tedious, interminable cycle of assertion and counter-assertion. In this disordered and contentious moral setting, which MacIntyre claims is *our* moral predicament, the casuists' goal of consensus based upon intuitive responses to cases might well appear to be a Panglossian dream.

One need not endorse MacIntyre's pessimistic diagnosis in its entirety to notice that many of our moral practices and policies bear a multiplicity of meanings; they often embody a variety of different, and sometimes conflicting, values. An ethical methodology based exclusively on the casuistical analysis of these practices can reasonably be expected to express these different values in the form of conflicting ethical conclusions. . . .

Conventionalism and Critique

. . . Eschewing any theoretical derivation of principles and insisting that the locus of moral certainty is the particular, the casuist asks "What principles best organize and account for what we have already decided?" Viewed from this angle, the casuistic project amounts to nothing more than an elaborate refinement of our intuitions regarding cases. As such, it begins to resemble the kind of relativistic conventionalism recently articulated by Richard Rorty (Rorty, 1989).

Obviously, one problem with this is that our intuitions have often been shown to be wildly wrong, if not downright prejudicial and superstitious. To the extent that this is true of *our own* intuitions about ethical matters, then casuistry will merely refine our prejudices. Any casuistry that modestly restricts itself to interpreting and cataloguing the flickering shadows on the cave wall can easily be accused of lacking a critical edge. If applied ethics might rightly be said to have purchased critical leverage at the expense of the concrete moral situation, then casuistry might be charged with having purchased concreteness and relevance at the expense of philosophical criticism. This charge might take either of two forms. First, one could claim that the casuist is a mere expositor of *established* social meanings and thus lacks the requisite critical distance to formulate telling critiques of regnant social understandings. Second, casuistry could be accused of ignoring the power relations that shape and inform the social meanings that its practitioners interpret. . . .

Reinforcing the Individualism of Bioethics

Analytical philosophers working as applied ethicists have often been criticized for the ahistorical, reductionist, and excessively individualistic character of their work in bioethics (Fox *et al.*, 1984; Noble, 1982; MacIntyre, 1982). While the casuistical method cannot thus be justly accused of importing a short-sighted individualism into the field of bioethics—that honor already belonging to analytical philosophy—it cannot be said either that casuistry offers anything like a promising remedy for this deficiency. On the contrary, it seems that the casuists' method of reasoning by analogy only promises to exacerbate the individualism and reductionism already characteristic of much bioethical scholarship.

Consider, for example, how a casuist might address the problem of heart transplants. He or she might reason like this: Our society is already deeply committed to paying for all kinds of "half-way technologies" for those in need. We already pay for renal dialysis and transplantation, chronic ventilatory support for children and adults, expensive open-heart surgery, and many other "high tech" therapies, some of which might well be even more expensive than heart transplants. Therefore, so long as heart transplants qualify medically as a proven therapy, there is no reason why Medicaid and Medicare should not fund them (Overcast *et al.*, 1985).

Notwithstanding the evident fruitfulness of such analogical reasoning in many contexts of bioethics, and notwithstanding the possibility that these particular examples of it might well prevail against the competing arguments on heart transplantation, it remains true that such contested practices raise troubling questions that tend not to be asked, let alone illuminated, by casuistical reasoning by analogy. The extent of our willingness to fund heart transplantation has great bearing on the kind of society in which we wish to live and on our priorities for spending within (and without) the health care budget. Even if we already fund many high technology procedures that cost as much or more than heart transplants, it is possible that this new round of transplantation could threaten other forms of care that provide greater benefits to more people; and we might therefore wish to draw the line here (Massachusetts Task Force, 1984; Annas, 1985).

The point is that, no matter where we stand on the particular issue of heart transplants, we *might* think it important to raise such "big questions," depending on the nature of the problem at hand. We might want to ask, to borrow from a recent title, "What kind of life?" (Callahan, 1990). But the kind of reasoning by analogy championed by the new casuists tends to reduce our field of ethical vision down to the proximate moral precedents, and thereby suppresses the important global questions bearing on who we are and what kind of society we want. The result is likely to be a method of moral reasoning that graciously accommodates us to any and all technological innovations, no matter what their potential long-term threat to fundamental and cherished institutions and values.

Conclusions

. . . It remains to be seen whether casuistry, as a program in practical ethics, will be able to marshall sufficient internal resources to respond to these criticisms. Whatever the outcome of that attempt, however, an equally promising approach might be to incorporate the insights and tools of casuistry into the methodological approach known as "reflective equilibrium" (Rawls, 1971; Daniels, 1979). According to this method, the casuistical interpretation of cases, on the one hand, and moral theories, principles and maxims, on the other, exist in a symbiotic relationship. Our intuitions on cases will thus be guided, and perhaps criticized, by theory; while our theories and moral principles will themselves be shaped, and perhaps reformulated, by our responses to paradigmatic moral situations. Whether we attempt to flesh out this method of reflective equilibrium or further develop the casuistical program, it should be clear by now that the methodological issue between theory and cases is not a dichotomous "either/or" but rather an encompassing "both-and."

In closing I would like to gather together my various recommendations, strewn throughout this paper, for the use of casuistry in bioethics education:

1. Use real cases rather than hypotheticals whenever possible.
2. Avoid schematic case presentations. Make them long, richly detailed, messy, and comprehensive. Make sure that the perspectives of all the major players (including nurses and social workers) are represented.
3. Present complex sequences of cases that sharpen students' analogical reasoning skills.
4. Engage students in the process of "moral diagnosis."
5. Be mindful of the limits of casuistical analysis. As a mere engine of moral argument, casuistry must be supplemented and guided by appeals to ethical theory, the history of ethics, and moral norms embedded

182   Getting Down to Cases

in our traditions and social practices. It must also be supplemented by critical social analyses that unmask the power behind much social consensus and raise larger questions about the kind of society we want and the kind of people we want to be.

Bibliography

Annas, G.: 1985, "Regulating heart and liver transplants in Massachusetts," *Law, Medicine and Health Care* 13(1), 4–7.

Beauchamp, T.L. and Childress, J.F.: 1989, *Principles of Biomedical Ethics*, 3rd edition, Oxford University Press, New York, New York.

Callahan, D.: 1990, *What Kind of Life?*, Simon and Schuster, New York, New York.

Carse, A.L.: 1991, "The "voice of care:" Implications for bioethics education," *Journal of Philosophy and Medicine* 16, 5–28.

Daniels, N.: 1979, "Wide reflective equilibrium and theory acceptance in ethics," *The Journal of Philosophy* 76, 256–82.

Fox, R.C. and Swazey, J.P.: 1984, "Medical morality is not bioethics—medical ethics in China and the United States," *Perspectives in Biology and Medicine* 27, 336–360.

Jonsen, A.R.: 1980, "Can an ethicist be a consultant?," in V. Abernethy (ed.), *Frontiers in Medical Ethics*, Ballinger Publishing Company, Cambridge, Massuchsetts, pp. 157–171.

Jonsen, A.R.: 1986a, "Casuistry and clinical ethics," *Theoretical Medicine* 7, 65–74.

Jonsen, A.R.: 1986b, "Casuistry," in J.F. Childress and J. Macgvarrie (eds.), *Westminster Dictionary of Christian Ethics*, Westminster Press, Philadelphia, Pennsylvania, pp. 78–80.

Jonsen, A.R. and Toulmin, S.: 1988, *The Abuse of Casuistry*, University of California Press, Berkeley, California.

MacIntyre, A.: 1981, *After Virtue*, University of Notre Dame Press, Notre Dame, Indiana.

Massachusetts Task Force on Organ Transplantation: 1984, *Report of the Massachusetts Task Force on Organ Transplantation*, Boston, Massachusetts.

Meilaender, G.: 1986, "The anencephalic newborn as organ donor: Commentary," *Hastings Center Report* 16, 22–23.

Noble, C.: 1982, "Ethics and experts," *Hastings Center Report* 12, 7–9.

O'Neill, O.: 1988, "How can we individuate moral problems?" in D.M. Rosenthal and F. Shehadi (eds.), *Applied Ethics and Ethical Theory*, University of Utah Press, Salt Lake City, pp. 84–99.

Overcast, D. *et al.*: 1985, "Technology assessment, public policy and transplantation," *Law, Medicine and Health Care* 13 (3), 106–111.

Pascal, B.: 1981, *Lettres écrites à un provincial*, A. Adam (ed.), Flammarion, Paris.

Rawls, J.: 1971, *A Theory of Justice*, Harvard University Press, Cambridge Massachusetts.

Rorty, R.: 1989, *Contingency, Irony, and Solidarity*, Cambridge University Press, Cambridge, England.
Toulmin, S.: 1981, "The tyranny of principles," *Hastings Center Report* 11, 31–39.
Warren, V.: 1989, "Feminist directions in medical ethics," *Hypatia* 4, 73–87.

Feminist and Medical Ethics
Two Different Approaches to Contextual Ethics

Susan Sherwin

Trained in philosophy at Stanford University during the early 1970s, Susan Sherwin currently teaches philosophy and women's studies at Dalhousie University. Her essay distinguishes feminist ethics from other inductive methods of analysis. Unlike casuistry and narrative ethics, feminist ethics sees its task as calling attention to the particular features of context that oppress women. In health care, this means exposing patriarchal features of medical practice.

Introduction

. . . In this paper, I shall explore the ways in which context is appealed to in both feminist and medical ethics, and I shall argue that particular sorts of details should be included in the recommended narrative approaches to ethical problems. In particular, I claim that incorporating an explicitly feminist political analysis in our discussion of context is critical to our ethical deliberations. . . .

The Role of Context in Feminist Ethics

Turning first to examine the role of context in feminist ethics, we must acknowledge the important influence of Carol Gilligan (1982). In identifying a female tendency to approach ethical problems in a personalized, contextual manner, Gilligan helped articulate the sense of alienation many women have experienced in trying to work within the structures of contemporary moral theory.[1] She identified distinct masculine and feminine voices in ethical reasoning, allowing us to recognize that mainstream ethical theory has been carried on in a voice that is overwhelmingly masculine—the voices of women have been largely excluded or ignored. Feminists stress that it is important in ethics, as in all fields, to include women's moral experiences and reasoning in the deliberations. Hence, most theorists seeking to develop a feminist approach to ethics have given serious consideration to the gender map which Gilligan has provided and have tried to incorporate many of her observations into their approach to ethics.[2]

In her research, Gilligan found that girls and women tend to approach ethical dilemmas in a contextualized, narrative way that looks for resolution in

Susan Sherwin. "Feminist and Medical Ethics: Two Different Approaches to Contextual Ethics." Abridged from *Hypatia*, Volume 4, Summer 1989, pp. 57–71. Reprinted by permission of the author.

particular details of a problem situation; in contrast, boys and men seem inclined to try to apply some general abstract principle without attention to the unique circumstances of the case. For instance, in Kohlberg's famous Heinz case, Gilligan found that males tended to answer in terms of the logical implications of a general rule, such as that stealing is wrong or that the duty to save a life outweighs other moral rules. In contrast, she found that female subjects tried to preserve relationships and to find new options through better communication and a presumption of co-operation; they tended to respond by seeking more information or by trying to re-conceive the terms set by the example. Gilligan recognized two different patterns of reasoning here: one which pursues universal rules in an endeavour to ensure fairness, and one which is focused on the actual feelings and interactions of those involved. The first approach, which she found to be associated with male moral thinking, she labelled an ethic of justice; the latter, which she found to be more commonly exercised by female subjects, she identified as an ethic of care.

The gender difference she describes is two-fold, characterized by differences in both scope and values: men seem to be preoccupied with developing comprehensive, generalizable, abstract ethical systems which are based on rights, while women seem to be concerned with understanding the specific human dynamics of a situation and, hence, concentrate on particular narrative details with the aim of avoiding hurt and providing care. As a result, we can identify distinct methodological differences between men and women in their approaches to morally troubling questions. But we should be cautious in interpreting the significance of the gender correlations of these differences; much of the discussion in feminist ethics has been occupied with evaluating the implications of developing what might be called a feminine ethics or a woman-centered ethics.[3] Since, in our sexist society, gender is inseparable from oppression, we should be sensitive to the fact that characteristics associated with gender are also likely to be associated with oppression. Obviously, it is important that women's distinctive moral reasoning be (at last) acknowledged as worthy of respect, but many feminists—including Gilligan herself—have expressed caution in interpreting the gender patterns her research reveals in the context of a society that systematically oppresses women. In particular, many feminists are wary of enthusiasm for virtues like caring which are associated with both gender and oppression.[4] Gilligan recommends that we work towards an androgynous ethics that could combine elements of both approaches, but other feminists have pointed out that notions of androgyny seem, themselves, to perpetuate the old gender system. . . .

The Role of Context in Medical Ethics

The theme of seeking a practical, context-specific approach to ethics is not restricted to feminist literature, however. The literature of medical ethics also contains frequent discussions about the inadequacy of abstract moral reasoning for resolving real moral dilemmas; there, too, we can find evidence of a widespread recognition that we must go beyond "mere theory." Further, there is frequent mention of the need to engage considerations of caring in medical ethics, usually couched in the language of the beneficence which is owed to patients. When placed in context (even if hypothetically), medical dilemmas are often discussed in terms that appear to rank sensitivity and caring ahead of applications of principle.[5]

In the "early days" of philosophical medical ethics (i.e., the 1970s), there was an attempt to try to fit responses to moral dilemmas into the general framework offered by standard moral theories, especially utilitarianism and Kantian deontology. It became apparent quite early on, however, that the simple appeal to theory and principle did not offer satisfying analyses of the sorts of dilemmas that arise in medical ethics. Case studies became a central element in influential journals, in many textbooks, and in individual articles. The texture and the details of cases have become important in trying to decide about perennial issues such as confidentiality, truth-telling, and euthanasia. Clear answers deduced from precise principles are not at hand for most of the topics addressed; many authors now accept the assumption that universal principles cannot be found which will govern such issues in all cases. . . .

Some philosophers still entrenched in mainstream moral theory have difficulty in seeing the distinction being cited here, since surely all moral theories are context sensitive to some degree. Kantian theory, for example, demands an interpretation of context in order to determine which maxim applies in a given case. But Kantian theory does assume that the maxims, once identified, will be universal and our policy on suicide, truth-telling, or confidentiality will be consistent across the full spectrum of relevant cases. It does not direct us to make our ethical assessments in terms of particular details of the lives of the individuals.

Utilitarianism is often espoused precisely as an antidote to such a rigid ethics. It certainly seems to be extremely sensitive to contextual features, in that it recommends we calculate relevant utilities for all possible options in a given set of circumstances. Nonetheless, it discounts some important features which medical ethics and feminist ethics consider important. Utilitarianism requires that we calculate the relevant utility values for all persons (or beings) affected by an action or practice and proceed according to a calculation of the relevant balances. In contrast, those engaged in doing feminist or medical ethics often reflect a desire to take account of the details of specific relationships and to give added weight to some particular utility-related qualities like caring and responsibility. Many of those engaged in feminist ethics diverge even further from standard utilitarianism, for they argue that the preferences of the oppressed ought to be counted differently from those of the dominant group. (Feminist objections to pornography, for instance, do not rely merely on the weighing of harms done against pleasure produced but reflect concern about the dehumanizing effect of the message of pornography whatever the utilities involved turn out to be.) In feminist and medical ethics, it is important to consider factors that do not carry any special weight in utilitarianism. There is need to look at the nature of the persons and the relationships involved in our analysis and not merely to record such values as preference satisfaction or pleasure or pain; while the latter values are specifically held, their importance comes from some abstract sum and not from their attachment to any particular persons in particular situations. Hence, neither Kantian nor utility theory satisfies the requirement of particularity as it is conceived in feminist and medical ethics. . . .

Some Requirements for a Feminist Ethics

For medical ethics to be thought feminist, it must also reflect a political dimension, but this is mostly lacking in the literature to date. Although there are currently many diverse attempts to characterize feminist ethics, all share some political analysis of the unequal power of women and men, of white people and people of colour, of first world and third world people, of rich and poor, of healthy and disabled, etc.[6] Ours is a world structured by hierarchies and a sense of supremacy on the part of the powerful; there are numerous social patterns which shape the people we are and the sorts of relationships we will have with one another. In attending to the quality of actual interactions among people in ethics, we need to account for the influence of social and political factors on the nature of those relationships. From either the caring or the justice perspective (to use Gilligan's language), we can see that empowerment of people who are currently victims of oppression is an ethical as well as a political issue, and ethical investigations of particular problem areas should reflect these dimensions. Many feminist critics have observed that current medical practice constitutes a powerful social institution which contributes to the oppression of women. They have demonstrated that the practice of medicine serves as an important instrument in the continuing disempowerment of women (and members of other oppressed groups) in society and thrives on hierarchical power structures. By medicating socially induced depression and anxiety, medicine helps to perpetuate unjust social arrangements. With its authority to define what is normal and what is pathological and to coerce compliance to its norms, medicine tends to strengthen patterns of stereotyping and reinforce existing power inequalities. It serves to legitimize practices such as woman battering or male sexual aggression that might otherwise be evaluated in moral and political terms.[7]

Nonetheless, the discussion in medical ethics to date has been largely myopic, failing to comment on this important political role of medicine. That is, the institution of medicine is usually accepted as given in discussions of medical ethics, and debate has focused on certain practices within that structure: for example, truth-telling, obtaining consent, preserving confidentiality, the limits of paternalism, allocation of resources, dealing with incurable illness, and matters of reproduction. The effect is to provide an ethical legitimization of the institution overall, with acceptance of its general structures and patterns. With the occasional exception of certain discussions of resource allocation, it would appear from much of the medical ethics literature that all that is needed to make medical interactions ethically acceptable is a bit of fine-tuning in specific problem cases.

A good indication of the legitimizing function of medical ethics can be seen by noting its gradual acceptance among those who are influential within the medical profession. Increasingly, medical practitioners seem to be recognizing the value of incorporating discussions of medical ethics within their own work, for they can thereby demonstrate their serious interest in moral matters. Such serious professional concern in matters of medical ethics serves to encourage the public to place even greater trust in their judgment. Keeping the scope of medical ethics narrowed to specific problems of interaction helps physicians maintain their supportive stance towards it.

Feminists must be critical of the fact that medical ethics has remained largely silent about the patriarchal practice of medicine. Few authors writing on medical ethics have been critical of practices and institutions that contribute to the oppression of women. The deep questions about the structure of medical practice and its role in a patriarchal society are largely inaccessible within the framework; they are not considered part of the standard curriculum in textbooks of medical ethics. Consequently, medical ethics, as it is mostly practiced to date, does not amount to a feminist approach to ethics. . . .

Notes

1. For an apt description of the "moral madness" women commonly experience when confronted with patriarchal ethical demands, see Morgan (1987).
2. See, for instance, the various discussions in the collection, *Women and Moral Theory*, Kittay and Meyers, 1987.
3. Nel Noddings (1984) has spelled out the full implications of pursuing the feminine approach to ethics exclusively in *Caring*. Though I would not classify her as a feminist, Noddings has given theoretical voice to the ethic of care described by Gilligan, rejecting all aspects of an ethics based in abstract principles in favour of an ethics concerned only with particular relationships based on caring.
4. See, for instance, the arguments put forward by Houston (1987) and Wilson (1988).
5. This tendency seems to me to be especially common in the contributions of physicians to medical ethics; it is less apparent in the philosophical discussions in the field.
6. I am well aware of the rich diversity of views clustered under the label of "feminist analysis," but I think that there are some core views that transcend the differences which divide feminists in their internal debates. For the purposes of this paper, I will focus only on the common themes which include a recognition that women are in a subordinate position in society, that oppression is a form of injustice and hence is intolerable, that there are further forms of oppression in addition to gender oppression (and that there are women victimized by each of these forms of oppression), that it is possible to change society in ways that could eliminate oppression, and that it is a goal of feminism to pursue the changes necessary to accomplish this. I believe that the argument presented in this paper is unchanged however we explain the cause of women's oppression and whatever we imagine is best for bringing about the desired changes. Therefore, I shall speak of a feminist analysis without being specific here about which particular variation I have in mind.

7. See Stark, Flitcraft, and Frazier (1983). For a more far ranging discussion, see the powerful indictment of medicine's contribution to the oppression of women in the survey by Ehrenreich and English (1979).

References

Ehrenreich, Barbara and Dierdre English. 1979. *For her own good: 150 years of the experts' advice to women.* Garden City, NY: Anchor Press, Doubleday.

Houston, Barbara. 1987. Reclaiming moral virtues: Some dangers of moral reclamation. In *Science, morality, and feminist theory.* Marsha Hanen and Kai Nielsen, eds. *Canadian Journal of Philosophy* (supplementary volume) 13.

Kittay, Eva Feder and Diana T. Meyers, eds., 1987. *Women and moral theory.* Totowa, N.J.: Rowman and Littlefield.

Morgan, Kathryn. 1987. Women and moral madness. In *Science, morality, and feminist theory.* Marsha Hanen and Kai Nielsen, eds. *Canadian Journal of Philosophy* (supplementary volume) 13.

Noddings, Nel. 1984. *Caring: A feminine approach to ethics and moral education.* Berkeley: University of California Press.

Stark, Evan, Anne Flitcraft, and William Fraxier. 1983. Medicine and patriarchal violence: The social construction of a "private" event. In *Women and health: The politics of sex in medicine.* Elizabeth Fee, ed. Farmingdale, N.Y.: Baywood Publishing Company.

Wilson, Leslie. 1988. Is a "feminine" ethics enough? *Atlantis* 5 (17):15–23.

Questions for Discussion
Part II, Section 2

1. According to Jonsen, what is casuistry and how does contemporary casuistry provide a useful method of ethical reasoning for medicine?

2. How does Hunter's narrative approach differ from the casuistic approach Jonsen defends? Can the two methods be used together in a consistent fashion to address ethical concerns in medicine?

3. As Sherwin notes, both casuistry and feminism pay careful attention to the contexts in which ethical problems arise. What special features of context are of concern to feminists? Do these differ from the features that interest casuists?

4. Arras doubts that casuistry is really theory-free and suggests that casuists make unstated theoretical assumptions in the resolution of ethical cases. Are such doubts warranted?

5. How can adherents of casuistic methods defend themselves against the charge that casuistry is nothing more than conventionalism, that is, an uncritical exposition of established social and moral meanings?

SECTION 3

DESCRIPTIVE METHODS

QUANTITATIVE AND QUALITATIVE
EMPIRICAL STUDIES

ह&

Attitudes toward Assisted Suicide and Euthanasia among Physicians in Washington State

Jonathan S. Cohen, Stephan D. Fihn, Edward J. Boyko,
Albert R. Jonsen, and Robert W. Wood

Cohen, Fihn, Boyko and Wood are physicians trained in general internal medicine; they are affiliated with the Seattle Veterans Affairs Medical Center (Cohen, Fihn, and Boyko) and the University of Washington School of Medicine (Wood). Dr. Jonsen is trained in Religious Studies and serves as chair of the Department of Medical History and Ethics at the University of Washington, Seattle. This interdisciplinary team studied the attitudes of physicians toward physician-assisted suicide and euthanasia. The study reveals that there is no general ethical consensus about the ethics of physician-assisted death among physicians in Washington state.

There is considerable public interest in the legalization of physician-assisted suicide and euthanasia.[1] By a margin of 54 to 46 percent, voters in Washington defeated Initiative 119, which would have legalized assisted suicide and euthanasia, in 1991. In 1992, voters in California defeated Proposition 161, a similar initiative, by the same margin. A Michigan law that forbids assisted

Jonathan S. Cohen, Stephan D. Fihn, Edward J. Boyko, Albert R. Jonsen, and Robert W. Wood. "Attitudes Toward Assisted Suicide and Euthanasia Among Physicians in Washington State." Reprinted from *The New England Journal of Medicine*, Volume 331, No. 2, 1994, pp. 89–94. Reprinted by permission of *The New England Journal of Medicine*. Copyright © 1994, Massachusetts Medical Society.

suicide is currently under court challenge.[2] Several organizations strongly support physician-assisted suicide and euthanasia, and efforts to legalize these practices are likely to continue.

The debate on these issues among professionals and academic physicians has been contentious,[3-12] and specific proposals for permitting assisted suicide or euthanasia have provoked controversy.[13-15] Despite extensive discussion, relatively little is known about the opinions of physicians on this subject. The available surveys of physicians concerning assisted suicide and euthanasia have been hampered by small samples,[16-19] low response rates,[16,19-22] limited generalizability,[16,17,19,21,22] ambiguous terminology,[17,19-22] and insufficiently detailed questions.[16,19,20,22] Most surveys have dealt with several ethical issues related to terminal care instead of focusing on assisted suicide and euthanasia. Few surveys have examined the beliefs underlying stated opinions or explored preferences for specific restrictions and safeguards.

We conducted a population-based survey of attitudes toward assisted suicide and euthanasia among randomly selected physicians practicing in Washington State. The study was designed to determine whether physicians believe assisted suicide and euthanasia are ethical, whether they believe either or both should be legalized, and whether physicians are willing to participate in these practices personally. We also investigated the reasons for physicians' positions and their views about the safeguards necessary in possible legislation permitting these practices.

Methods

Respondents

We selected potential respondents from a Washington State Medical Association data base that includes both members of the organization (62 percent) and nonmembers (38 percent) and that incorporates data supplied by the Washington State Division of Licensing, the American Medical Association, county medical societies, insurance companies, hospitals, and clinics. We excluded retired physicians, trainees, and physicians practicing outside the state. We randomly selected 250 physicians from each of the following fields: general internal medicine, family practice, general surgery, psychiatry, and a combination of all the other specialties except hematology and oncology, for a total of 1250 physicians. We also included 166 hematologists and oncologists: 98 from the medical-society data base and 68 from address lists of the American Society of Hematology, the American Society of Clinical Oncology, and the University of Washington faculty. The final sample thus totaled 1416 physicians.

Questionnaire

Our questionnaire was based on earlier surveys,[19-22] discussions of issues in the literature,[3-9] interviews with leading proponents and opponents of legalized assisted suicide and euthanasia in Washington, and extensive pilot testing. The survey consisted of 48 questions about the characteristics of the respondents, their attitudes toward assisted suicide and euthanasia, their opinions of possible legalization related to these practices, their willingness to participate in assisted suicide or euthanasia, the reasons for their positions, and their views about safeguards or restrictions that might be part of any legislation governing assisted suicide or euthanasia. Membership in the Washington State Medical Association was not ascertained. Responses were given in the form of ratings, on a five-point scale, of the degree of agreement with a variety of statements, ranging from "strongly agree" to "strongly disagree." For clarity, we collapsed the responses into three categories: strongly agree or agree, neutral, and disagree or strongly disagree.

To avoid ambiguity, we did not use the terms "assisted suicide" and "euthanasia" in the survey. Instead of "physician-assisted suicide," we used the following phrase: "prescription of medication [e.g., narcotics or barbiturates] or the counseling of an ill patient so he or she may use an overdose to end his or her own life." Instead of "euthanasia," we used the phrase "deliberate administration of an overdose of medication to an ill patient at his or her request with the primary intent to end his or her life." Although other actions may arguably be considered assisted suicide or euthanasia, these descriptions provide a clear indication of intent and action, reflect the consensus of experts in the field, and are consistent with the definitions proposed by the American Medical Association[23] and the American College of Physicians.[24] For simplicity, we have used the terms "assisted suicide" and "euthanasia" in reporting our findings.

We mailed questionnaires to the physicians in the sample in December 1992. Although the survey was anonymous, return envelopes were coded to permit the identification of nonrespondents, to whom we sent additional surveys in February 1993 and again in March 1993. (Copies of the questionnaires are available from the authors.) To measure potential response bias, we randomly selected a 10 percent subsample of the physicians who had not responded by March 1993, mailed them an anonymous questionnaire containing 12 items from the initial survey, and telephoned them to encourage them to respond. Because the responses in the survey were anonymous, the study was exempt from review by the University of Washington Human Subjects Committee.

Statistical Analysis

For each item, we computed the frequency or mean response, with 95 percent confidence intervals,[25] and compared means between subgroups using the unpaired-samples t-test.[25] To adjust for the oversampling of some specialties, we performed a weighted analysis to reflect the actual distribution of specialists among physicians in Washington State. The results of the weighted analysis were nearly identical to those obtained with unadjusted data. Only the unadjusted results are therefore presented.

We used logistic regression to assess the independent effects of specialty, age, sex, and practice characteristics (the independent variables) on attitudes toward assisted suicide and euthanasia (the dependent variables)[26] and estimated odds ratios for each independent variable. For comparisons between specialties, general internal medicine was used as the reference category. All P values are two-tailed.

To determine which medical conditions were considered by physicians to create a situation in which euthanasia or assisted suicide might be appropriate, we analyzed separately the replies of physicians who believed that both euthanasia and assisted suicide are sometimes ethical. To investigate which specific safeguards and restrictions physicians considered important, we analyzed separately the responses of physicians who supported legalizing both euthanasia and assisted suicide.

Results

Of the 1416 physicians surveyed, 61 were found to be ineligible because of address changes or retirement. Of the remaining 1355 physicians, 938 (69 percent) completed surveys. The characteristics of the respondents are shown in Table 1. The differing proportions of respondents in the various specialties reflect the composition of our sample and the varying response rates. Women represented a higher proportion of the responding internists (30 percent) and family practitioners (25 percent) than of the hematologists or oncologists (16

TABLE 1   Characteristics of the 938 Respondents to the Survey.*

Characteristic	Value
Age (yr)	46 ± 10
Male/female (%)	81/19
Medical specialty (%)	
Family practice	20
Psychiatry	18
General surgery	14
Hematology and oncology	12
General internal medicine	10
Other	26
No. of terminally ill patients seen during previous month	7 ± 16
Affiliated with student, resident, or fellowship training program (%)	42
Size of population where practice is located (%)	
<10,000	8
10,000–19,999	4
20,000–49,999	20
50,000–99,999	12
≥100,000	56

*Plus–minus values are means ± SD

percent) or surgeons (5 percent). The mean number of terminally ill patients seen in the previous month was 7; this figure ranged from 2 for psychiatrists to 28 for hematologists and oncologists. Forty-two percent of the respondents were affiliated with a student, residency, or fellowship training program (range, 33 percent for family practitioners to 64 percent for hematologists and oncologists).

Attitudes toward Assisted Suicide and Euthanasia

Forty-eight percent of respondents said they agreed with the statement that euthanasia is never ethically justified, and 42 percent disagreed. Fifty-four percent thought euthanasia should be legal in some situations, but only 33 percent stated that they would be willing to perform euthanasia themselves. There was slightly more support for physician-assisted suicide. Thirty-nine percent of respondents agreed with the statement that assisted suicide is never ethically justified, and 50 percent disagreed. Fifty-three percent thought assisted suicide should be legal in some situations, but only 40 percent stated that they would be willing to assist a patient in committing suicide.

Differences among Groups of Physicians

Attitudes toward assisted suicide and euthanasia varied significantly among the specialties (Fig. 2). Of the groups surveyed, psychiatrists were most supportive of these two practices, and hematologists and oncologists were least supportive. These differences in attitudes persisted after logistic-regression models were used to adjust for potential confounding by sex and affiliation with a training program.

Physicians affiliated with a training program were less likely than those who were not so affiliated to view euthanasia as unethical (odds ratio, 0.74; 95 percent confidence interval, 0.6 to 1.0; P = 0.04) or to view assisted suicide as unethical (odds ratio, 0.72; 95 percent confidence interval, 0.5 to 1.0; P = 0.03); they were more willing to perform euthanasia themselves (odds ratio, 1.4; 95 percent confidence interval, 1.0 to 1.9; P = 0.03) and assist in suicide (odds ratio, 1.5; 95 percent confidence interval, 1.1 to 2.0; P = 0.009). Men were more likely than women to regard assisted suicide as unethical (odds ratio, 1.7; 95 percent confidence interval, 1.1 to 2.4; P = 0.01). There was no significant difference between the sexes about the ethics of euthanasia (data not shown).

Reasons for Attitudes toward Assisted Suicide and Euthanasia

We analyzed the reasons physicians gave for their attitudes by grouping respondents with similar positions on euthanasia and assisted suicide and excluding those who either felt differently about the two forms of physician-assisted dying or were neutral toward either. Fifty-six percent of the 318 respondents who

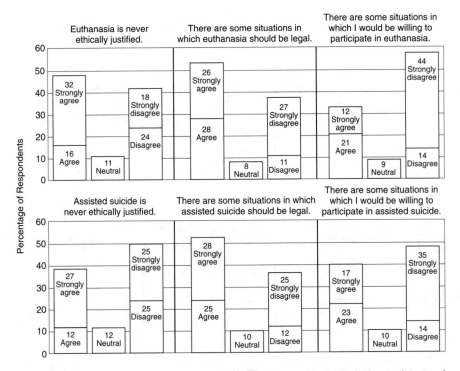

Figure 1   Physicians' Responses to Six Statements Expressing Attitudes toward Assisted Suicide and Euthanasia.

The values shown are the percentages of total responses in each category. The statements are paraphrases of those in the questionnaire. Because of rounding, percentages for some categories do not total 100.

agreed that euthanasia and assisted suicide are never ethically justified stated that they were influenced by religious beliefs, as compared with 15 percent of the 343 respondents who disagreed with those statements. Seventy-four percent of those who opposed euthanasia and assisted suicide considered these practices inconsistent with the physician's role in relieving pain and suffering. In contrast, 91 percent of those who believed the practices to be ethical considered them consistent with the physician's role. Eighty percent of those who opposed euthanasia and assisted suicide cited the potential for abuse. Thirty-two percent of those who considered the practices unethical believed that currently available treatments may be inadequate to eliminate pain and suffering, as compared with 80 percent of those who believed that these practices are ethical. Ninety-seven percent of those who supported assisted suicide and euthanasia said that patients' right to self-determination should be respected, and 91 percent said that the availability of assisted suicide and euthanasia might reduce patients' fears of losing control or of a painful death.

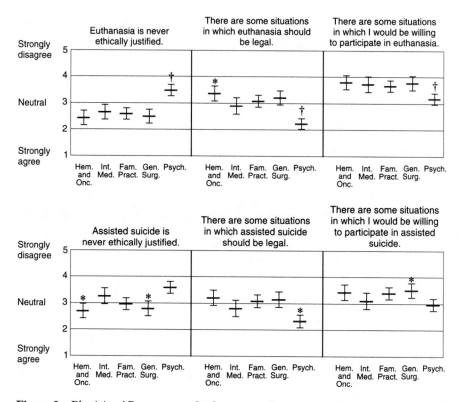

Figure 2 Physicians' Responses to Six Statements Expressing Attitudes toward Assisted Suicide and Euthanasia, According to Medical Specialty.

The values shown are means and 95 percent confidence intervals; they correspond to the degree of agreement with each statement (paraphrased from the questionnaire), on a five-point scale: 1 indicates strong agreement, 3 a neutral attitude, and 5 strong disagreement. The mean response for each specialty was compared with the mean response for physicians in internal medicine by the unpaired-samples t-test. The asterisk indicates $P < 0.05$, and the dagger $P < 0.01$ (both two-tailed). Hem. and onc. denotes hematology and oncology, int. med. internal medicine, fam. pract. family practice, gen. surg. general surgery, and psych. psychiatry.

Situations in Which Euthanasia or Assisted Suicide May Be Appropriate

Among the 343 physicians who believed that both euthanasia and assisted suicide are sometimes ethical, 88 percent thought that a poor quality of life, despite adequate pain control, might be sufficient justification for these practices; paradoxically, 51 percent thought that a patient's pain should be beyond control in order to justify euthanasia or assisted suicide, and 64 percent believed that a patient's life expectancy should be less than six months. Thirty-one percent agreed with the statement that if a "patient has a good quality of life at present, but has an illness which will cause severe mental and/or physical deterioration in the future, fatal overdose may still be appropriate." Twenty-one percent agreed that euthanasia or assisted suicide may be appropriate if external factors (such as not wanting to burden the family or not wanting to deplete savings) led to the patient's request, despite adequate pain control and quality of life.

Restrictions and Safeguards

Among the 432 physicians who favored the legalization of both assisted suicide and euthanasia, the safeguard supported most strongly was the requirement that the patient's request be witnessed by an independent person who would not benefit from the patient's death (Table 2). Other favored safeguards included confirming the patient's mental competence, requiring that two physicians agree with the decision, and requiring that the physician administering or prescribing a fatal overdose have an established relationship with the patient.

Survey of Nonrespondents

Of 40 physicians who did not respond to the initial questionnaire whom we surveyed after March 1993, 29 responded; 2 others had moved out of state, and 1 had retired. The attitudes of the nonrespondents, as measured by the briefer questionnaire, did not differ significantly from those obtained in the initial survey.

Discussion

Physicians in Washington have sharply polarized attitudes toward assisted suicide and euthanasia, which mirror the sharp divisions among voters in Washington and California. Only about 10 percent of physicians stated that they were neutral on the questions of euthanasia and assisted suicide. Only a minority of physicians expressed a willingness to participate in assisted suicide or euthanasia or believed these practices to be ethical. A slight majority, however, favored their legalization. In general, attitudes toward physician-assisted suicide were more favorable than those toward euthanasia, although the percentages of physicians favoring legalization of the two practices were similar.

There were wide variations in the responses according to specialty, sex, and affiliation with a training program. These variations could not be attributed to age, contact with terminally ill patients, or other practice characteristics. Hematologists and oncologists had the most exposure to terminally ill patients and were also the strongest opponents of euthanasia and assisted suicide. Psychiatrists, who had the least contact with terminally ill patients, were the strongest proponents of the two practices. One explanation for these findings may be that many hematologists and oncologists believe that more effective use of available treatments to relieve pain and suffering would obviate the need for euthanasia

TABLE 2   Responses to Statements about Legal Restrictions and Safeguards among 432 Respondents Who Supported the Legalization of Assisted Suicide and Euthanasia*

Statement	Strongly Agree or Agree	Neutral	Disagree or Strongly Disagree
	percent		
The patient's request should be witnessed by an independent person (or people) who will not benefit from the patient's death.	90	7	3
The physician administering or prescribing a fatal overdose should have an established relationship with the patient.	84	12	4
Available alternatives (e.g., hospice care, treatment of depression) to a drug overdose to end the patient's life should have been fully utilized.	84	9	7
Two physicians should be in accord with the decision.	81	13	6
The patient should be mentally component.	81	10	9
There should be a specified waiting period between the time a patient requests a drug overdose to end his or her life and the time such a request is granted.	78	15	7
Psychiatric consultation should be obtained to rule out treatable psychiatric illness that may be underlying a patient's request to end his or her life.	60	21	19
The patient's immediate family should be in accord with the decision.	58	28	18
The patient should not be depressed.	56	24	20
A hospital ethics committee should review and be in accord with the decision.	51	24	26
A patient should request an overdose to end his or her life on two separate occasions before such a request is granted.	49	34	18
Hastening death should be restricted to the adult population.	33	22	46

*Only the 432 respondents who strongly agreed or agreed that both euthanasia and physician-assisted suicide should be legal are included in this analysis. Because of rounding, percentages for some statements do not total 100.

and assisted suicide. Further study of these issues is needed to clarify these divergent views.

Our study has several strengths. To enhance its validity, we used terminology in the questionnaire that was unlikely to be ambiguous, and we focused exclusively on assisted suicide and euthanasia. To enhance the generalizability of our findings, we randomly sampled a wide cross section of physicians in a variety of medical specialties, practice settings, and geographic locations. In addition, public debate about the ballot initiative in Washington that would legalize euthanasia and assisted suicide has presumably made physicians in the state better informed than average about the issues, perhaps with the result that their responses are more thoughtful than might be the case elsewhere.[27] The rate of response to our survey (69 percent) was relatively high. Moreover, in a small survey of physicians who did not complete the initial questionnaire we did not find evidence of a response bias.

Our study also has several limitations. First, the results of a survey of physicians in Washington may not be applicable to other regions of the country. Second, the Washington State Medical Association opposed Initiative 119, which would have legalized euthanasia and assisted suicide, and sent a newsletter outlining these views to its members, who make up 75 percent of the licensed physicians in the state. The views of the medical association may have influenced the attitudes of respondents. We did not ask respondents whether they were members of the association or whether the association's position had influenced their views. Finally, the fixed-response format of the questionnaire may have limited the amount of information obtained and the level of detail in the responses.

The results of this study have important implications for patients, physicians, and policy makers. The polarized attitudes of physicians will make it difficult to formulate and implement laws and policies concerning assisted suicide and euthanasia. Despite the lack of consensus on these issues, a substantial number of physicians believe that currently available treatments may be inadequate to eliminate pain and suffering for terminally ill patients and were dissatisfied with their legal options. To receive support from a large number of physicians, legislation permitting assisted suicide or euthanasia would have to contain ample safeguards. There was strong support among our respondents for previously proposed safeguards for physician-assisted suicide,[14] which include the restriction of such suicides to mentally competent, terminally ill patients with a poor quality of life; the required exhaustion of all other reasonable treatment options; and the requirement that there be an established relationship between physician and patient.

The wide public interest in assisted suicide and euthanasia indicates clearly that physicians should work to improve the care of terminally ill patients. These efforts should include better communication with patients, maximal use of advance directives, effective control of pain and other symptoms, and development of hospices and similar programs for terminally ill patients.[28] Whether assisted suicide and euthanasia have a role in the care of such patients remains an issue for further debate.

References

1. Blendon RJ, Szalay US, Knox RA. Should physicians aid their patients in dying? The public perspective. JAMA 1992;267:2658–62.
2. Supreme Court will hear assisted suicide cases. Detroit Free Press. June 7, 1994:6B.
3. Battin M. Voluntary euthanasia and the risks of abuse: can we learn anything from the Netherlands? Law Med Health Care 1992;20:133–43.
4. Cassel CK, Meier DE. Morals and moralism in the debate over euthanasia and assisted suicide. N Engl J Med 1990;323:750–2.
5. Hendin H, Klerman G. Physician-assisted suicide: the dangers of legalization. Am J Psychiatry 1993;150:143–5.
6. Misbin RI. Physicians' aid in dying. N Engl J Med 1991;325:1307–11.
7. Singer PA, Siegler M. Euthanasia—a critique. N Engl J Med 1990;322:1881–3.
8. Wanzer SH, Federman DD, Adelstein SJ, et al. The physician's responsibility toward hopelessly ill patients: a second look. N Engl J Med 1989;320:844–9.
9. Weir RF. The morality of physician-assisted suicide. Law Med Health Care 1992;20:116–26.
10. CeloCruz MT. Aid-in-dying: should we decriminalize physician-assisted suicide and physician-committed euthanasia? Am J Law Med 1992;18:369–94.
11. Kamisar Y. Are laws against assisted suicide unconstitutional? Hastings Cent Rep 1993;23:32–41.
12. Annas GJ. Physician-assisted suicide—Michigan's temporary solution. N Engl J Med 1993;328:1573–6.
13. Benrubi GI. Euthanasia—the need for procedural safeguards. N Engl J Med 1992;326:197–9.
14. Quill TE, Cassel CK, Meier DE. Care of the hopelessly ill: proposed clinical criteria for physician-assisted suicide. N Engl J Med 1992;327:1380–4.
15. Brody H. Assisted death—a compassionate response to a medical failure. N Engl J Med 1992;327:1384–8.
16. Crosby C. Internists grapple with how they should respond to requests for aid in dying. The Internist. March 1992:16.
17. Caralis PV, Hammond JS. Attitudes of medical students, housestaff, and faculty physicians toward euthanasia and termination of life-sustaining treatment. Crit Care Med 1992;20:683–90.
18. Fried TR, Stein MD, O'Sullivan PS, Brock DW, Novack DH. Limits of patient autonomy: physician attitudes and practices regarding life-sustaining treatments and euthanasia. Arch Intern Med 1993;153:722–8.
19. Overmeyer M. National survey: physicians' views on the right to die. Physician's Manage 1991;31:40–60.
20. The Center for Health Ethics and Policy. Withholding and withdrawing life-sustaining treatment: a survey of opinions and experiences of Colorado physicians. Denver: University of Colorado at Denver Graduate School of Public Affairs, 1988.
21. Heilig S. The SFMS euthanasia survey: results and analyses. San Francisco Med 1988;61(5):24–6, 34.
22. Washington State Medical Association. Informal survey of WSMA members on 'death with dignity' initiative complete. WSMA Leadership Memo. March 14, 1991.

23. American Medical Association, Council on Ethical and Judicial Affairs. Decisions near the end of life. JAMA 1992;267:2229–33.
24. American College of Physicians ethics manual. 3rd ed. Ann Intern Med 1992;117:947–60.
25. Snedecor GW, Cochran WG. Statistical methods. 7th ed. Ames: Iowa State University Press, 1980:93–5, 121.
26. Kleinbaum DG, Kupper LL, Morgenstern H. Epidemiologic research: principles and quantitative methods. Belmont, Calif.: Lifetime Learning, 1982:419, 491.
27. Converse PE. The nature of belief systems in mass publics. In: Apter DE. ed. Ideology and discontent. New York: Free Press, 1964:206–61.
28. Quill TE. Doctor, I want to die. Will you help me? JAMA 1993;270:870–3.

Survival after Cardiopulmonary Resuscitation in the Hospital

*Susanna E. Bedell, Thomas L. Delbanco, E. Francis Cook,
and Franklin H. Epstein*

Susanna Bedell, a physician in the Division of General Medicine and Primary Care, Beth Israel Hospital, and physician colleagues Thomas Delbanco, Francis Cook, and Franklin Epstein studied prospectively the outcomes after in-hospital resuscitation for 294 consecutive patients who were resuscitated in a university teaching hospital. They found that certain prognostic factors, such as pneumonia, hypotension, renal failure, cancer, and a home-bound life style were significantly associated with in-hospital mortality. These empirical findings raise important ethical issues, including the question of whether or not resuscitation should be offered to patients who present with these prognostic factors.

Since the introduction of external cardiac massage in 1960,[1] cardiopulmonary resuscitation has frequently been attempted in community and university hospitals.[2-5] At the Beth Israel Hospital in Boston, physicians perform cardiopulmonary resuscitation in 3 of every 10 patients who die. However, in contrast to out-of-hospital arrest, a subject that has received extensive study,[6-10] little is known about the characteristics of patients resuscitated in-hospital, the predictors of outcome, or the quality of life for the survivors. In the hospital setting the patient, family, physician, and nurse may debate the decision to perform or withhold cardiopulmonary resuscitation.[11-13] To evaluate in-hospital resuscitation on the basis of fact, in addition to emotion and philosophy, knowledge of both the history of patients who have been resuscitated and the outcome of resuscitation is imperative. Therefore, we conducted a study to address the following questions: What are the demographic and clinical characteristics of patients who have been resuscitated in-hospital? What are the outcomes for these patients? What are the predictors of outcome? What is the quality of survival for patients who survive to be discharged from the hospital?

Methods

We evaluated prospectively all patients resuscitated at Beth Israel Hospital, a university teaching hospital, during the 18-month period from January 1, 1981,

Susanna E. Bedell, Thomas L. Delbanco, E. Francis Cook, and Franklin H. Epstein, "Survival After Cardiopulmonary Resuscitation in the Hospital." Reprinted from *The New England Journal of Medicine*, Volume 309, 1983, pp. 569–574. Reprinted by permission of The New England Journal of Medicine. Copyright © 1983, Massachusetts Medical Society.

through June 30, 1982. For the purpose of this study, cardiac arrest was defined as the sudden cessation of circulation or respiration, resulting in documented loss of consciousness and requiring initiation of cardiopulmonary resuscitation. Arrests were identified through the records of the central-page operators and in regular rounds in the cardiac and pulmonary intensive-care units. Each resuscitation was conducted by the patient's own ward or unit team with the assistance of a senior medical resident and an anesthesiologist. For the purposes of this study, we excluded patients in whom cardiac arrest occurred before admission to the hospital.

For the 28 patients who required cardiopulmonary resuscitation on more than one occasion, we examined only the initial effort at resuscitation. We recorded demographic and clinical information for each patient on a data form containing 193 entries. These covered the patient's primary and secondary diagnoses, the functional status before hospitalization, the medical history before cardiac arrest, and the clinical condition 24 hours before and after cardiopulmonary resuscitation. We also reviewed all death certificates from the hospital during the 18-month study period to obtain information about the patients for whom no attempt at resuscitation was made.

After obtaining informed consent, we interviewed each patient who survived to the time of discharge from the hospital. We conducted the initial interview in the hospital during the three days before discharge. We also reinterviewed all patients who were still alive six months after leaving the hospital. The follow-up interview took place in the patient's home. We administered four questionnaires to provide a comprehensive assessment of the patient's quality of life: the Wechsler memory scale,[14] which measures memory and attention; the Center for Epidemiologic Studies' depression scale,[15] a validated self-reporting scale for depression; a scale from the Philadelphia Geriatric Center that measures the activity of daily living;[16] and our own questionnaire, which was designed to evaluate the patient's subjective response to the arrest itself and his or her desire for resuscitation in the future (available on request). The interviews were designed to last one hour but averaged two hours because of questions initiated by the patients.

Statistical Analysis

We analyzed all variables in the data base to compare patients who died in the hospital after cardiopulmonary resuscitation with those who were discharged from the hospital. Categorical variables were analyzed by the usual chi-square test for association. Continuous variables were analyzed by Student's two-sample t-test and the Wilcoxon rank-sum test.[17] By selecting clinically appropriate cutoff points, such as less than or more than 65 years of age, we also analyzed continuous variables as categorical variables, using the chi-square test.

We used two different types of multivariate analysis to examine how the many variables that were significant by univariate analysis interacted to predict outcome after cardiopulmonary resuscitation. We used stepwise logistic regression[18] to identify variables that had a significant "independent" relation with outcome. We used recursive partitioning[19,20] to identify concise subgroups of patients with different risks of death after cardiopulmonary resuscitation. Both types of multivariate analyses were repeated three times in order to take into account the information available to the physician at three separate points in the patient's hospital course: before the onset of cardiac arrest, at the time of the arrest, and after the effort at resuscitation.

Results

Clinical Course

Figure 1 summarizes the outcome of cardiopulmonary resuscitation in the study population. During the year-and-a-half study period, 294 patients had a cardiopulmonary arrest (the study group). Thirty subsequent episodes of arrest occurred in this group. After the initial resuscitation, the pulse and blood pressure were restored in 128 of the 294 patients (44 per cent), and 166 (56 per cent) died. Thirty-one of the 128 survivors died within 24 hours after cardiopulmonary resuscitation, and another 56 survivors died before leaving the hospital. Thus, 41 patients, or one third of the initial survivors and 14 per cent of the total study group, were discharged from the hospital. At follow-up six months after discharge, 33 of the 41 patients (80 per cent) were still alive. From the perspective of a practicing physician caring for critically ill patients, it is also meaningful to examine the survival of patients who live longer than 24 hours after cardiopulmonary resuscitation. On the basis of this criterion, 97 patients (33 per cent) survived resuscitation initially; 42 per cent of them were discharged from the hospital, and 34 per cent were still alive six months later.

Demographic Information

The cohort of 294 patients consisted of 160 men and 134 women. Their mean age was 70 years, with a range of 18 to 101. The majority (86 per cent) were

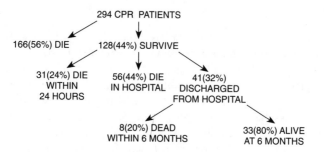

Figure 1. Outcomes of 294 Attempts at Resuscitation during the 18-Month Study Period.

admitted to the hospital from their own home, and the rest from a nursing home. Half were married (51 per cent), and half were single, widowed, or divorced (49 per cent). Twenty-eight patients (10 per cent) were employed full- or part-time before hospitalization; the remainder were retired or unemployed.

Of the 265 patients for whom we could determine the level of activity before hospitalization, 128 had engaged in activities outside the home, and 137 had confined their lives to the home or nursing home for at least six months before hospitalization.

Clinical Characteristics

The most common clinical diagnosis in the study group of 294 patients was coronary-artery disease. Before cardiac arrest, 41 per cent of the patients had an acute myocardial infarction in the hospital, 73 per cent had a history of congestive heart failure, and fully 20 per cent had a history of prior cardiac arrest and resuscitation one or more times before the current hospitalization.

Among noncardiac diagnoses, renal failure (defined as a level of blood urea nitrogen higher than 50 mg per deciliter [18 mmol per liter]) predominated, occurring in 26 per cent of the cases. Twenty-four per cent of the patients had diabetes, 20 per cent had pneumonia, 20 per cent had a history of cancer (excluding cancers of the skin), and 5 per cent had an acute stroke resulting in a neurologic deficit.

The median duration of hospitalization for the patients who died in the hospital was 6 days, with a range of 1 to 61. For the patients discharged from the hospital, the median duration of hospitalization was substantially longer (26 days; range, 8 to 61).

For 39 of the 128 patients (31 per cent) who initially survived cardiopulmonary resuscitation, there were written orders not to repeat resuscitation in the event of a subsequent arrest.

Characteristics of the Arrest

We examined five major characteristics of the arrest that are commonly thought to influence the outcome of cardiopulmonary resuscitation (Table 1): location, mechanism, duration, initial arterial blood gases, and need for intubation.[21-24] Resuscitation was performed most frequently in the intensive-care unit (in 42 per cent of the cases) or on the general ward (in 35 per cent). The most common mechanism of arrest was ventricular tachycardia or fibrillation (occurring in 33 per cent of the cases), followed closely by primary respiratory arrest (in 27 per cent). There was a wide range in the duration of the effort at resuscitation (from 2 to 180 minutes), but in the majority of patients (82 per cent) the effort lasted longer than 15 minutes, and in 61 per cent it lasted longer than 30 minutes. Cardiopulmonary resuscitation was initiated within five minutes after arrest in 89 per cent of the cases. Eighty-seven per cent of the patients were intubated.

TABLE 1   Characteristics of the Arrest.

	No. of Patients (%)
Location	
Intensive-care unit	124 (42)
General ward	103 (35)
Emergency ward	56 (19)
Other unit	11 (4)
Mechanism	
Ventricular tachycardia/ fibrillation	97 (33)
Respiratory	79 (27)
Asystole	53 (18)
Electromechanical dissociation	49 (16)
Complete heart block	11 (4)
Not known	5 (2)
Initial arterial PO$_2$ and pH*	
PO$_2$ $\leq$ 40	78 (27)
PO$_2$ > 40	201 (68)
PO$_2$ not known	15 (5)
pH $\leq$ 7.0	16 (5)
pH > 7.0	262 (90)
pH not known	16 (5)
Intubation required	
Yes	255 (87)
No	39 (13)
Duration	
$\leq$15 minutes	48 (16)
>15 minutes	241 (82)
Not known	5 (2)

*PO$_2$ denotes partial pressure of oxygen.

The initial partial pressure of oxygen was higher than 40 in 68 per cent of the cases, and the initial pH was higher than 7.0 in 90 per cent.

Predictors of Outcome after Cardiopulmonary Resuscitation

Clinical variables at the onset of cardiopulmonary resuscitation, during the arrest, and after resuscitation were compared in the group of patients who died and in the group of survivors who were discharged from the hospital. Table 2 lists the salient univariate variables that did not attain multivariate significance. Table 3 lists the significant predictors, according to the logistic regression multivariate analysis. The variables before, during, and after arrest, discussed below, are those identified in the multivariate analysis.

TABLE 2 Salient Univariate Predictors of Survival to Discharge from Hospital.*

Category	No. of Patients	No. of Survivors (%)
Demographic Information		
Sex		
Male	160	15 (9)
Female	134	26 (19)
Clinical information before resuscitation		
Renal failure (creatinine, mg/dl)		
≤2.5	214	38 (18)
>2.5	64	3 (5)
Not known	16	0 (0)
Coronary-artery disease		
History of angina		
Yes	165	34 (21)
No	118	7 (6)
Not known	11	0 (0)
Circulatory failure		
Congestive heart failure (class)		
I or II	25	14 (56)
III or IV	88	7 (8)
Not recorded	101	20 (20)
Urinary output (ml/24 hr)		
<300	87	0 (0)
≥300	115	31 (27)
Not recorded	92	10 (11)
S_3 *gallop*		
Yes	59	1 (2)
No	156	32 (21)
Not recorded	79	8 (10)
Sepsis		
Yes	42	0 (0)
No	243	39 (16)
Uncertain	9	2 (22)
Arrest factors		
Intubation		
Yes	255	22 (9)
No	39	19 (49)
Type		
Ventricular tachycardia/fibrillation	97	26 (27)
Other	192	15 (8)
Not recorded	5	0 (0)
After resuscitation		
No subsequent resuscitation†		
Yes	39	2 (5)
No	89	39 (44)

*$P < 0.01$.

†Written order not to resuscitate in case of subsequent cardiac arrest.

TABLE 3   Independently Significant Predictors of In-Hospital Mortality after Cardiopulmonary Resuscitation, by Logistic Regression Analysis.*

Characteristic	Estimated Coefficient
Before arrest	
Hypotension (blood pressure, <100 mm Hg)	2.69
Pneumonia	2.85
Renal failure (blood urea nitrogen, >50 mg/dl [18 mmol/l])	2.75
Cancer	2.06
Homebound life style	2.13
During arrest	
Arrest duration >15 minutes	2.51
Intubation	2.35
Hypotension (blood pressure, <100 mm Hg)	2.70
Pneumonia	2.48
Homebound life style	2.24
After resuscitation	
Coma	2.40
Need for pressors	2.16
Arrest duration >15 minutes	1.87

*Factors selected by three separate stepwise analyses (P < 0.05).

Variables before the Arrest   One important prognostic factor at the onset of cardiopulmonary resuscitation was circulatory failure, especially as indicated by hypotension (blood pressure, less than 100 mm Hg for at least one day before the arrest). Among the 110 patients who had hypotension before the arrest, only two survived (2 per cent). Both became homebound, and one remained severely depressed until his death seven months later. Of the 87 patients with a urinary output under 300 ml per 24 hours on the day before the arrest, none survived. Despite the univariate significance (P < 0.001) and 92 per cent mortality associated with Class III or IV congestive heart failure, this variable did not attain multivariate significance, probably because the majority (60 per cent) of patients with this characteristic also had hypotension before the arrest.

Renal failure, characterized by a blood urea nitrogen level higher than 50 mg per deciliter (18 mmol per liter), was an important predictor of mortality. Only 2 of the 75 patients (3 per cent) with renal failure survived. Neither of these patients had required dialysis.

Among patients in our hospital who die without efforts having been made to resuscitate them, those with cancer are most common (30 per cent). In our study population patients with cancer also had a low survival rate after resuscitation. Of the 59 patients with cancer, 4 (7 per cent) survived. None of them had metastatic disease, and in two patients with a history of carcinoma that had been resected more than 10 years earlier there was no pathological confirmation of disease.

A striking and unexpected finding was that none of the 58 patients who had pneumonia before resuscitation survived.

Finally, the patient's level of activity before hospitalization proved to be an important marker for the outcome after cardiopulmonary resuscitation. Patients who had been confined to home before hospitalization were much less likely to survive after resuscitation than were those who had been active outside the house. Only 6 of the 137 homebound patients (4 per cent) survived, as compared with 35 of the 128 patients (27 per cent) who had pursued activities outside the home before their acute illness ($P < 0.0001$).

For the patients with hypotension, renal failure, pneumonia, cancer, or a homebound life style, the mortality rate was 95 per cent. In contrast, the mortality rate for patients with none of these characteristics was 34 per cent ($P < 0.0001$).

In addition to the foregoing five characteristics, there were several disease categories in which no patient survived. Most notably, none of the 42 patients with sepsis and none of the 16 with a history of acute stroke accompanied by neurologic deficit were discharged from the hospital. In contrast, seven of eight patients (88 per cent) with a ventricular arrhythmia in the configuration of torsade de pointes[25] survived.

The patient's age and the electrocardiographic location of acute myocardial infarction—two characteristics previously considered to be predictors of poor outcome after cardiopulmonary resuscitation[22,26]—were not significant predictors in our cohort (Fig. 2). Although women were almost twice as likely to survive as men ($P = 0.01$), this difference was not significant in the context of a multivariate analysis based also on the patient's underlying disease and level of activity. Finally, it is of interest that the outcome of resuscitation in the 60 patients who had a history of prior cardiopulmonary arrest did not differ significantly from the outcome in the patients undergoing their first arrest.

Variables at the Time of Arrest   Significant variables at the time of the arrest were prolonged duration of the resuscitative effort and need for intubation. Patients who required intubation had a 91 per cent mortality, as opposed to a 51 per cent mortality for the patients who were not intubated ($P < 0.0001$). Among the 241 patients whose arrest lasted longer than 15 minutes, 95 per cent died. In contrast, mortality declined to 44 per cent overall for the patients who were resuscitated within 15 minutes after arrest ($P < 0.0001$). For the subset of patients who were resuscitated within 15 minutes and who had pursued activities outside the house before the arrest, mortality declined to 17 per cent. None of the surviving patients had an arrest that lasted longer than 30 minutes.

Within the framework of a logistic regression analysis, neither the location of the arrest in the hospital nor its mechanism differentiated between patients who died in-hospital and those who were discharged ($P > 0.5$).

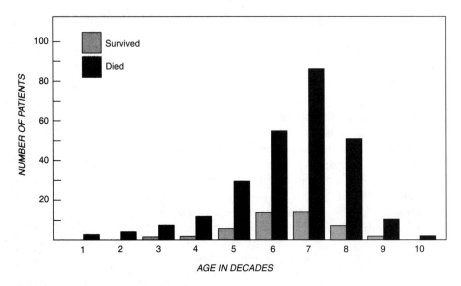

Figure 2. Age Distribution, in Decades, of the Cohort of 294 Patients. Age had no influence on survival.

Variables after the Arrest   The 128 patients who were still alive 24 hours after cardiopulmonary resuscitation can be divided into two prognostic groups (good and poor) on the basis of their level of consciousness, the need for pressors to maintain blood pressure, and the duration of the arrest. The patients who were successfully resuscitated within 15 minutes after arrest, were alert, and did not require pressors 24 hours after resuscitation had a survival rate of 92 per cent. In contrast, patients whose arrest lasted longer than 15 minutes, who were comatose, or who required pressors had a survival rate of 18 per cent (P < 0.0001). Only 1 patient of the 52 who were still in a coma 24 hours after cardiopulmonary resuscitation left the hospital. She remained lethargic at the time of discharge and died two months later.

Follow-up of Surviving Patients

Patient Responses to Arrest and Resuscitation   Thirty-eight of the 41 survivors of cardiopulmonary resuscitation described the experience of their arrest. The majority remembered nothing, but two patients recalled receiving a "hard bang" on the chest before losing consciousness. Several patients described vividly a "look of terror in the eyes of the doctors and nurses," and others recalled hearing physicians telling people to "get out of the room." No one remembered the experience of intubation or prolonged cardiac massage. Contrary to numerous reports about the psychic experiences of dying patients,[27] there was only one patient who described a "near-death" experience. For him the arrest "was peaceful, beautiful, and accompanied by angels over my head. It would have been an easy death."

All the patients remembered a sore chest on awakening. As one patient said, "They really beat the hell out of me." Several volunteered that they were frightened as they regained consciousness but that the doctors and nurses around the bed reassured them that they were all right. They reported that the hardest part of their subsequent hospital course was adjusting to "feeling sick" and dealing with the new loss of independence.

We asked the 38 mentally competent survivors whether they would choose to be resuscitated in the future, if it were necessary. Twenty-one (55 per cent) said yes, 16 (42 per cent) said no, and one was ambivalent. At follow-up six months later, three patients had changed their minds: two no longer desired resuscitation, and one said that she would choose it.

Evaluation of Mental Status   At discharge from the hospital, 28 of the 41 surviving patients (68 per cent) had an intact mental status on the basis of normal age-adjusted scores on the Wechsler memory scale[28] (Table 4). Of the remaining 13 patients, 10 (24 per cent) were alert and oriented but could not be tested formally because they were fatigued or did not speak English. Two were demented but had also been so before the arrest. Gross impairment of mental status, characterized by lethargy and minimal responsiveness to voice, occurred for the first time in only one patient. She returned to her nursing home and died two months after discharge from the hospital.

Evaluation of Depression   What is perhaps even more striking is the psychological adaptation of the survivors to their acute illness (Table 4). At the time of discharge, these patients were severely depressed, as reflected both by clinical affect and mean score on the Center for Epidemiologic Studies' depression scale. The mean score at discharge was 21, which is between the scores for acutely and chronically depressed control populations.[15] However, six months later the mean depression score had fallen significantly ($P < 0.0001$) and was within the range of scores for a normal community population.

Evaluation of Functional Status   Each patient reported a decrease in functional status, though the extent of impairment varied widely (Table 4). For some patients, decreased function meant only that activities were pursued more slowly than before the arrest or that hobbies, such as fishing, were abandoned. During the course of the six-month follow-up, 22 of the 41 patients (54 per cent) required one or more hospitalizations for acute illness. The majority of rehospitalizations (14 of 22) occurred within the first two months after discharge from the hospital. In addition, five patients who had lived at home before the cardiac arrest required institutionalization after it. Of nine patients who had been em-

TABLE 4   Follow-up Evaluation of Patients Who Were Discharged after Cardiopulmonary Resuscitation.*

	No. of Patients	
	at Discharge	at Six Months
Mental status	41	33
Alert, oriented, appropriate	38	31
Normal score on Wechsler memory scale	28	23
Tested only on orientation on Wechsler scale	10	8
Longstanding dementia	2	2
Newly abnormal mental status after CPR	1	0

	No. of Patients	Mean Score
Depression†		
CPR survivors		
At discharge	38	21
At six-month follow-up	31	11
Controls		
Community population	3992	9
Acutely depressed hospitalized patients	148	38
Recovered from depression	87	15

No. of Patients		
Functional status at six months		
(n = 33)		
New institutionalization	5	
New retirement	5 (of 9 employed before CPR)	
Newly homebound	10	
Total homebound	14	

*CPR denotes cardiopulmonary resuscitation.

†Score on the Center for Epidemiologic Studies' depression scale. Control data are from the Center for Epidemiologic Studies.

ployed before the arrest, five retired and two reduced their work schedules to half-time after the arrest.

In addition to the 4 patients confined to home before the arrest, 10 became homebound for the first time after it. A salient characteristic of at least half these patients was their incapacitation by fear, to a degree well beyond the limitations imposed by organic disease. Although this finding could not be documented retrospectively by standardized scales, many of these patients said that fear of another arrest led them to regulate their daily lives and limit their activities to ensure immediate access to medical care.

Discussion

Our study was undertaken to identify the characteristics of patients who were resuscitated in the hospital and to compare those who survived to be discharged with those who died. Fourteen per cent of the patients who underwent cardiopulmonary resuscitation were discharged from the hospital, and 11 per cent were still alive six months later. Though other series have reported success rates ranging from under 5 per cent[29] to over 20 per cent,[30] our figures do not vary substantially from the majority of reports over the past 20 years.[5] In addition, the present report details the functional status of the patients who survived to be discharged from the hospital. Our findings should prove helpful to patients who have been resuscitated, to their families, and to the professional staff caring for the patients.

Given the consistently high mortality for all patients with cardiogenic shock,[31] it is not surprising that we, like others, found a high (98 per cent) mortality rate among patients with severe left ventricular dysfunction before the cardiopulmonary arrest.[26,32] Similarly, the 96 per cent mortality rate among patients with cancer (100 per cent for patients with metastatic disease) is perhaps to be expected because of the multiorgan system failure so often associated with cancer in its late stages.[33] Also consistent with other reports[4] was the very high (98 per cent) mortality among patients with renal failure. Less expected, and to our knowledge not previously reported, was the uniformly poor outcome for patients with pneumonia, all of whom died in the hospital after cardiopulmonary resuscitation. It is also striking that the patient's activity level before hospitalization was an important predictor of survival after resuscitation.

The electrocardiographic mechanism of arrest has been considered a major determinant of survival. Our findings are consistent with the observations of other workers[2,4,22,24] that patients are more likely to survive when ventricular fibrillation, rather than asystole or electromechanical dissociation, is the initial rhythm. However, our multivariate analysis suggests that the duration of arrest is an even stronger predictor than the mechanism of arrest. Patients whose arrest lasted less than 15 minutes had a far better outcome than those whose arrest lasted longer than 15 minutes. Since efforts at resuscitation lasting more than 30 minutes appear to be uniformly unsuccessful, they should be abandoned except in unusual circumstances.[3,24,34] In addition, we found that in a hospital setting, where patients received prompt, supervised resuscitation, the location of arrest did not affect the outcome.

Our findings concerning the level of consciousness after cardiopulmonary resuscitation confirm the detailed evaluations of Caronna and Finklestein[35] and of Levy et al.,[36] and suggest that consciousness regained within one day after arrest predicts neurologic recovery and discharge from the hospital. The one surviving patient who remained semicomatose 24 hours after cardiopulmonary resuscitation was in a vegetative state at the time of discharge and died two months later.

a thorough consideration of the history of patients undergoing cardiopulmonary resuscitation should go far to dispel unnecessary anxiety and guilt, and will provide perspective when a decision must be made whether to attempt resuscitation in the event of a cardiac arrest.

References

1. Kouwenhoven WB, Jude JR, Knickerbocker GG. Closed-chest cardiac massage. JAMA 1960; 173:1064–7.
2. Hollingsworth JH. The results of cardiopulmonary resuscitation: a three-year university hospital experience. Ann Intern Med 1969; 71:459–66.
3. Jeresaty RM, Godar TJ, Liss JP. External cardiac resuscitation in a community hospital: a three-year experience. Arch Intern Med 1969; 124:588–92.
4. Johnson AL, Tanser PH, Ulan RA, Wood TE. Results of cardiac resuscitation in 552 patients. Am J Cardiol 1967; 20:831–5.
5. Lemire JG, Johnson AL. Is cardiac resuscitation worthwhile?: a decade of experience. N Engl J Med 1972; 286:970–2.
6. Baum RS, Alvarez H, Cobb LA. Survival after resuscitation from out-of-hospital ventricular fibrillation. Circulation 1974; 50:1231–5.
7. Kannel WB, Doyle JT, McNamara PM, Quickenton P, Gordon T. Precursors of sudden coronary death. Circulation 1975; 51:606–13.
8. Kuller L, Cooper M, Perper J. Epidemiology of sudden death. Arch Intern Med 1972; 129:714–9.
9. Liberthson RR, Nagel EL, Hirschman JC, Nussenfeld SR. Prehospital ventricular defibrillation N Engl J Med 1974; 291:317–21.
10. Schaffer WA, Cobb LA. Recurrent ventricular fibrillation and modes of death in survivors of out-of-hospital ventricular fibrillation. N Engl J Med 1975; 293:259–62.
11. Jackson DL, Younger S. Patient autonomy and death with dignity: some clinical caveats. N Engl J Med 1979; 301:404–8.
12. Lo B, Jonsen AR. Clinical decisions to limit treatment. Ann Intern Med 1980; 93:764–8.
13. Miles SH, Cranford R, Schultz AL. The do-not-resuscitate order in a teaching hospital: considerations and a suggested policy. Ann Intern Med 1982; 96:660–4.
14. Wechsler D. A standardized memory scale for clinical use. J Psychol 1945; 19:87–95.
15. Weissman MM, Sholomskas D, Pottenger M, Prusoff BA, Locke BZ. Assessing depressive symptoms in five psychiatric populations: a validation study. Am J Epidemiol 1977; 106:203–14.
16. Jarvick LF. Psychiatric symptoms and cognitive loss in the elderly evaluation and assessment techniques. New York: Halsted Press, 1979.
17. Brown BW, Hollander M. Statistics: a biomedical introduction. New York: John Wiley, 1977.
18. Harrell F. Statistical analysis system. North Carolina: SAS Institute, 1980.
19. Friedman JH. A recursive partitioning decision rule for nonparametric classification. IEEE Trans Comput C-26 1977; 404:404–8.
20. Gordon L, Olshen RA. Consistent nonparametric regression from recursive partitioning schemes. J Multivar Anal 1980; 10:611–27.

21. Camarata SJ, Weil MH, Hanashira PK, Shubin H. Cardiac arrest in the critically ill. I. A study of predisposing causes in 132 patients. Circulation 1971; 44:688–95.

22. Castagna J, Weil MH, Shubin H. Factors determining survival in cardiac arrest. Chest 1974; 65:527–9.

23. Filmore SJ, Shapiro M, Killip T. Serial blood gas studies during cardiopulmonary resuscitation. Ann Intern Med 1970; 72:465–9.

24. Stemmler EJ. Cardiac resuscitation: a one-year study of patients resuscitated within a university hospital. Ann Intern Med 1965; 63:613–8.

25. Smith WM, Gallagher JJ. Les torsades de pointes: an unusual ventricular arrhythmia. Ann Intern Med 1980; 93:578–84.

26. Robinson JS, Sloman G, Mathew TH, Goble AJ. Survival after resuscitation from cardiac arrest in acute myocardial infarction. Am Heart J 1965; 69:740–7.

27. Saborn MB. Recollections of death: a medical investigation. New York: Harper & Row, 1981.

28. Hulicka IM. Age difference in Wechsler memory scale score. J Genet Psychol 1966; 109:135–45.

29. Peschin A, Coakley CS. A five year review of 734 cardiopulmonary arrests. South Med J 1970; 63:506–10.

30. Coskey RL. Cardiopulmonary resuscitation. JAMA 1971; 217:79–80.

31. Friedberg CK. Cardiogenic shock in acute myocardial infarction. Circulation 1961; 23:325.

32. Gregory JJ, Grace WJ. Resuscitation of the severely ill patient with acute myocardial infarction. Am J Cardiol 1967; 20:836–41.

33. Swenson E, Matsuura J, Martinson IM. Effects of resuscitation for patients with metastatic cancers and chronic heart disease. Nurs Res 1979; 28:151–3.

34. Cane RD, Buchanan N. Length of survival after cardiac resuscitation in an intensive care unit. S Afr Med J 1978; 53:594–6.

35. Caronna JJ, Finklestein S. Neurological syndromes after cardiac arrest. Stroke 1978; 9:517–20.

36. Levy DE, Bates D, Caronna JJ, et al. Prognosis in nontraumatic coma. Ann Intern Med 1981; 94:293–301.

37. Grace WJ, Minogue WF. Resuscitation for cardiac arrest due to myocardial infarction. Dis Chest 1966; 50:173–5.

38. Sandoval RG. Survival rate after cardiac arrest in a community hospital. JAMA 1965; 194:675–7.

39. Naismith LD, Robinson JF, Shaw GB, MacIntyre MM. Psychological rehabilitation after myocardial infarction. Br Med J 1979; 1:439–42.

40. Mumford E, Schlesinger HJ, Glass GV. The effects of psychological intervention on recovery from surgery and heart attacks: an analysis of the literature. Am J Public Health 1982; 72:141–51.

41. Rahe RH, Ward HW, Hayes V. Brief group therapy in myocardial infarction rehabilitation: three to four-year follow-up of a controlled trial. Psychosom Med 1979; 41:229–42.

42. Shaw LW. Effects of a prescribed supervised exercise program on mortality and cardiovascular morbidity in patients after a myocardial infarction: the national exercise and heart disease project. Am J Cardiol 1981; 48:39–46.

43. Messert B, Quglieri CE. Cardiopulmonary resuscitation: perspectives and problems. Lancet 1976; 2:410–2.

44. Stephenson HE. Cardiac arrest and resuscitation. St. Louis, CV Mosby, 1958.
45. Peatfield RC, Taylor D, Sillet RW, et al. Survival after cardiac arrest in hospital. Lancet 1977; 2:1223–5.
46. Saphir R. External cardiac massage: prospective analysis of 123 cases and review of the literature. Medicine (Baltimore) 1968; 47:73–87.

Limitation of Medical Care
An Ethnographic Analysis

William Ventres, Mark Nichter, Richard Reed, and Richard Frankel

These authors represent the fields of family and community medicine (Ventres and Reed); anthropology (Nichter); and internal medicine (Frankel). Their empirical study uses in-depth discussions with doctors to evaluate the efficacy of a form used by the University of Arizona College of Medicine to elicit patients' preferences about treatment. The study demonstrates how empirical methods of analysis can provide essential information for evaluating the usefulness of institutional policies and practices.

In December of 1989, the University Medical Center (UMC) Bioethics Committee at the University of Arizona College of Medicine introduced a Limitation of Medical Care form. This form was developed, in part, to facilitate discussions between residents and patients about resuscitation issues. Its other purposes were: to give clear and timely guidance to involved health-care workers; to ensure consistency of treatment; to establish accountability for resuscitative decision making; and to protect the rights of patients to determine the course of their treatment.[1] The form was designed by the bioethics committee during the two years preceding its introduction. Over one-half of this committee's 17 members were physicians from the University of Arizona College of Medicine; the remainder were either faculty members from other departments at the University of Arizona, ancillary personnel at UMC, or community residents of Tucson.

The purpose of this study is to examine the use of the Limitation of Medical Care form in the context of actual hospital practice. Needed to accomplish this examination of DNR [do-not-resuscitate] communication and decision making is a research approach different from the strategies characterized by survey questionnaires,[2] hypothetical scenarios,[3] descriptive epidemiology,[4] and simulated discussions.[5] This study uses ethnographic methods drawn from the discipline of cultural anthropology. Several authors have recommended this research methodology to evaluate interactive elements of the resuscitation decision.[6] They suggest that clinically based ethnographic investigations should be used to explore what is said when discussing code status, how information is communicated among the parties involved, and the meaning that underlies this communication. In the context of this study, this method entails extensively analyzing the conduct and outcome of discussions in which doctors used the Limitation of Medical Care form to broach DNR orders with patients and their families.

Methods

We utilized three anthropologic techniques to gather information pertinent to this discussion: participant observation,[7] informant interviews, and microanalysis of discourse.[8] From February to May of 1990, the principal author attended morning rounds at the University of Arizona's family-practice inpatient service three days a week. The residents on the service identified from their newly admitted patients those with whom they chose to have discussions regarding resuscitation ($N = 8$). Written consent for inclusion in the study was obtained from the medical team members and those patients and families targeted for DNR discussion.

In three cases, the principal author observed discussions regarding DNR orders between doctor, patient, and family. These discussions were audiotaped, and a written description of nonverbal communication was recorded. Both prior to and following the above discussions, semistructured interviews regarding the discourse and process of decision making were conducted. Following this protocol, the principal author interviewed physicians, patients, involved family members, nurses, social workers, and members of the clergy. Selected informants were interviewed one to three months following each patient's hospital discharge or death. All primary observational and interview data, as well as secondary interpretive data, were recorded in journal or transcript form.

The next stage of the investigation involved the analysis of discourse and ethnographic data. The DNR discussions were transcribed according to standardized sociolinguistic convention, intended to capture important features of speech production as they occur from moment to moment.[9] Analysis of this communication centered on issues of control, giving and withholding information,[10] and attentiveness between participants.[11] Two people, the principal author and a sociolinguist (RF), blinded to all but necessary case information, reviewed these tapes in order to enhance reliability of interpretive content. Other informant interviews were transcribed without sociolinguistic notations.

Primary and secondary data were reviewed weekly with a medical anthropologist (MN) and a psychiatrist involved with behavioral aspects of medical care in the family-practice service. This reevaluation by colleagues served as a triangulation procedure to cross-check data and arrive at a consensus regarding interpretations.[12] To enhance credibility, member checks were conducted; that is, interpretations were discussed and tested with both professional and lay participants in the study.[13]

Results

The following cases were drawn from this examination. They describe how two family physicians in training used the Limitation of Medical Care form. The use of the form is placed in the context of the interaction between the medical team and the patients with their families. Each case also illustrates specific themes relating to the social and cultural aspects of the doctor-patient-family relationship.

Case 1

Sarah Jones[14] is a 51-year-old white woman from Ohio who came to Tucson with her husband in order to attend a local convention. A trip to this convention and Tucson's warm winter weather had become an annual event for the couple. The trips served as an important respite for Mrs. Jones. In Ohio, she was always exceedingly busy "cooking, cleaning, and looking after" her husband and teen-age son, the last of five children left at home; in addition she managed a household store. Mr. Jones stated that she smoked heavily and drank alcohol in between customers as a means of "controlling her depression." After witnessing a significant weight loss, Mr. Jones recognized something was seriously wrong. He encouraged her to stay in Ohio while he traveled. Mrs. Jones insisted on making the trip. Her husband, chronically dependent on his wife, passively agreed.

A few days after arriving in Tucson, Mrs. Jones became febrile and developed a productive cough with chest pain and shortness of breath. Taken to the UMC emergency room, Mrs. Jones noted that she had lost 25 pounds over the last six months. A physical exam revealed wheezes over the right lung field with decreased breath sounds superiorly; radiographs confirmed a necrotizing lobar pneumonia. She also had a marked enlargement of her liver [hepatomegaly]. Admission laboratory tests were performed, revealing an elevated white blood-cell count; elevated liver-function tests and a disorder of blood coagulation suggested chronic liver damage. The family-practice residents were called to admit her.

Upon seeing Mrs. Jones, the residents were struck by her frailness and weight loss. One later commented, "When we walked into the emergency room, I just looked at her and said to myself, this woman has cancer. I don't care if she has pneumonia." Nonetheless, Mrs. Jones immediately began receiving broad-spectrum antibiotics for the pneumonia and was placed on oxygen. The residents also started measures to avert alcohol withdrawal and initiated a diagnostic workup to detect the presumed underlying cancer.

Mrs. Jones's physical and mental status rapidly deteriorated. On the ward she became increasingly short of breath and had frequent short episodes of delirium. Given this rapid decline and the presumption of cancer, the residents considered discussing code status. They proceeded with this discussion after receiving the results of an abdominal ultrasound that showed hepatomegaly with multiple echogenic lesions, suggestive of metastatic disease. They explicitly based their decision to discuss DNR on the unlikely statistical chance of survival with pneumonia and metastases should Mrs. Jones require resuscitation. The residents knew of no previously established advance directives for Mrs. Jones's care.

The intern, Dr. Jim Adams, approached Mr. and Mrs. Jones on the evening of her second hospital day. At the time, Mrs. Jones was agitated. She was pulling on her two intravenous (IV) lines, tugging at her oxygen mask. The alarm on her pulse oximeter was sounding regularly. In a later interview, Dr. Adams reflected on the situation:

> I remember when I walked in there . . . . I said, this room is out of control. In fact, I told Mrs. Jones. I've been to a lot of hospital rooms, but when I went in there I just felt like it was like Romper Room gone berserk. It was like a bad day at Romper Room when I looked in. There were nurses all over. There was stool all over the floor. It was a bad sign.

Because of Mrs. Jones's apparent disorientation, Dr. Adams addressed his comments to her husband. The transcript of Dr. Adams's conversation with Mr. Jones follows:

Dr. A.:   Well, Mr. Jones, basically what I'd like to talk to you about is, is her condition.
Mr. J.:   Mmh hmh.
Dr. A.:   And I need to ask you some very direct questions. Um, she originally came in and we know that she has pneumonia.
Mr. J.:   Mmh hmh.
Dr. A.:   But as I mentioned when she first came in, I feel that there is something going on underneath the pneumonia.
Mr. J.:   Mmh hmh.
Dr. A.:   Because her 20-, her 25-pound weight loss, the way she looks overall is very thin.
Mr. J.:   Yes.
Dr. A.:   And now with her acting in a real disorganized manner, um, it makes—I'm fairly certain that there's something else going on, although as yet we don't have a diagnosis. Sometimes it takes a while.
Mr. J.:   Mmh.
Dr. A.:   Um, to be honest, after I—reviewing the results of her ultrasound and looking at her chest film I think that there is a good chance that she has cancer, and I'm not sure where it came from.

After a short exchange during which Mr. Jones responded that his wife was always putting off physical examinations, the discussion continued.

Dr. A.:   So I guess the, um, the thing that we need to talk about right now in this setting is have you given any thought to what would happen with Sarah, or what you would like to have done in the event that she is in a grave [condition]?

Mr. J.: [Mmh hmh.] Well, yes, yes, I would like to get her back to Ohio.
Dr. A.: Okay.
Mr. J.: Because definitely, like all her family is there. I don't have any family, but all hers is there.
Dr. A.: Okay. Okay. If something should happen to her during this hospitalization, have you given any thought, and have you discussed with your wife [what you would like to do?]
Mr. J.: [No.]
Dr. A.: You haven't discussed that?
Mr. J.: No, I don't even want to.
Dr. A.: Okay.
Mr. J.: I don't want to alarm her. . . .

Three issues characterized the remainder of the interview. First, the content continued along the lines of the above discourse. Dr. Adams asked specific questions about intubation, defibrillation, and pressor medication, using lay terminology. Mr. Jones replied in each case that he wanted the measures undertaken to ensure her return to Ohio. Second, the conversation remained dyadic, between Dr. Adams and Mr. Jones. The patient herself was drawn into the conversation only to confirm her husband's wishes, which she appeared to do even though confused. Third, an unspoken sense of ambiguity pervaded the discussion. Neither Dr. Adams nor Mr. Jones seemed to sense the meaning of what the other was saying during the interview. As a result of this discussion, no Limitation of Medical Care form was filled out. Mrs. Jones remained a full code.

Follow-up ethnographic interviews confirmed these characterizations of the initial discussion regarding CPR. Shortly following his conversation with Mr. Jones, Dr. Adams recounted to researchers his need to gather information about the specific aspects of the resuscitative process as delineated in the Limitation of Medical Care form, even though his gut feeling told him that Mrs. Jones would not survive a code and that neither she nor her husband truly wanted her to undergo unsuccessful resuscitative efforts. Even when reviewing the narrow concerns of medical viability, he recognized the existence of conflict when each resuscitative measure was taken out of global context:

> I feel that overall, that if this woman was to code, she would not come back. That's basic. But when you get down to particular things, for example, defibrillation, I think her heart's strong, I think it would come back, okay? So I think, yeah, she could probably withstand that. If it comes down to respirator, she's got one good lung! So, I can't argue with that. When it comes down to pressor agents, again, her heart is strong enough. So sure, she could have that. She's already getting antibiotics and IV fluids, and nutrition is not necessarily an issue right now. So in other words, although my overall feeling is that I would like this patient to be a no code, because I really don't think in the long run she's going to make it, when you break it down item by item, I can't argue with his decision on any one of them.

On the other hand, Dr. Adams noted that the Limitation of Medical Care form did allow him a structure with which to approach the interview, making it easy for him to cover major medical contingencies. What it lacked was "room to say the *patient* does not want resuscitation" and why. Dr. Adams understood Mr. Jones's desire that his wife return home and his insistence that resuscitative efforts be instituted if necessary; he lacked the institutional authority to recognize formally these patient needs.

Mr. Jones later recalled that his concern throughout the interview was that if the UMC physicians were to discover a cancer and operate, he believed his wife would die suddenly. His mother had recently died rapidly from lung cancer, without anyone knowing she was ill. A passive man, Mr. Jones was afraid he would be blamed for his wife's death if he did not encourage resuscitation. Yet no one else in the family even knew she was hospitalized.

For her part, Mrs. Jones occupied herself during the DNR conversation with efforts to pull out her IV lines. It was only the following morning, when Dr. Adams returned with the rest of the family-practice team to examine Mrs. Jones, that her understanding could be assessed. Her night had been restless, and she now wore soft restraints. She was lucid, however, when Dr. Adams asked her to recollect the previous evening's talk.

> **Dr. A.:** Mrs. Jones, do you remember the discussion that I had yesterday with you and your husband? At that time we were discussing what you would like us to do in the event that you become gravely ill, and we would need to do things like start your heart, or have you be on a breathing machine.
>
> **Mrs. J.:** Right. I remember that.
>
> **Dr. A.:** You remember that? Could you just tell us a little bit about how you, how did you feel about that conversation?
>
> **Mrs. J.:** If it was my heart?
>
> **Dr. A.:** Mmh hmh.
>
> **Mrs. J.:** If it was my heart, go ahead. If it was cancer, I don't want anything done.
>
> **Dr. A.:** If you have cancer, you don't want us to do anything for your body?
>
> **Mrs. J.:** No.

In contrast to the night before, Mrs. Jones showed only a few signs of confusion and agitation. Her responses to direct questions were clear. During an interview with researchers held immediately following the above discussion, the senior resident recognized this cognitive change in Mrs. Jones as well as the apparent conflict in resuscitative choice between husband and wife:

> During this interview, Mrs. Jones was the most lucid I've seen her, and even though it was a directed interview, no one directed it to the point of saying, "This is what we think you should do." We basically gave her an open-ended question and said, "In this circumstance what would you do?" She in her own mind separated the heart

from cancer. We didn't separate that for her, and she was fairly clear about what she wanted to do, so. . . . I think she's told us her wishes.

Before making any changes in code status, the medical team opted to wait for the results of further investigative studies to confirm the suspected cancer. The remainder of Mrs. Jones's course at UMC was rocky. The following day a CT [computerized tomography] head scan revealed a 100 cc left-hemispheric subdural hemorrhage, for which she was transferred to the intensive care unit (ICU). She also developed an upper gastrointestinal (GI) bleed, evidenced by black, tarry stools. Laboratory results confirmed *Staphylococcus aureus* as the cause of her lung infection and associated bacteremia; they also documented a decrease in fibrinogen [a globulin that is produced in the liver that is converted to fibrin during clotting of blood] and the development of fibrin split products, suggestive of impending disseminated intravascular coagulation. Her clinical course paralleled these distressing data. She initially had difficulty articulating words, then began hallucinating. Her respiratory status deteriorated as her fevers continued.

After two days in the ICU, she dramatically improved. Her delirium cleared. Her physical status was still tenuous, but she was stable enough to be transferred back to the ward. Further investigations documented no clear evidence of cancer as a direct etiology for the constellation of ailments afflicting her. After two weeks at UMC she was transferred to an Ohio hospital by air ambulance, with instructions for completion of her antibiotic course, observation of her intracranial and gastrointestinal bleeding, and alcohol treatment. She was back working six weeks after transfer.

Case 2

Martin Reyes is a 35-year-old Native American who grew up not on the nearby reservation, but in Minneapolis, where his father had worked. His past medical history was significant for surgical removal of the left-upper lobe of his lung for tuberculosis at the age of three. Subsequently, he had multiple traumatic accidents but no major illnesses. Upon returning to Arizona, he avoided the reservation and lived in Tucson with his Anglo girlfriend. She characterized him as a happy-go-lucky person who found pleasure in singing in a rock band and solace in drinking.

He was admitted to the family-practice service with a GI bleed and altered mental status. Two weeks prior to his admission he had begun binge drinking and developed jaundice, nausea, and vomiting. His cognitive abilities progressively deteriorated to the point of admission, when he was agitated but unresponsive.

Examination in the emergency room demonstrated jaundice, enlargement of his liver, and heme-positive stool. Laboratory examination revealed marked anemia, electrolyte imbalances, renal insufficiency, and a disorder affecting coagulation of the blood. Mr. Reyes was admitted to the ICU for his upper GI bleed. Endoscopy showed enlarged veins in the esophagus; sclerotherapy was performed. The patient was transfused. Because of his mental status changes, the patient was intubated to protect his airway.

Mr. Reyes was extubated two days later. As his mental status gradually improved and his hematocrit remained stable over the next few days, he was transferred to the ward. During the hospitalization, the patient's urine output fell. Serial examinations showed worsening renal function, in spite of massive intravenous hydration and diuretics. Together with his poor liver status, this information suggested the patient had developed hepatorenal syndrome with its associated dismal prognosis. While the patient's mental status improved, it never returned to baseline.

At the point when the ward team decided that no further diagnostic or therapeutic studies would change this diagnosis of hepatorenal syndrome, the intern, Dr. Bob Smith, called the family together to discuss code status. Family members included Mr. Reyes's mother, two adult sisters who lived on a nearby reservation, and his girlfriend . . . team consensus was that the family believed Mr. Reyes was improving and would have no problems leaving the hospital. The ward resident reviewed with Dr. Smith the importance of communicating how serious Mr. Reyes's illness was before reviewing his resuscitative disposition.

The discussion regarding resuscitation was conducted at Mr. Reyes's bedside. The four family members faced Dr. Smith, who was partially turned away from the patient. Dr. Smith began the interview by reviewing the course of this hospitalization and the development of hepatorenal syndrome. Step by step, he told the family of Mr. Reyes's liver dysfunction, bleeding in his stomach, and kidney failure. He noted how these problems were due to drinking. . . .

Dr. Smith next reviewed why it was important for the family to participate in the decision making, suggesting that Mr. Reyes was not competent to "make all the decisions that have to be made." In response to the family's questions about his physical condition, he again reviewed the causative elements of hepatorenal syndrome and the poor prognosis awaiting Mr. Reyes, noting that he would likely steadily get worse and live only a short time. Dr. Smith then continued:

Dr. S.: So, that said, I'd like to just bring up some issues that, that we can talk about now, and that you can talk among yourselves, and you can talk to Martin about, about how we're going to react to problems that he's going to have in the future. And what exactly you want us as the, as the doctors to do for Martin. Some things that we, we have to decide, are—if, if he gets worse, for instance, and you need to have, uh, what we call life support, you need to be intubated, and put on the ventilator, we'd like to know how you'd feel about that. We'd also like to know, if Martin has ever talked about that, has ever talked about being on life [support systems].

Friend: [I don't think] he'd want it, anything.

Dr. S.: Has he ever mentioned it to [you?]

Friend: [Yeah.]

Dr. S.: What did he say?

Friend: He just, we've talked about, you know, if he'd been sick in the hospital, if, you know, you couldn't do anything, there wasn't any chance, that we wouldn't want to prolong it.

Sister: Indians don't care for life support.

Dr. S.: Don't care for life support?

Sister: Uh-huh. (indicating affirmative)

Dr. S.: Okay, um, there are, there are a lot of issues, and, and one of them is, is, uh, quality of life versus quantity of life. There's a chance that it will come to a point where we could keep Martin physically alive, but, uh, but he wouldn't, he wouldn't necessarily be conscious. He couldn't necessarily communicate. And he might not be comfortable. So it might come to a point where we have to decide whether to make, uh, Martin comfortable, or to extend his life to give him more time, even though that treatment might make him uncomfortable. . . . So that's a question that, it sounds like Martin has already talked to you some, and you already have some ideas about how you feel about that . . . But we would like to, to have an idea of, of, uh, how far you'd like us to go, or if you'd want him to be on a respirator, what you'd want us to do if his heart went bad, if you want us to do chest compressions, that type of thing. How would you feel if his heart, his heart stopped? How would you feel about the chest compressions we could do? About medicine, or electroshock that we give to restart the heart?

Each of the family members was offered a chance to ask questions; each responded. One sister, a nurse's assistant, asked how to spell hepatorenal. Another reaffirmed that resuscitation was not appropriate in Indian culture, and she related stories of relatives who had chosen not to undergo resuscitation. Mr. Reyes's mother, the designated decision maker in the family, asked if he would need to be shocked multiple times if his "heart attacked."

The conversation concluded when Dr. Smith suggested the family consider the issues among themselves. A second family conference was scheduled for later that evening. Following the discussion, Dr. Smith expressed his satisfaction with the way things had gone in an interview with the researchers. He had accomplished his goals in the conversation. As he expressed it:

> I think it's important for the physician to lay out the situation, the patient's clinical status, his prognosis, and his treatment options. And then I think it's important for the physician to ask the patient and the family to clarify that they understand what the situation is, that they understand the options, and that they share what their views are as to quality-of-life issues and how they view the basic treatment and support issues.

He had been explicit in his description of hepatorenal syndrome. He had heard their questions about resuscitative measures. He had allowed them time to consider this important decision.

The family members, however, had different concerns that they expressed in interviews with the researchers following Dr. Smith's visit. The eldest daughter wondered why Dr. Smith proceeded to describe in technical detail the resuscitative measures, even after they had made it clear that none were desired. She felt that he really didn't trust their decision. Mr. Reyes's girlfriend began to ruminate over the patient's lack of participation in the discussion, questioning how they could talk about him in his presence, without acknowledging his feelings. In an interview with researchers one month after Mr. Reyes's death, his mother reflected upon the pain she thought he was experiencing. . . .

Following the DNR discussion, the family members left the room and talked among themselves. Several expressed their concern that Mr. Reyes would give up all hope after hearing his prognosis. They confirmed that neither did he want resuscitative efforts, nor was it culturally appropriate. When they met again with Dr. Smith and his attending physician, they again communicated their desire not to have resuscitative efforts performed. The Limitation of Medical Care form was filled out, indicating that no intubation, chest compression, defibrillation, or pressor agents would be used should the patient arrest. The following morning, in his sleep, Mr. Reyes died of a massive gastrointestinal hemorrhage.

Discussion

While the styles of the two physicians differed, their agendas dominated the discussions regarding resuscitation. Dr. Adams listened to the calls by Mrs. Jones's husband to return to Ohio, but redirected the conversation back to issues of intubation, defibrillation, and pressor medicines. His task was to fulfill the requirements of the Limitation of Medical Care form. Dr. Smith, on the other hand, followed a prestructured strategy that paralleled the form's content. When the patient's family explicitly disclosed that resuscitation was incompatible with both their cultural and personal beliefs, Dr. Smith proceeded to address the mechanical aspects of CPR, without acknowledging the family members' expressed concerns.

These cases suggest that the requirements of the Limitation of Medical Care form shaped the structure of the physicians' conversations with patients about resuscitation. For doctors in training, these guidelines on how to conduct a code discussion are reassuring. They provide a framework for handling a difficult situation, one with which they have little previous instruction. If they fill out the form for the attending physician's signature, the residents believe they have adequately accomplished the job of discussing code status with patients and families.

Without reference to context or guidelines for use, the Limitation of Medical Care form represents a framework that limits exploration of the patient's values and beliefs. The form narrowly lists the needs of physicians considering DNR orders, and it offers no intent to document the wishes of the patient or family. It also reduces the decision to only part of a whole. Rather than asking for global decisions regarding resuscitation, it stipulates particular treatment modalities. Medical residents, mindful of time and emotional pressures, are quick to recognize the narrow limits of their responsibilities, in this case a responsibility to check off the declined treatments on the form. The decision-making process in these two cases was thus intervention-specific,[15] narrowly focusing on the particulars of resuscitation without taking into account the social, emotional, or family context in which decisions were being made.

Patients and families make decisions based on other factors. At the same time that doctors talk about the possible mechanical interventions, patients and families are thinking about other decisions, in the context of their past experiences. Mr. Jones interpreted the intern's presentation of resuscitation to mean that aggressive diagnostic interventions soon awaited his wife. Reflecting on the process of his mother's death and how he wanted to avoid being blamed for his wife's death, he decided Mrs. Jones needed to return home before she died. Any resuscitative measures at UMC were justified to ensure this outcome. The mother of Mr. Reyes, the identified decision maker in the family, thought of medical interventions only as they related to the pain her son experienced as a young child. She did not want him to endure any more suffering. In each of the two cases reported, the doctors confused patients or families by not explaining the logic behind their statements and queries. While following procedure, they left people uninformed and doubtful that their concerns were heard.

That doctors and patients think and talk in different interactive frames is well known.[16] These frames of reference represent divergent world experiences and beliefs that are respectively communicated through the "voice of medicine" and the "voice of the life world."[17] As Kleinman has noted, patients and doctors often view sickness and the roles and responsibilities associated with it in terms of different explanatory models.[18] Each has different beliefs on the etiology of disease, resolution of infirmity, and management of a good death.[19]

In the context of DNR decision making, divergent explanatory models can lead to conflicting and confusing demands on doctors, patients, and families. The need of clinicians to "get a code status" reduces the life-and-death decision regarding in-hospital resuscitation to mechanistic criteria, and doctors often fail to use these criteria to clarify important patient and family desires based on other experiential and cultural contingencies. It is difficult to shift frames of reference, given the existing structure of physicians' and patients' interactions, which are based around significantly different objectives. The need of physicians to objectify and decontextualize information makes them unable to discover the meanings their patients and families intend to offer.[20] The normative bias of clinical ethics and the medicalization of DNR decision making preferentially favor the demands of clinicians over the wants of patients and families. A focus on treatments replaces a focus on goals.

While the Presidential Commission on Biomedical Ethics and others have recognized patient's rights to decide their own choice of medical interventions in terminal situations,[21] the bureaucratic transformation of ethical decision making, as embodied in the Limitation of Medical Care form, has tended to remove control from patients and their families when no advance directive is in place. . . .

Summary

This ethnographic study has shown how one attempt to apply ethical principles through a routine procedure failed to fit the clinical context and, in the two cases studied, served to counteract the very foundation these principles were based on—that patients or their families have the right to determine life-and-death decisions regarding code status. The results suggest that the use of well-meaning forms that are intended to facilitate decision making can, in the absence of appropriate guidelines, routinize the doctor-patient discourse to meet bureaucratic needs, narrowing rather than expanding understanding and communication. Bioethical principles implemented in abstraction, apart from the complex intricacies of the doctor-patient-family relationship and the sociocultural influences upon which this relationship is dependent, may be counter-productive to patient interests.

As bioethicists and clinicians work to implement the demands of the Patient Self-Determination Act,[22] they will undoubtedly try to forestall legal problems, assure ethical consistency, facilitate auditing, and promote documentation by creating forms. They may look to create inventories, such as the Limitation of Medical Care form described here, or turn to other, less explicit, means of documentation.[23] This study suggests that, in these efforts, genuine attention should be given to patient concerns, not just to the ethical or institutional needs of medicine. This shift in focus from outcome to process can enhance patient and clinician satisfaction, help resolve difficulties in reaching consensus between involved decision makers, and return the power in DNR decision making to patients and families.

References

1. D. Mattheiu, "Advance Directives" (Paper presented at the University of Arizona College of Medicine, Tucson, 25 May 1990).
2. D. Crane, "Decisions to Treat Critically Ill Patients: A Comparison of Social versus Medical Considerations," *Milbank Memorial Fund Quarterly* 53 (Winter 1975): 1–33; D.A. Schwartz and P. Reilly, "The Choice Not to Be Resuscitated," *Journal of the American Geriatrics Society* 34 (1986): 807–11; C.J. Stolman, J.J. Gregory, D. Dunn, and J.L. Levine, "Evaluation of Patient, Physician, Nurse, and Family Attitudes toward Do Not Resuscitate Orders," *Archives of Internal Medicine* 150 (1990): 653–58; D. Frankel, R.K. Oye, and P.E. Bellamy, "Attitudes of Hospitalized Patients toward Life Support: A Survey of 200 Medical Inpatients," *American Journal of Medicine* 86 (1989): 645–48.
3. M. Kohn and G. Menon, "Life Prolongation: Views of Elderly Outpatients and Health Care Professionals," *Journal of the American Geriatrics Society* 36 (1988): 840–44; R.H. Shmerling, S.E. Bedell, A. Lilienfeld, and T.L. DelBanco, "Dis-

cussing Cardiopulmonary Resuscitation: A Study of Elderly Outpatients," *Journal of General Internal Medicine* 3 (1988): 317–21.

4. R.F. Uhlmann, W.J. McDonald, and T.S. Inui, "Epidemiology of No-Code Orders in an Academic Hospital," *Western Journal of Medicine* 140 (1984): 114–16; S.E. Bedell, D. Pelle, P.L. Maher, and P.B. Cleary, "Do-Not-Resuscitate Orders for Critically Ill Patients in the Hospital," *Journal of the American Medical Association* 256 (1986):233–37; C.J. Stolman, J.J. Gregory, D. Dunn, and B. Ripley, "Evaluation of the Do Not Resuscitate Orders at a Community Hospital," *Archives of Internal Medicine* 149 (1989): 1851–56; K. Gleeson and S. Wise, "The Do-Not-Resuscitate Order: Still Too Little Too Late," *Archives of Internal Medicine* 150 (1990): 1057–60.

5. A. Miller and B. Lo, "How Do Doctors Discuss Do-Not-Resuscitate Orders?" *Western Journal of Medicine* 143 (1985): 256–58; S.H. Miles, S. Bannick-Mohrland, and N. Lurie, "Advance-Treatment Planning Discussions with Nursing Home Residents: Pilot Experience with Simulated Interviews," *The Journal of Clinical Ethics* 1 (1990): 108–12.

6. Schwartz and Reilly, "The Choice Not to Be Resuscitated"; H. Brody, "Commentary to M.H. Ebell, M.A. Smith, K. Seifert, and K. Polsinelli: 'The Do-Not-Resuscitate Order: Outpatient Experience and Decision-Making Preferences,' " *Journal of Family Practice* 31 (1990): 630–36.

7. J.P. Spradley, *The Ethnographic Interview* (New York: Holt, Rinehart, and Winston, 1979), 32–34.

8. R.M. Frankel and H.B. Beckman, "Conversation and Compliance with Treatment Recommendations: An Application of Micro-Interactional Analysis in Medicine," in *Rethinking Communication*, vol. 2, *Paradigm Exemplars*, ed. B. Dervin, L. Grossberg, B.J. O'Keefe, E. Wartella (Beverly Hills, Calif.: Sage, 1989), 60–74; J. Nessa and K. Malterud, "Discourse Analysis in General Practice: A Sociolinguistic Approach," *Family Practice* 7 (June 1990): 77–83.

9. Frankel and Beckman, "Conversation and Compliance with Treatment Recommendations."

10. H. Waitzkin, "Information Giving in Medical Care," *Journal of Health and Social Behavior* 26 (1985): 81–101.

11. E.G. Mishler, J.A. Clark, J. Ingelfinger, and M.P. Simon, "The Language of Attentive Patient Care: A Comparison of Two Medical Interviews," *Journal of General Internal Medicine* 4 (1989): 325–35.

12. E.G. Guba, "Criteria for Assessing the Trustworthiness of Naturalistic Inquiries," *Education and Communication and Technology Journal* 29 (1981): 75–91.

13. Y.S. Lincoln and E.G. Guba, *Naturalistic Inquiry* (Beverly Hills, Calif.: Sage, 1985), 314–16.

14. All names are pseudonyms.

15. A.S. Brett, "Limitations of Listing Specific Medical Interventions in Advance Directives," *Journal of the American Medical Association* 266 (1991): 825–28.

16. D.A. Evans, M.R. Block, E.R. Steinberg, and A.M. Penrose, "Frames and Heuristics in Doctor-Patient Discourse," *Social Science & Medicine* 22 (1986): 1027–34.

17. E. Mishler, *Interrupting the Voice of Medicine: A Radical Analysis,* "The Discourse of Medicine: Dialectics of Medical Interviews" (Norwood, N.J.: Ablex, 1984), 95–135.

18. A. Kleinman, *Patients and Healers in the Context of Culture* (Berkeley: University of California Press, 1980), 104–11; A. Kleinman, *The Illness Narratives: Suffering, Healing, and the Human Condition* (New York: Basic Books, 1988), 43–55.
19. W.B. Ventres, "Communicating about Resuscitation: Problems and Prospects," *Journal of the American Board of Family Practice* 6 (1993): 137–41.
20. A.V. Cicourel, "Hearing Is Not Believing: Language and Structure of Belief in Medical Communication," in *The Social Organization in Doctor-Patient Communication*, ed. S. Fisher and A.D. Todd (Washington, D.C.: Center for Applied Linguistics, 1983), 221–39.
21. President's Commission for the Study of Ethical Problems in Medicine and Biomedical and Behavioral Research, *Deciding to Forego Life-Sustaining Treatment: A Report on the Ethical, Medical and Legal Issues in Treatment Decisions* (Washington, D.C.: U.S. Government Printing Office, 1983); S.H. Wanzer, S.J. Adelstein, R.E. Cranford, *et al.*, "The Physician's Responsibility toward Hopelessly Ill Patients," *New England Journal of Medicine* 310 (1984): 955–59; AMA Council on Ethical and Judicial Affairs, "Guidelines for the Appropriate Use of Do-Not-Resuscitate Orders," *Journal of the American Medical Association* 265 (1991): 1868–71.
22. J.C. Fletcher, "The Patient Self-Determination Act: Yes," *Hastings Center Report* 20 (September–October 1990): 33–35; A.M. Capron, "The Patient Self-Determination Act: Not Now," *Hastings Center Report* 20 (September–October 1990): 86; J. La Puma, D. Orentlicher, and R.J. Moss, "Advance Directives on Admission: Clinical Implications and Analysis of the Patient Self-Determination Act of 1990," *Journal of the American Medical Association* 266 (1991): 402–5; M.L. White and J.G. Fletcher, "The Patient Self-Determination Act: On Balance, More Help Than Hindrance," *Journal of the American Medical Association* 266 (1991): 410–12.
23. F. Davila, E.V. Boisaubin, and D.A. Sears, "Patient Care Categories: An Approach to Do-Not-Resuscitate Decisions in a Public Teaching Hospital," *Critical Care Medicine* 14 (1986): 1066–67; Stolman, Gregory, Dunn and Ripley, "Evaluation of the Do Not Resuscitate Orders at a Community Hospital."

Should Medical Encounters Be Studied Using Ethnographic Techniques?

Cynthia J. Stolman

Cynthia J. Stolman is a clinical ethicist at Children's Hospital of New Jersey and a member of the faculty of the Department of Pediatrics, New Jersey Medical School, Newark.
In this essay she compares the advantages of quantitative and qualitative methods of conducting empirical research. Stolman argues that although both kinds of empirical research provide vital information for ethical analysis, there are certain insights about medical culture that can be gained only by using qualitative techniques.

In "Limitation of Medical Care: An Ethnographic Analysis," William Ventres, Mark Nichter, Richard Reed, and Richard Frankel state that an approach other than "survey questionnaires, hypothetical scenarios, descriptive epidemiology, and simulated discussions" is called for in order to evaluate their institution's Limitation of Medical Care form. The ethnographic interview technique that the authors use is not commonly seen in the medical literature. Margaret Mead's detailed study of the culture of a Samoan village is probably the most widely known example of the use of the ethnographic interview technique. Scientific and medical research, with the exception of the individual case report, tend to employ descriptive or inferential statistics. Since ethnographic research and conventional techniques that use inferential statistics are very different methods of research, a closer look at the purpose and procedures of these techniques is relevant before proceeding.

Ethnographic research in its purest form is the study of a particular culture from the perspective of those who live within that culture. Specific research questions and hypotheses are not formulated. The purpose of the enterprise is to discover and accurately describe how people view the subject under study. The research moves from the particular to the general, where major themes are identified, a thesis is stated, and eventually a comparison is made to other cultures. Data collection should include random sampling of discourse. Sampling proceeds until the ethnographer is satisfied that no new information is being found and that the widest range of data has been collected for a particular category. The ethnographer should apply standardized rules for recording conversations, and other researchers should confirm interpretations. At some point, the researcher makes an intuitive leap from the many particular statements, in which a great deal of ethnographic information is synthesized, to the general statement. The task of communicating ethnographic research is done through specific examples of incidents that illustrate the generalizations. This type of research can lead to the generation of hypotheses for later testing, but the purpose of the enterprise is to become familiar with the particular culture. The ethnographer searches for meaningful questions to describe the culture that is under study, and often the questions change as the research progresses. The validity and reliability of the methodology is established through random sampling and standardized procedures for transcribing and interpreting discourse. Results are reported in narrative form.[1]

In contrast to this methodology, survey and epidemiologic research define the terms and the relevant questions to be asked in the form of hypotheses to be tested. For survey research, questionnaires are subject to pretest procedures to assure the validity and reliability of test instruments. Investigators follow specific procedures for choosing a research design, sampling the population, and deciding upon the sample size. All this is done to assure that the results are valid, reliable, and reproducible. Data are subject to standardized procedures to avoid biasing the results, and analyzed using statistical tests appropriate to the type of data, research design, and hypotheses to be tested. The research results appear in quantitative form and are subject to tests of significance according to a preset standard. If appropriate procedures are followed, inferences can be made to the larger population, and patient-care and policy decisions can be made.[2]

The central question that is raised by the study by Ventres *et al.* is: How well does the ethnographic technique answer the authors' stated purpose—"to examine the use of the Limitation of Medical Care form in the context of actual hospital practice"? While the methodology of cultural anthropology appears attractive because of the rich descriptive exchanges that occur between participants, there are a number of problems with the way the authors apply this technique to the stated purpose of the study.

The authors mention a sample of eight patients who were identified for DNR discussion. However, they provide no discussion of these cases. We are told that data were collected for only three patients, but the study displays partial data for only two patients. The authors do not indicate what criteria were used to select the two reported cases, and they do not explain how or why passages were selected for inclusion in the study. For example, there is one seemingly gratuitous passage included, where Dr. Adams reflects on entering Mrs. Jones's room and finding it "like a bad day at Romper Room." There is no comment in the discussion that would help the reader appreciate why this passage was chosen for inclusion and other passages were not. The reader is not shown important sections of dialogue that form the basis for the reported conclusions; therefore, the reader must rely upon the researchers' report and interpretation.

Glaser and Strauss state that it is never sufficient to study one incident in one group. Many incidents are needed to arrive at categories and describe their properties.[3]

The authors have included two statements that are not supported in any way by the data that they present. They state that the Limitation of Medical Care form lacked "room to say the *patient* does not want resuscitation and why." Clearly, the form does contain a place to indicate the patient's stated wishes. The physician is able to include a written statement of what the patient wants under Section 3c, where the form states: "the reasons why certain medical therapy is now inappropriate." The authors' second unsupported statement is as follows: "Dr. Adams understood Mr. Jones's desire that his wife return home and his insistence that resuscitative efforts be instituted if necessary; he lacked the institutional authority to recognize formally these patient needs." This statement contradicts the Limitation of Medical Care policy, which states in the first sentence: "The presumption in every patient is that full cardiopulmonary resuscitation and medical support will be provided unless changed by a specific order signed and dated by the responsible attending physician." According to this policy, there is no need to recognize formally that the patient desires to be resuscitated, since this will be done automatically unless there is an order to the contrary.

The authors imply in the discussion section that the residents were given little preparation for how to perform the interview other than that they were told to use the Limitation of Medical Care form. In the second reported case, we are told that Mr. Reyes's sister was upset that the resident continued to read through a list of resuscitation procedures after the family had indicated that they did not want resuscitation. It is reasonable to assume that, lacking prior instruction, the resident may have thought that the aim of the exercise was to document the patient's and/or the surrogate's feelings about the specific items listed on the form. If the resident had received instruction regarding how to conduct an interview on forgoing life-sustaining treatment, then we would expect to see some signs of familiarity with the process and sensitivity to the patient's and/or family's responses. Conducting discussions of forgoing life-sustaining treatment are difficult even for experienced physicians; they are certainly not part of the experience of the average resident. As the authors point out, to conduct these interviews compassionately and effectively requires instruction and guided practice. Without considering the ethical issues, most would agree that it would be a waste of time to study the ability of two surgical interns to perform a successful bowel resection independently without prior instruction. Similarly, it is unreasonable to expect untutored residents to engage in sensitive interviews without prior instruction.

The ethnographic techniques used in this study provide insight into the lack of experience of two residents in conducting a special type of interview. It is certainly not valid to draw the conclusion that the policy or the hospital form are at fault. We might easily predict that any resident—or, for that matter, even a member of the bioethics committee—who, without prior instruction, is given a hospital form that deals with a sensitive issue (such as permission for autopsy or organ donation) requiring consent from a patient or his family, would not be able to use the form appropriately. In fact, the New Jersey Organ Tissue Sharing Network specifically asks to be called by hospital personnel for all potential organ donations, so that their professionals can conduct the interviews.

Survey research and epidemiological studies display raw data in a report including the survey questions and details of the methodology that can then be manipulated or duplicated by the reader. The ethnographic techniques used in this study cannot be reviewed since the reader has not been offered access to the raw data. Questions of validity, reliability, and reproducibility of research results are easily asked and answered for survey and epidemiologic research. In this ethnographic study, we must rely upon the researcher for assurance that standardized procedures were used for collecting, analyzing, and reporting data and that results are valid, reliable, and reproducible.[4]

One or two randomly chosen cases that are subject to careful qualitative analysis and reporting procedures can reveal valuable insights and information about the nature of the subject being studied. However, this study fails to provide key passages of dialogue that would support the authors' conclusions. In the case of Mr. Reyes, the authors describe the family's reaction, but they do not provide the dialogue for important interactions. Unfortunately, the conclusions are obvious, since untutored residents are unable to assimilate the complexities and subtleties of conducting discussions regarding forgoing life-sustaining treatment.

It is important to know if the two cases that are described in this report are representative of other cases that involve discussions of limitations of life support and if these failed interviews were representative of all other interviews that were conducted by residents in this setting using this form. Qualitative research can provide rich insights into human behavior and can be revealing of exact problems encountered in the doctor-patient relationship, but generalizations to larger settings and relationships cannot be made unless large numbers of instances are studied. Quantitative methods allow for generalizations to larger populations, but this is done at the cost of sacrificing the rich expressive information provided during interviews. The challenge of gaining a better understanding of physician-patient interactions can no doubt be aided by ethnographic techniques. But, when the methods employed do not adhere to basic tenets of ethnographic research, the reader remains unconvinced.

The hospital environment—complete with health-care professionals who speak a foreign language ("medspeak") and engage in providing "patient care"— constitutes a separate culture every bit as worthy of study as the culture Margaret Mead encountered on a Samoan island. Rigorous methodology should be applied to study these encounters, and the research questions should evolve from this process. Much has been written about the nature of the doctor-patient relationship, and failure in communication is the single most important reason for patient dissatisfaction and malpractice suits in the United States. This type of qualitative research can raise important questions that form the basis for further study where quantitative methodology can serve as verification.

References

1. J.P. Spradley, *The Ethnographic Interview* (New York: Harcourt Brace Jovanovich, 1979), 206–30; B.G. Glaser and A.L. Strauss, *The Discovery of Grounded Theory: Strategies for Qualitative Research* (New York: Aldine Publishing, 1967), 61–62.
2. S. Isaac and W.B. Michael, *Handbook in Research and Evaluation* (San Diego, Calif.: Edits, 1979), 13–27.
3. Glaser and Strauss, *The Discovery of Grounded Theory*, 62.
4. H. Waitzkin, "On Studying the Discourse of Medical Encounters: A Critique of Qualitative Methods and a Proposal for Reasonable Compromise," *Medical Care* 28 (June 1990): 473–88.

Questions for Discussion
Part II, Section 3

1. Why are quantitative empirical methods important to the study of ethical problems in medicine? For example, how might the Findings of Cohen et al. shape the way in which ethicists approach the ethical problems of assisted suicide and euthanasia in their institutions?

2. How do quantitative approaches of the sort used by Bedell et al. differ from the qualitative method employed by Stolman?

3. What are the strengths and weaknesses of each of these two empirical methods?

4. What is ethnography? How does Stolman utilize this approach to evaluate discussions of do-not-resuscitate measures?

CULTURAL ASSUMPTIONS IN BIOETHICAL METHODS

ક્ર

Medical Morality Is Not Bioethics
Medical Ethics in China and the United States

Renée C. Fox and Judith P. Swazey

Renée C. Fox received a doctorate in sociology from Radcliffe College in 1954 and has spent her research and teaching career at the University of Pennsylvania's Departments of Sociology, Psychiatry and Medicine. Judith P. Swazey is currently president of the College of the Atlantic in Bar Harbor, Maine. These authors compare the tenets of Chinese medical morality and American bioethics to illustrate that Western values are not embraced by all societies. They go on to argue that American bioethicists tend to be unaware of their cultural assumptions and of the "American-ness" of the value concerns they raise.

Introduction to Chinese Medical Morality

In the summer of 1981, we spent 6 weeks doing medical sociology fieldwork in the People's Republic of China, primarily in the city of Tianjin. Our trip was arranged by the program of scientific exchanges created by the American Association for the Advancement of Science in Washington, D.C., and the China Association of Science and Technology (CAST) in Beijing. The focal point of our work was a mini-ethnographic study of a profoundly Chinese urban hospital that is energetically committed to modern scientific and technological medicine. . . .

The hospital that our Chinese colleagues chose as the base for our research

Renée C. Fox and Judith P. Swazey. "Medical Morality Is Not Bioethics—Medical Ethics in China and the United States." Abridged from *Perspectives in Biology and Medicine*, Volume 27, 1984, pp. 336–360. Copyright © 1984 by University of Chicago Press.

and teaching proved to be the center of medical modernization that we had asked to study—and more. It contained the only free-standing Critical Care Unit in China [1], conducted hemodialysis for acute renal failure, included a bioengineering-oriented absorbent artificial kidney group, and had made some forays into the transplantation of human organs. It was also highly active in matters pertaining to our work in medical ethics—an interest which we had not thought of pursuing in a Chinese setting.

In retrospect, it seems far from accidental that the hospital we were sent to turned out to be as notable for its leadership in what the Chinese term medical morality as in the "fourth modernization" of (medical) science and technology. We soon learned that the First Central Hospital's intensive involvement in medical ethics was partly due to the influence of its vice-director, Madame She Yun-zhu, a remarkable 75-year-old woman who is one of the pioneers of modern nursing in China. . . .

But even without the dynamic presence of Madame She, we probably would have been introduced to medical morality as representatives of what our Chinese colleagues conceived to be medical sociology and expected from it—albeit in a somewhat more tentatively conceptualized and less vigorously uplifting way. For, in a number of medical and nursing schools that we visited or about which we were told, first steps were being taken to develop courses that were alternately called "Medical Sociology," "Medical Psychology," and/or "Medicine, Morals, and Society." As the last course title suggests, in China, medical sociology and medical ethics are not only interrelated—they are virtually synonymous. Social relationships and a conception of what one of our hosts termed "the individual as a social community" are at the heart of what the Chinese have always defined as ethics. And ethics is the center of the Chinese world view—its very core and essence in Chinese society today as it has been for thousands of years. What is more, participant observation—which the Chinese recognized as a guiding principle as well as a major technique of our research—is also inherent to their own inductive, humanistic approach to ethics. For them, thinking in an entirely abstract or speculative way about moral or social questions runs the risk of what Chinese scholars historically have called "playing with emptiness." What seems to them more "practical" and "right," as well as comfortably familiar, is to work from everyday, empirically observable human reality, focusing particularly on the relationship between specific, identifiable persons, and on their "lived-in," reciprocal existence.

It was both surprising and satisfying to learn in a firsthand way that, despite the thousands of geographical miles and historical years that separate Chinese society and our own, and their very different cosmic outlooks, these aspects of Chinese thought are compatible with the conceptual and methodological framework in which we observe, analyze, interpret, and evaluate as sociologists. . . .

Medical morality is "the kind of morality that doctors and nurses should have." It is concerned with three sets of interconnected goals and with the obligation of "medical workers," individually and collectively, to do everything possible—"sparing no effort"—to attain these goals. Repairing the moral and intellectual as well as the economic and political damage of the Cultural Revolution (1966–1976) is one of the primary objectives of medical morality. Supreme importance is given to restoring the basic "order" that was "smashed" by the Cultural Revolution (and its personification in the Gang of Four): the "task of straightening things out in every field of [medical] work" that must be accomplished, especially the reteaching of "what is right and wrong." A second basic aim of medical morality is to "scale the heights" of modern medicine and thereby achieve the "golden-dream" benefits that come from applying advanced science and technology to problems of health, illness, and the care of patients. This is the medical facet of the national policy of "Four Modernizations" (agriculture, industry, defense, science and technology) that currently prevails in China. In turn, "order" and "modernization" are part of the third general goal of medical morality: the dynamic and creative continuation of the "Great Liberation," the revolution that established the People's Republic of China in 1949.

As this implies, medical morality fits into a larger societal frame. "Work ethics" and "civic virtues" and their relationship to the integrity and development of the whole society are constantly stressed, ideologically and politically, in every sphere of Chinese life. Nationwide campaigns like the civic virtues month and the *Wujiang Simei* ("Five Efforts" and "Four Beauties") movement have been organized around these themes. Workers of all kinds are continually reminded that they are expected to pay attention to morality. Medical workers are among those who have special ethical responsibilities because their job is to care for patients, "relieve them from pain," help them to recover from their illnesses, and "save them from death." Leading nurses and doctors, in particular, are exhorted to demonstrate "the highest level of ethics" in their own behavior—to be "the first to observe the principles and disciplines" entailed—and thereby to set an example that is "a silent order" to those who work with them.

Medical morality is rooted in a conception of the individual in relation to statuses and roles, enmeshed in the network of human relationships that this involves. In this conception, the individual steadfastly strives to meet his responsibilities and carry out his duties ever more totally and perfectly, guided by certain principles, inspired by particular maxims and exemplars, and in conformity with concrete rules. At the vital center of this morality is the continuous effort that each person is expected to make to perfect his at once individual and social self through relationships to significant others and the fulfillment of obligations to these persons. The relationships encompassed by medical morality include those of physicians, nurses, other medical workers, and hospital administrators with each other and with patients and their families. It also concerns the relations between the unit or *danwei* [2] to which medical workers belong and the local bureaucrats and Communist party officials associated with their professional activities. The bedrock and point of departure of medical morality lie in the quality of these human relationships: in how correct, respectful, harmonious, complementary, and reciprocal they are. . . .

. . . But medical morality and its attainment require more. In the words of Dr. Wang Chin-ta (director of the Critical Care Unit of Tianjin First Central Hospital): "No matter how good doctors and nurses are technically, if they do not have noble thinking, they cannot serve the patient, the people, and the country."

"Noble thinking" is an epigrammatic way of referring to the moral virtues that good medical professionals are ideally expected to demonstrate in their work and work relations. Foremost among these medically relevant virtues are the following:

Humanity, compassion, kindness, helpfulness to others;
Trust in others;
A spirit of self-sacrifice;
A high sense of responsibility;
A good sense of discipline, good order;
Hard, conscientious work that is also systematic, careful, precise, punctual, and prudent;
Devotion, dynamic commitment;
Courage to think, act, innovate, blaze new trails, overcome difficulties;
Alertness, high spirits, optimism, a positive attitude;
Patience;
Modesty;
Self-control, a sense of balance and equilibrium;
Politeness, good manners, proper behavior;
Cleanliness, tidiness, good hygiene, keeping healthy;
Lucidity, clarity, intelligence, wisdom;
Honesty, integrity;
Self-knowledge, self-examination, self-criticism, self-cultivation, self-improvement;
Frankness about difficulties, limitations, shortcomings, and mistakes—admitting them, and working to overcome them.

Seen as a whole, these virtues have a number of patterned characteristics. They are relatively concrete ethical qualities, close to the empirical reality of medical practice and patient care. They are formulated as responsibilities and duties, generally stated as positive "musts" and "can do's," rather than as admonitory "must nots" and "do nots." They are punctuated by aphorisms and proverb-like political slogans. A "we shall overcome" moralistic optimism pervades the outlook that they represent. But seen in closer detail, the dynamic nature of these moral virtues is a product of the balancing and blending of the active and passive, traditional and innovative, intellectual and emotional, personal and interpersonal, individual and collective qualities that their fulfillment requires. They are as neo-Confucian as they are Maoist, and more of both than they are Marxist or Leninist.

Particular individuals are singled out because they personify the virtues of medical morality. They are considered to be models whose "example will inspire and encourage others to follow them. . . ."

In the particular settings where nurses, physicians, and their co-workers carry out their medical duties, the principles and virtues of medical morality are translated into specific sets of rules. The ethical importance of these rules is aesthetically expressed through the high quality of their calligraphy, the care with which they are framed, and the prominence with which they are displayed. Here, for example, are the rules of the Critical Care Unit of Tianjin First Central Hospital. Composed by the members of the unit out of their shared experiences, they are written in elegant black script under the title, "Regulations of the Critical Care Unit," which is written in contrasting red ink. Enclosed in an ornate green frame, they hang alone on a wall adjacent to the unit's doorway. The nine sets of regulations are explicit and detailed statements of the unit's work norms, and also of the problematic attitudes and behaviors—the persistent "shortcomings" at work—that have been identified as needing improvement:

1. Patients in this room need critical care. When they are better, they should be transferred to the recovery ward.
2. Care should be given to these patients day and night.
3. The work should be done strictly by the medical workers. They should cooperate. In these ways, they will be able to serve the people wholeheartedly.
4. Medical workers must check the equipment, drugs, and machines on every shift, e.g., ventilator, EKG, tracheal tubes, IV, catheters, abdominal dialyzer, suction, extension cord. Everything must be kept in its place. Do not lend things out.
5. Adhere strictly to regulations. Visiting doctors should make rounds twice a day, in the morning and in the afternoon. Doctors on duty should carefully observe the patients. They should make careful observations at the bedside in order to discover any developments, and be prepared to give emergency treatment if necessary.
6. The staff on one shift should tell the staff on the next shift about any changes that have taken place with the patients. Explain things clearly for continuing with the next shift.
7. For emergency treatment, use Western and Chinese medicine together. There are four principles to follow in administering Chinese medicine— four things that must be done in time:
   a. Prescription;
   b. Fetching of drugs;
   c. Cooking of prescription;
   d. Administering of prescription.
8. Check regulations, and carry them out strictly, in time. Carry out the doctor's orders, to do well and avoid complications.
9. Perform a case history in time.

The First Central Hospital's various sets of rules, regulations, and requirements are now being organized into a centralized system of total quality control (called TQC) under the direction of the hospital's medical administration office

242Medical Morality Is Not Bioethics

and the Party dialectician who is attached to it. The TQC is an elaborate moral accountancy system, designed principally to apply to nurses and doctors and to raise the overall level of medical care. One of its major features is a "shortcomings control" classification scheme which identifies and categorizes various kinds of "technical" and "responsibility" errors and mistakes that physicians and nurses can make in giving care. It then attaches quantitative weights to them according to how major or minor they are considered to be. "Responsibility shortcomings" are viewed largely as moral errors. They are therefore defined as more grave than are shortcomings judged to be primarily technical in nature and are correspondingly subject to more severe penalties and punishments. Eventually, First Central Hospital hopes to translate the variables of its TQC system into a computer program for calculating individual and group "medical quality scores" in a sophisticated, modern way. The hospital regards the computer not only as an important technological tool in this effort but also as a powerful empirical and symbolic expression of the medical modernization toward which it strives. . . .

The "Chinese-ness" of Medical Morality

. . . The central status that medical morality attaches to the primary ethical importance of fulfilling one's duties to specified others in commonplace settings and in everyday acts, and to the continual improvement and perfecting of self in and through these relations and duties, is . . . anciently and quintessentially Chinese. These are core ideas in the traditional morality: of how striving to perfect one's individual and social being expresses the principle of immanent order in the cosmos and contributes to a society that embodies it.

The "noble" ethical virtues emphasized by medical morality are also closely related to the Confucian virtues that structured the ongoing ethical effort required by traditional Chinese morality (*ren* [humanity], *li* [sense of rites], *yi* [sense of duties], *zhi* [wisdom]). Rules were one of the principal forms in which these ethical obligations were made explicit, as is the case with medical morality. In China's past, they were often developed out of the group experience of a guild or a clan and were posted in temples, clan halls, and schools in a manner comparable to the way that medical morality rules are currently displayed in First Central Hospital.

The stylistic features and ambience of medical morality—with its emphasis on orthodoxy, righteousness, and propriety, its concern about "moral sympathy," its stress on the power of didacticism, its ritualization and bureaucratization, and its preeminently public nature—all have their counterparts and origins in Chinese tradition.

Tianjin First Central Hospital's TQC system has significant antecedents in Chinese history and tradition. It could be said that ancestral versions of TQC existed in the "morality books" (*shanshu*) and the "ledgers of merit and demerit" (*gongguoge*) that were kept by individuals and families in the sixteenth- and early seventeenth-century years of China's Ming dynasty [3, pp. 193–196, 197, 4]. These were moral account books, based on the self-examination of conscience, the written confession of wrongdoing, and the recording of both good and bad thoughts and acts. Not only were thoughts and deeds morally classified in this positive and negative way, but they were sometimes weighted by a point system. In some ledgers, good points were recorded in red ink, bad ones in black ink. (Since at least the time of the Han dynasty, red had been the color of positive numbers and black of negative ones.) At periodic intervals, the person keeping this moral audit added up the points, thereby arriving at a quantitative score of his current state of ethicality and his cumulated "moral capital." Sinologists identify Taoist and Buddhist influences in these morality books, including concepts of judgments meted out by a "cosmic bureaucracy" that involved one's present life, life span, and rebirth [5].

This is not to imply that medical morality is a pure emanation of Confucianism, Taoism, and Chinese Buddhism, or that Marxism-Leninism-Maoism has played a negligible role in shaping its form and content. Certain precepts of medical morality constitute radical departures from the concepts on which the traditional system of Chinese ethics was built. Most notable are the ways in which the egalitarian and universalistic principles of Marxism have strongly influenced the tenets of medical morality. Doctors and nurses are urged to unite, to work closely together professionally and "transprofessionally," and to treat colleagues equally. This egalitarian view runs counter to the traditional Chinese thesis that morality and public order consist of, and depend on, a series of hierarchically structured relationships and the fulfillment of the duties associated with them. The archetype and the ethical keystone of these superordinate-subordinate relationships was that between father and son; filial piety (*xiao*) was regarded as the model and the source of all other virtues. . . .

. . . In contradistinction to American bioethics, as already indicated, Chinese medical morality is not preoccupied with social and ethical problems associated with the advancement of medical science and technology. At the present time, medical modernization—enriched by its incorporation of traditional Chinese medicine—is viewed as morally good, socially desirable, economically necessary, and politically obligatory. Substantive issues that *do* fall under the aegis of medical morality include the population's response to the new, one-child-per-family policy; the wisdom of telling or not telling seriously ill patients (particularly those with cancer) about the gravity of their illness; the role that the family ought and ought not to play in the care of ill relatives who are hospitalized; the causes, prevention, and treatment of suicide attempts; and the problem of obtaining blood donations. All are issues that are encountered by nurses and doctors in the various medical milieus where they currently work. Prominent bioethical concerns, such as human experimentation, the "gift of life" and "quality of life," the termination of treatment, and questions about the allocation of scarce resources associated with therapeutic innovations like organ transplantation and hemodialysis in our own society, are not yet considered to be problems in China. Chinese nurses, physicians, and relevant officials are aware that, as the process of medical modernization goes forward, they may face comparable difficulties. But, in accord with Chinese pragmatism, they are disinclined to

244 Medical Morality Is Not Bioethics

engage in abstract speculation about hypothetical problems that may (or may not) develop, and about how they should be handled if they do. It is not until the Chinese face such issues in a firsthand way, and can meet and analyze them as "lived-in experiences," that these matters will become part of their medical morality.

From all the foregoing, it is amply clear that medical morality is not bioethics. It is as Chinese as bioethics is American. We now turn to bioethics, an arena in which we have worked and observed since the mid-1960s. In the final analysis, as we shall see, American bioethics and Chinese medical morality are so culturally dissimilar that they are not sufficiently related to form a yin-yang (opposing, but complementary) pair.

American Bioethics

In contrast to medical morality, the phenomena with which bioethics is primarily concerned are related to some of the ways in which modern, Western, American medicine has already *succeeded* in what the Chinese call "scaling the high peaks" of science and technology. Bioethics is focused on what we consider serious *problems* associated with these advances, rather than on the achievements they represent or the "golden dream" promises that they hold forth [6]:

> Actual and anticipated developments in genetic engineering and counseling, life support systems, birth technology, population control, the implantation of human, animal, and artificial organs, as well as in the modification and control of human thought are principal [areas] of concern. Within this framework, special attention is concentrated on the implications of amniocentesis, abortion, *in vitro* fertilization, the prospect of cloning, organ transplantation, the use of the artificial kidney machine, the development of an artificial heart, the modalities of the intensive care unit, the practice of psychosurgery, and the introduction of psychotropic drugs. Cross-cutting the consideration . . . given to these general and concrete [spheres] of biomedical development, there is marked preoccupation with the ethicality of human experimentation under various conditions. . . .

Bioethics has also been concerned with the proper definition of life and death and personhood and with the humane treatment of "emerging life and life that is passing away" [7]—especially with the justifiability of forgoing life-sustaining forms of medical therapy. One of the most significant general characteristics of this ensemble of bioethical concerns is the degree to which they cluster around problems of natality and mortality, at the beginning and at the end of the human life cycle.

The chief intellectual and professional participants in American bioethics are philosophers (above all, those who are called "ethicists" in the United States, and "moral philosophers" in Europe), theologians (predominantly Catholic and Protestant), jurists, physicians, and biologists. Lately, the thought and presence of economists have been strongly felt in the field; but relatively few other social scientists are actively involved or notably influential in bioethical discussion, research, writing, and action. The limited participation of anthropologists, sociologists, and political scientists in bioethics is a complex phenomenon, caused as much by the prevailing intellectual orientations and the weltanschauung of present day American social science as by the framework of bioethics [8].

The disciplinary backgrounds of bioethicists contrast sharply with those of the key participants in medical morality because of historic differences in the American and Chinese cultures as well as current differences in our respective political and economic systems. For example, although one could argue that there are functional parallels between the role of a Chinese dialectician and that of an American theologian, one would hardly expect a theologian trained in the Judeo-Christian tradition to define value and belief issues and make decisions in the same way as someone whose world view is shaped by Confucian, Taoist, and Buddhist thought. Nor does the pivotal place of lawyers and judges in bioethics have its counterpart in medical morality. The status and role of jurists in bioethics are integrally connected with the singular importance that Americans attach to the principle as well as to the fact of being "a society under law, rather than under men."

On the other hand, the control in degree and kind over medical morality exercised by the central government in Beijing is not only an emanation of the Chinese Communist party, its present-day leadership, and its current doctrine. It is thoroughly compatible with the at once profane and sacred power over the order and organization of the entire society accorded to the emperor and his imperial bureaucracy throughout all the dynasties of Chinese history. In the United States, quite to the contrary, the fact that bioethical questions, with their moral and religious connotations, have been appearing more frequently and prominently in national and local political arenas—in our legislatures, courts, and in specially created commissions—constitutes a societal dilemma. Although ours is a "society under law," it is also a nation founded on the separation of church and state as one of its sacredly secular principles. What ought we to do, then, about the fact that bioethics (like Mr. Smith) has gone to Washington? In the light of the religious and even metaphysical, as well as moral, nature of bioethical issues, is it legitimate or wise for our government to deal with them? If so, at what level, through what branch, using what mechanisms? If not, are there other means through which we can try to resolve such matters of our collective conscience, on behalf of the whole society? These are distinctly American questions that are decidedly not Chinese.

The pluralism of American society and its voluntarism have contributed to the development of the numerous centers, institutes, and associations of varying orientations that have been organized around bioethical activities in the United States over the course of the past 20 years, both inside and outside university settings. Most of the persons who are professionally active in the field of bioethics belong to one or several of such groups and participate in their interconnected and to some extent overlapping activities (discussions, research, teaching, consultations, meetings, publications, etc.). In this sense, they form a sort of "invisible college," although not a unified school of thought.

Such a plethora of voluntary associations, organized around common interests, but with somewhat different origins, auspices, memberships, and outlook, is a very American configuration. It embodies a set of culture patterns and social traits, not confined to bioethics, that always have been strikingly characteristic of American society and its conception of democracy. As early as the 1830s, Alexis de Tocqueville, the astute French observer-analyst of our new nation-state, identified our tendency to form and join voluntary associations as one of our most notable societal attributes. Again, for reasons broader, deeper, and older than the particular contemporaneous circumstances that have given rise to bioethics and medical morality, this is not a pattern that exists in China or that one would expect to find there.

But above all, it is in the values and beliefs emphasized and deemphasized by bioethics, and in its cognitive framework and style, that its Western and American orientation is both most evident and most fully articulated.

To begin with, as already indicated, individualism is the primary value-complex on which the intellectual and moral edifice of bioethics rests. Individualism, in this connection, starts with a belief in the importance, uniqueness, dignity, and sovereignty of the individual, and in the sanctity of each individual life. From this flows the assumption that every person, singularly and respectfully defined, is entitled to certain individual rights. Autonomy of self, self-determination, and privacy are regarded as fundamental among these rights. They are also considered to be necessary preconditions for another value-precept of individualism: the opportunity for persons to "find," develop, and realize themselves and their self-interests to the fullest—to achieve and enjoy individual well-being. In this view, "individuals are entitled to be and do as they see fit, so long as they do not violate the comparable rights of others" [9]. "Paternalism" is defined as interfering with and limiting a person's freedom and liberty of action for the sake of his or her own good or welfare. It is regarded as ethically dubious because, however beneficent its intentions or outcome, it restricts autonomy, involves coercion, implies that someone else knows better what is best for a given individual, and may insidiously impair that individual's ability to decide and act independently.

The notion of contract plays a major role in the way relations between autonomous individuals are conceived in bioethics. Self-conscious, rational, specific agreements by persons involved in interaction with one another, that explicitly delineate the scope, content, and conditions of their joint activities, are presented as ethical models. They are considered to be exemplary expressions of the way that moral relationships, protective of individual rights, can be structured. The archetype of such contractual relations is the kind of informed, voluntary consent agreement between subjects and investigators in medical research which the field of bioethics helped to formulate and that is now required by all federal and most private agencies funding this research. The informed consent contract, though mutual, is asymmetric. It is principally concerned with the rights and welfare of one of the two partners—the human subject, often a patient—because he is the most vulnerable, disadvantaged, and least powerful of the pair. The special contractual obligation to watch over and safeguard the rights of the person(s) most susceptible to exploitation or harm in this type of exposed and unequal situation is a part of the bioethics conception of individualism and of moral relations between individuals. But little mention is made by bioethicists of what sociologist Emile Durkheim termed the "noncontractual aspects of contract": that is, the more implicit and informal commitment, fidelity, and trust aspects of social relationships that reciprocally bind persons to live up to their promises and their responsibilities to one another.

Veracity and truth-telling, the "faithfulness" dimension of relationships on which bioethics fixes its attention, is more specific and circumscribed than the Durkheimian concept. In keeping with the overall orientation of bioethics, what is stressed is the right of patients or research subjects to "know the truth" about the discomforts, hazards, uncertainties, and "bad news" that may be associated with medical diagnosis, prognosis, treatment, and experimentation. The physician's obligation to communicate the truth to the patient or subject is derived from and based on the latter's presumed right to know. Discerning what is the truth and what is a lie is seen as relatively unproblematic. And there is a decided tendency to look on the use of denial by the patient as an undesirable defense, because it complicates truth-telling and blocks truth-receiving. Here, the affirmation that patients have the right to know the truth veers toward insistence that they ideally ought to face the truth consciously and deal with it rationally (in keeping with the particular definitions of "truth" and of "rationality" inherent to bioethics).

Another major value preoccupation of bioethics—and one that it has increasingly emphasized since the mid-1970s—concerns the allocation of scarce, expensive resources for advanced medical care, research, and development. What proportion of our national and local resources should be designated for these purposes, in what ways, and according to what principles and criteria? The resources with which bioethics is chiefly concerned are material ones, mainly economic and technological in nature. The allocation of nonmaterial resources such as personnel, talent, skill, time, energy, caring, and compassion is rarely mentioned. Bioethics situates its allocation questions within a rather abstract, individual rights-oriented notion of the general or common good, assigning greater importance to equity than to equality. The ideally moral distribution of goods is defined as one that all rational, self-interested persons are willing to accept as just and fair, even if goods are allotted unequally. "Cost containment" is also an essential value-component of this view of rightful distribution. In the bioethical calculus, it is not just a practical or necessary response to an empirical situation of economic scarcity. It has become a more categorical moral imperative.

Finally, what is usually referred to as "the principle of beneficence" or "benevolence" is also a key value of bioethics. This enjoinder to "do good" and to "avoid harm" is structured and limited by the supremacy of individualism. The benefiting of others advocated in bioethical thought is circumscribed and constrained by the obligation to respect individual rights, interests, and autonomy. Furthermore, rather than being seen as an independent virtue, doing good is generally conceived to be part of a "benefit-harm ratio" in which, ideally, benefits should outweigh costs. "Minimization of harm" rather than "maximization of good" is more strongly emphasized in this bioethical equation.

These values are predominant in American bioethics and are considered to be the most fundamental. They are accorded the highest intellectual and moral significance and are set forth with the greatest certainty and the least qualification. Other values and virtues and principles and beliefs that are part of the ethos of bioethics occupy a more secondary and less secure status. They are less frequently invoked and when introduced into ethical discussion and analysis are likely to elicit debate or require special justification. . . .

The emphasis that bioethics places on individualism and on contractual relations freely entered into by voluntarily consenting adults tends to minimize and obscure the interconnectedness of persons and the social and moral importance of their interrelatedness. Particularly when compared with Chinese medical morality, it is striking how little attention bioethics pays to the web of human relationships of which the individual is a part and to the mutual obligations and interdependence that these relations involve. Concepts like reciprocity, solidarity, and community, which are rooted in a social perspective on our moral life and our humanity, are not often employed. Characteristically, bioethics deals with the "more-than-individual" in terms of the "general good," the "common good," or the "public interest." In the bioethical use of these concepts, the "collective good" tends to be seen atomistically and arithmetically as the sum total of the rights and interests, desires and demands of an aggregate of self-contained individuals. The fair and just distribution of limited collective resources is the major dimension of commonality that is stressed, often to the exclusion of other aspects, and usually with a propensity to define resources as material (primarily economic), and quantitative. In this view, private and public morality are sharply distinguished from one another in keeping with the underlying essential dichotomy between individual and social. Social and cultural factors are largely seen as external constraints that limit individuals. They are rarely presented as enabling and empowering forces, *inside* as well as outside of individuals, that are constituent, dynamic elements in making them human persons. . . .

These assumptions about what is and is not purely moral are integrally related to the major cognitive characteristics of bioethical thought: to how participants in bioethics actually *do* think, and especially, to what they define as ideal standards of ethical thinking. A high value is placed on logical reasoning—preferably based on a general moral theory and concepts derived from it—that is systematically developed according to codified methodological rules and techniques around select, analytically designated variables and problems. Rigor, precision, clarity, consistency, parsimony, and objectivity are regarded as earmarks of the intellectually and ethically "best" kind of moral thought. Flawed logical and conceptual analysis is considered to be not only a concomitant of moral error but also, to a significant degree, responsible for producing it. This way of thought also tends toward dichotomous distinctions and bipolar choices. Self versus others, body versus mind, individual versus group, public versus private, objective versus subjective, rational versus nonrational, lie versus truth, benefit versus harm, rights versus responsibilities, independence versus dependence, autonomy versus paternalism, liberty versus justice are among the primary ones. Even the field's own self-defining conception of what is and is not a moral problem is formulated in a bipolar, either/or fashion.

Bioethics is an applied field that brings its theory, methods, and knowledge to bear on phenomena and situations deemed ethically problematic. It seeks to identify and illuminate points of moral consideration and provide a way of thinking about them that can contribute to their practical moral resolution through concrete choices and specific acts. Bioethics attempts this by proceeding in a largely deductive manner to impose its mode of reasoning on the phenomenological reality addressed. The amount of detailed investigation of the actual situations in which the ethical problems occur varies. But what philosophers call "thought experiments" are more often conducted in bioethics than is empirical, in situ research. . . .

Within its rigorously stripped-down analytic and methodological framework, bioethics is prone to reify its own logic and to formulate absolutist, self-confirming principles and insights. These tendencies are associated with the disinclination of bioethics to critically examine its own moral epistemology: to searchingly identify and evaluate the presuppositions and assumptions on which it rests. In a scholastic sense, the field of bioethics is knowledgeably aware of the traditions of Western thought on which it draws (e.g., act and rule utilitarianism and various theories of justice). But there is a more latent level on which it nevertheless considers its principles, its style of reasoning, and its perceptions to be objective, unbiased, and reasonable to a degree that not only makes them socially and culturally neutral but also endows them with a kind of universality. Paradoxically, these very suppositions of bioethical thought contribute to its inadvertent propensity to reflect and systematically support conventional, relatively conservative American concepts, values, and beliefs.*

These value, belief, and thought patterns of bioethics have developed within an interdisciplinary matrix. But particularly since the mid-1970s, when philosophers began "arriving by the score" in bioethics (and "in applied ethics more broadly") [10], moral philosophy has had the greatest molding influence on the field. It is principally American analytic philosophy—with its emphasis on theory,

---

*Several major critiques of the emergence of the new philosophical subdiscipline of applied ethics on the American scene have been published in the *Hastings Center Report* which coincide in numerous respects with our characterization of bioethics, particularly its "seeming indifference to history, social context, and cultural analysis" [10–12].

methodology, and technique, and its utilitarian, Kantian, and "contractarian" outlooks—in which most of the philosophers who have entered bioethics were trained. Defined as "ethicists" who are specialized experts in moral problems associated with biomedicine, they have established themselves, and their approach to matters of right and wrong, as the "dominant force" [12] in the field.

This is not to say that all analytic philosophers who actively participate in bioethics think and write in a uniform way, or that every philosopher-bioethicist is grounded in this analytic tradition. Major contributors to bioethics, for example, also include a number of highly esteemed philosopher-scholars whose work incorporates more phenomenological, social, and religious dimensions rooted in the traditions of moral theology and American social ethics. The respect that such individuals are accorded notwithstanding, the perspective that they represent has had far less influence on the predominant ethos of bioethics than has analytic philosophy. . . .

Bioethics Is Not Just Bioethics

In our sociological view, the paradigm of values and beliefs, and of reflections on them, that has developed and been institutionalized in American bioethics is an impoverished and skewed expression of our society's cultural tradition. In a highly intellectualized but essentially fundamentalistic way, it thins out the fullness of that tradition and bends it away from some of the deepest sources of its meaning and vitality. . . .

Bioethics has "sprung loose from that broader [religious] framework" [13] in which the values of our cultural tradition are historically embedded. In turn, the particular forms that the secularism, the rationality, and the individualism of bioethics take, and the ways in which they interact with each other, contribute to another of the field's constricting features: its provincialism. Bioethics is sealed into itself in such a way that it tends to take its own characteristics and assumptions for granted. It is relatively uncritical of its premises and unaware of its cultural specificity. It is this sort of parochialism, with its mix of naiveté and arrogance, that makes it difficult for bioethicists not only to recognize medical morality and its Chinese-ness when they encounter it but also to perceive the "American-ness" of their particular value-concerns and of how they approach them. . . .

References

1. Fox, R. C., and Swazey, J. P. Critical care at Tianjin's First Central Hospital and the fourth modernization. *Science* 217:700–705, 1982.
2. Henderson, G. E. Danwei: the Chinese work unit: a participant observation study of a hospital. Dissertation submitted in partial fulfillment of the requirements of the Ph.D. (Sociology) at the University of Michigan, Ann Arbor, 1982.
3. Gernet, J. *Chine et Christianisme*. Paris: Gallimard, 1982.
4. Berling, J. Religion and popular culture: the management of moral capital in *The Romance of the Three Teachings*. In untitled work edited by A. Nathan, D.

Johnson, and E. Rawski. Berkeley and Los Angeles: Univ. California Press, forthcoming.

5. Sivin, N. Ailment and cure in traditional China (unpublished manuscript).

6. Fox, R. C. Ethical and existential developments in contemporaneous American medicine: their implications for culture and society. In *Essays in Medical Sociology.* New York: Wiley, 1979.

7. Bok, S. In discussion at the Conference on the Problem of Personhood, organized by Medicine in the Public Interest (MIPI). New York City, April 1–2, 1982.

8. Fox, R. C. Advanced medical technology—social and ethical implications. In *Essays in Medical Sociology.* New York: Wiley, 1979.

9. Gorovitz, S. *Doctors' Dilemmas: Moral Conflicts and Medical Care.* New York: Macmillan, 1982.

10. Callahan, D. At the center: from "wisdom" to "smarts." *Hastings Cent. Rep.* 12:4, 1982.

11. Noble, C. N. Ethics and experts. *Hastings Cent. Rep.* 12:7–9, 15, 1982.

12. Callahan, D. Minimalistic ethics. *Hastings Cent. Rep.* 11:19–25, 1981.

13. De Craemer, W. See [7].

Yes, There Are African-American Perspectives on Bioethics

Annette Dula

Annette Dula received a doctorate in education and is currently on the faculty of the University of Colorado, Boulder. In this essay she considers how exploitation and oppression experienced by African American women give rise to a unique perspective on bioethics. She concludes that the context of unequal relationships stands in the way of meeting basic ethical requirements, such as informed consent.

Reproductive Rights and Sterilization

Issues centering around birth control and reproduction are central to many bioethical discussions today. Among these are family planning, sterilization, and genetic screening—questions of particular interest to African-American women because we have been exploited in each of these areas. Therefore, we may see these issues differently from white women. If we look at the history of birth control in North America, we can understand the source of one of these different perspectives.

The birth control movement in the United States is marked by three phases. The middle of the eighteenth century witnessed the beginning of the first phase of the birth control movement.[1] "Voluntary motherhood" was the rallying cry of the early feminists. Essentially, voluntary motherhood meant that women ought to be able to say no to their husbands as a means of limiting the number of children they bore. The irony of voluntary motherhood was that while white feminists were refusing their husbands' sexual demands, African-American women did not have the same right to say no to the husbands of those same early feminists. This is to say nothing of the fact that African-American women had been exploited as breeding wenches in order to produce a stock of slaves.

The second phase of the birth control movement actually gave rise to the phrase "birth control," which was coined by Margaret Sanger in 1915.[2] Initially, this stage of the movement led to the recognition that reproductive rights and political rights were intertwined. The practice of birth control would give white women the freedom to pursue new opportunities, which their subsequent right to vote would soon make possible.[3] White women could go to work while

Annette Dula. "Yes, There Are African-American Perspectives on Bioethics." Abridged from *African-American Perspectives on Biomedical Ethics* , 1992, pp. 193–203. Reprinted by permission of Georgetown University Press.

African-American women cared for white children and did house work in white homes.

Unfortunately, the second stage of the birth control movement coincided with the eugenics movement in the first two decades of this century. When the white birth rate began to decline, eugenicists chastised middle-class white women for contributing to the suicide of the white race. As Paul Popenoe notes: "Continued limitation of offspring in the white race simply invites the black, brown, and yellow races to finish work already begun by birth control, and reduce the whites to a subject race."[4]

Eugenicists proposed two methods for curbing race suicide. On the one hand, middle-class white women had a moral obligation to have large families; on the other hand, poor immigrant women and African-American women had a moral obligation to restrict the size of their families because they were likely to be of inferior stock. On the basis of this argument, Guy Irving Burch of the American Eugenics Society advocated birth control for African-American and immigrant women. He notes: "We must prevent the American people from being replaced by alien or Negro stock, whether it be by immigration or by overly high birth rates among others in this country."[5] In addition, poor people created a drain on the taxes and charity of the wealthy.[6]

The woman's movement then adopted the ideals of the eugenicists regarding poor and minority women. Margaret Sanger saw the chief issue of birth control as "more children from the fit and less from the unfit."[7]

The 1940s marked the beginning of the third phase of birth control which was renamed, "Planned Parenthood."

In the 1950s, several states tried to extend sterilization laws to include compulsory sterilization of mothers of illegitimate children.[8] In the 1960s, the government began subsidizing family planning clinics. The purpose of these subsidies was to reduce the number of people on welfare by checking the transmission of poverty from generation to generation. The number of family planning clinics in an area was proportional to the number of African-Americans and Hispanics in the areas.[9] In Puerto Rico, by 1965, a third of the women had been sterilized.[10] In 1972 it was reported that there was a sevenfold rise in hysterectomies over the previous year at Los Angeles Hospital. These policies were influential in arousing African-American suspicions that there were racist motives behind family planning efforts.[11]

In 1973 two sisters, twelve-year-old Mary Alice Relf and fourteen-year-old Minnie Lee were surgically sterilized without consent. In the same town where they lived, eleven other young girls about the same ages as the Relf sisters had also been sterilized. Ten of these girls were African-American. In South Carolina, of thirty-four deliveries paid for by Medicaid, eighteen included sterilizations and all eighteen were young black women.[12] In 1972, Carl Schultz, Director of HEW's Population Affairs Office, estimated that between 100,000 and 200,000 sterilizations had been funded by the government.[13]

Thus, the first phase of the woman's movement completely ignored black women's sexual subjugation to white masters. And in the second phase, the movement adopted the racist policies of eugenics philosophy. The third stage saw a number of coercive measures supported by governmental policy to contain the population of African-Americans and poor people. While birth control per se was perceived as a benefit, African-Americans have historically objected to birth control as a method of dealing with poverty. . . .

The Answer Is Yes

Yes, we do have an African-American perspective on bioethics. . . .

There is a shocking history of medical abuse against powerless people. Often the form of the abuse is violation of informed consent. Indeed, the examples that I have presented share the two common elements of powerlessness and the absence of the informed consent. Consequently, I have suggested that in unequal relationships, informed consent does not work. . . .

Though there may be an acknowledged African-American perspective on bioethics, that does not mean that our perspectives have been fully articulated. Rather we need to organize professionally to articulate our views further. . . .

References

1. Linda Gordon, *Woman's Body, Woman's Right: Birth Control in America* (New York: Penguin Books, 1976).
2. Ibid.
3. Angela Davis, *Women, Race and Class* (New York: Vintage Books, 1981).
4. Paul Popenoe, *Conservation of the Family* (Baltimore: Williams and Wilkins, 1926), 144.
5. Gordon, *Woman's Body, Woman's Right*, 283.
6. Ibid.
7. Gordon, *Woman's Body, Woman's Right*, 281.
8. Joseph L. Morrison, "Illegitimacy, Sterilization, and Racism: A North Carolina Case History," *Social Science Review* 39 (1965): 1–10.
9. Ketayun H. Gould, "Black Women in Double Jeopardy: A Perspective on Birth Control," *National Association of Social Workers* (1984): 96–105.
10. Bonnie Mass, *Population Target: The Political Economy. Population Control in Latin America* (Toronto: Women's Press, 1976).
11. Davis, *Women, Race and Class*.
12. Herbert Aptheker, "Racism and Human Experimentation," *Political Affairs* 53, 2 (1974): 27–60.
13. Les Payne, "Forced Sterilization for the Poor," *San Francisco Chronicle*, 26 Feb 1974.

Questions for Discussion
Part II, Section 4

1. What do Fox and Swazey regard as the salient differences between Chinese medical morality and American bioethics?

2. Do you think that every society has a different moral perspective on ethical problems in medicine? If so, do you think these different moral perspectives are incompatible?

3. Dula suggests that American bioethics fails to represent the moral concerns of all Americans, and instead represents primarily the concerns of a limited and privileged set of Americans. What support does she provide for this claim?

4. What cultural assumptions do you bring to the study of bioethics?

5. Does bioethics incorporate your cultural perspective?

PART III

The Practice of Bioethics

Introduction to the Practice of Bioethics

Robert A. Pearlman

D uring the latter half of this century, health care professionals and society
faced ethical questions about withholding and withdrawing medical treatment (Fox and Swazey, 1974). The development of technologies in which marginal benefits were accompanied by significant burdens forced patients and
health care providers to struggle with ethical choices. Three principal responses
characterized society's efforts to apply ethical reasoning to the new challenges
presenting in the health care setting. These responses were the formation of
ethics committees, the emergence of ethics consultants, and the formulation of
ethics-related policies and guidelines.

The Historical Development of Ethics Advisory Committees

During the early 1960s the development of long-term hemodialysis permitted
treatment of persons with chronic kidney failure. To Dr. Belding Scribner, the
principal inventor, this posed several ethical concerns related to patient selection,
termination of treatment by the physician or the patient, and death with dignity
(Scribner, 1964). The Seattle Artificial Kidney Center's Admission and Policy
Committee was formed to develop guidelines for the nonmedical screening and
selection of dialysis candidates, anticipated to be more numerous than available
dialysis machines. Membership on the committee was intended to reflect broad
representation from the community. Despite these intentions, the majority of
members reflected white, upper-middle-class sociodemographics. The criteria
that emerged in the early challenging and psychologically exhausting deliberations about selection of dialysis candidates reportedly included factors such as
sex, martial status, education, income, occupation, past performance, and future
potential. These "social worth" criteria were criticized as prejudicial after publication and review of the workings of the committee (Alexander, 1962). One
criticism stated, "The Pacific Northwest is no place for a Henry David Thoreau
with bad kidneys" (Snaders and Dukeminier, 1968). This early committee experience highlighted two important lessons. First, diversity in committee membership is a safeguard to avoid the introduction of bias against classes of persons.
Second, public review of policies and procedures may help identify unexpected
problems.

  During the 1970s, ethics committees with a very different function were
formed, owing partly to the decision of the New Jersey Supreme Court in the

Furthermore, the outcomes in our study suggest that, contrary to the fears of many, most patients who die do so within the first few days after resuscitation. The long-lingering death after cardiopulmonary resuscitation appears to be the publicized exception rather than the common occurrence, as also noted by Grace and Minogue[37] for a more select group of patients resuscitated after acute myocardial infarction.

The evaluation of efforts at resuscitation must extend beyond the time of hospitalization itself. Conclusions about patients' long-term functional status after resuscitation have been unsubstantiated and vague[2,38] or have focused on changes in clinical status, such as the changes in class of heart failure documented by Lemire and Johnson.[5] Our finding that patients who survived cardiopulmonary resuscitation usually had an intact mental status is reassuring and offers hope for patients and families whose attention may focus on the tragic exception—the patient maintained in a comatose state for years. An inherent limitation in a study such as ours is the absence of a prearrest evaluation and thus the inability to detect subtle changes in mental status that may in fact occur after resuscitation. Whatever these relative changes may have been in our patients, the extent of neurologic recovery was almost uniformly remarkable.

Since depression is commonly observed after other illnesses, such as myocardial infarction, it is probable that the depression documented in our patients at the time of discharge from the hospital was a consequence of acute illness rather than a result of cardiopulmonary resuscitation itself.[39] Our finding of nearly uniform alleviation of this depression within six months after discharge allows the physician to convey optimism to the patient—an attitude that may in itself promote recovery.

The major residual disability for the patients who survived after cardiopulmonary resuscitation was their limitation in functional status and confinement to home. It was our clinical impression that over half these patients were limited by fear rather than by a change in physical capabilities. Whether restrictions were imposed by their physicians or reflected primarily the patients' fear of recurrence of sudden arrest cannot be determined. Since it has been shown that simple interventions after other acute illnesses, such as myocardial infarction, can favorably influence the functional outcome, we expect that similar maneuvers may help patients who have survived after resuscitation.[40–42]

Many have asked whether it is appropriate to resuscitate elderly patients. Camarata et al.,[21] Castagna et al.,[22] Messert and Quglieri,[43] and Stephenson[44] suggest that age is an important determinant of survival after cardiopulmonary resuscitation. However, our findings suggest that age does not affect the prognosis for survival after resuscitation, nor does it appear to influence adjustment to chronic illness or level of functioning after discharge from the hospital. What determines prognosis is the underlying disease, not the year of birth.[45,46]

Our findings clearly require validation in a larger sample and in a variety of settings. At the very least, however, they may serve as a helpful guide to physicians and to patients and their families who are concerned about the likelihood of a successful outcome after an attempt at resuscitation. We believe that case of Karen Ann Quinlan. In Quinlan, the Court stated that if the hospital ethics committee agreed that "there is no reasonable possibility of Karen's ever emerging from her present comatose condition to a cognitive, sapient state," the request of her parents, guardians, and attending physicians to remove life-sustaining treatment could be acted upon without fear of civil or criminal liability (*In re Quinlan*, 1976). Thus, early ethics committees functioned as prognosis committees, helping to ensure that patients in whom life-sustaining treatment was withheld or withdrawn qualified by virtue of being in a persistent vegetative state.

By the 1980s, the role of ethics committees expanded. Court cases pertaining to decision making for severely brain-damaged patients (including newborns) led to federal regulations to prevent discrimination on the basis of handicap and a recommendation by the President's Commission for the Study of Ethical Problems in Medicine and Biomedical and Behavioral Research (*Barber v. Superior Court*, 1983; *Infant Doe v. Baker*, 1982; Nondiscrimination on the Basis of Handicap, 1984; President's Commission for the Study of Ethical Problems in Medicine and Biomedical Research, 1983s). In *Deciding to Forego Life-Sustaining Treatment*, the Commission suggested institutional reviews, such as ethics committees, as a mechanism to protect the interests of patients who lack decision-making capacity and to ensure their well-being and self-determination. This recommendation was grounded in the premise that the possibility of errors in the process of decision making for mentally incapacitated patients could be reduced with judicious use of a review process. The so-called Baby Doe regulations also strongly encouraged hospitals caring for newborn infants to establish infant care review committees to develop policies, monitor adherence through retrospective record review, and review cases on an emergency basis when withholding or withdrawing treatment was being considered.

Subsequent debate and policy initiatives extended the competent patient's right to accept or reject recommended treatment to all circumstances of mental incapacity (Faden, Beauchamp, King, 1986). For example, family members of mentally incapacitated patients could speak for the previously competent patient and request the withholding or discontinuation of life-sustaining treatment even if the patient was not in a persistent vegetative state (Buchanan and Brock, 1989). This made the need for prognosis committees moot. The need for ethics committees, however, did not abate (Cranford and Doudera, 1984).

Roles of Hospital Ethics Committees

Ethics committees serve multiple purposes. Veatch (1977) and Macklin (1988) review these purposes in articles included in Part III. In the broadest sense ethics committees link societal values to medical practice. More specifically, they protect the rights and welfare of patients by promoting shared decision making. In 1983, the President's Commission outlined four functions of ethics committees that remain prominent for many ethics committees today (President's Commission for the Study of Ethical Problems in Medicine and Biomedical Research, 1983):

- to review cases to confirm the responsible physician's diagnosis and prognosis of a patient's medical condition (which took on less importance as discussed above)
- to provide a forum for discussing broader social and ethical concerns raised by a particular case, and in so doing, teach professional staff how to identify, frame, and resolve ethical problems
- to formulate policy and guidelines regarding such decisions
- to review decisions made by others about the treatment of specific patients or make such decisions themselves

In responding to this charge many ethics committees today are instrumental in developing educational programs for clinicians and patients (e.g., about patient rights and responsibilities), developing or reviewing ethics-related policies (e.g., decision making for patients who lack decision-making capacity and HIV testing and counseling, respectively), and providing case consultations and retrospective case reviews. To accomplish these tasks, ethics committee members must develop and maintain sufficient expertise.

When ethics committees initially are formed there may be debate about what type of training and education develops the necessary expertise and skills to conduct ethical analysis in the clinical setting. Committees may consider whether or not an ethicist is necessary to conduct consultations (Singer, Pellegrino, and Siegler, 1990). However, three lines of argument cast doubt on the need for and wisdom of recommending a professional ethicist for every health care facility. First, physician educators worry about giving the message that ethical analysis and problem resolution are activities requiring outside expertise. As a result, physician trainees might not learn how to engage proficiently in these activities and thereby develop into morally responsible providers. Moreover, reliance on an expert might foster singular views about contentious issues and limit moral discourse. Second, the experience of committees demonstrates that although skills in ethical analysis and critical thinking are important, other skills are necessary. These other skills include adequate understanding of clinical medicine and decision making, as well as communication and interpersonal interaction (see the paper by La Puma and Schneidermayer [1991] included in Part III). Adequate knowledge of health care law, public policy, and cultural and religious traditions are also recommended as desirable attributes (Fletcher and Hoffmann, 1994). Third, few individuals have all of the aforementioned knowledge and skills, and as a result, ethics committees usually require more than one person. To ensure adequate knowledge, skills, and sensitivity to differences among people, the typical ethics committee is comprised of health care professionals from many disciplines, people with expertise in law and religious traditions, and representatives from the community that health care institutions serve.

Ethics Education

Ethics committee members require sufficient education to teach other professionals about the ethical issues in health care so as to influence attitudes and behavior, and ultimately improve the quality of care to patients. Education also serves to prevent or minimize threats to optimal ethics committee functioning. (The paper, "Behind Closed Doors," included in Part III, discusses threats to optimal functioning.) Despite its advantages, education can be difficult to implement because the time and energy required to educate members of an ethics committee frequently takes longer and is greater than anticipated for several reasons. First, the diversity of its members' backgrounds often translates into appreciable differences in (a) baseline knowledge about ethics and clinical medicine, (b) understandings of concepts invoked in ethical discourse, and (c) weights given to cultural values. Second, committee members are often volunteers with an interest in ethics, but without discretionary use of time to participate in ethics committee activities. Third, some committee members are designated by their administrative superiors to participate, and both their time and their interest are limited. The time and energy required to educate an ethics committee is tantamount to teaching or having a class design a course for itself over a one- to three-year period.

Other challenges in educating ethics committee members include making resource materials accessible, addressing topics of interest, retaining a grounding in clinical reality, developing tools for rigorous analysis, promoting consistency across different cases, and identifying morally justifiable reasons for inconsistent recommendations. In addition, ethics committee members can benefit from education about barriers to effective interprofessional communication; respectful communication among professionals, patients, and families; the art of listening; and negotiation.

An early educational task for most ethics committees is exploring the nature of ethics and ethical decision making. Thus, many ethics committee members learn key principles such as beneficence, nonmaleficence, autonomy, and justice, as well as ethical theories and methods of moral inquiry. Equally important for committee members is to become familiar with a systematic approach to case analysis. One common approach is the *four-box* method of identifying relevant case information (Jonsen, Siegler, and Winslade, 1992). According to this approach, information is collected and organized into the following categories: medical indications, patient (or surrogate) preferences, quality of life assessments, and contextual features. Although this approach does not articulate a specific strategy for normative ethical analysis, it forces consistent consideration of certain topics in case deliberations.

Another approach to ethical case analysis that some ethics committee members learn is the application of subjective expected utility theory from cognitive psychology (Lusted, 1968). This approach relies heavily on the diversity, integrity, and honesty of ethics committee members. The first step in this approach is to have the ethics committee clearly articulate the ethical question (e.g.,

"Should she treat?", or "Should she not treat?"). This often is a difficult and worthwhile task that forces agreement about which question needs to be answered first. On each side of this question supportive arguments, possibly reflecting principles, outcomes, values, and legal concerns, are identified. The next task in the analysis is for the members to argue and debate the merits of each and ultimately to weigh these factors. By an inductive process, a morally acceptable course of action is identified. At this point in the process, recommendations can be reviewed for potential legal liability or institutional barriers.

After educating itself, the committee usually engages in or organizes educational activities for other members of the health care institution. The principal objective for most committees is to improve the quality of care for patients by augmenting the ability of clinicians to recognize, understand, and help resolve common and challenging ethical issues in clinical practice. Ethics education also attempts to help health care professionals examine their own personal and professional moral commitments; equip themselves with sufficient philosophical, social, and legal knowledge to aid in clinical reasoning; and develop interactional skills to facilitate effective listening and communication with patients, families and other professionals. Less frequently the goals of educational activities are to influence the organizational culture, promoting concepts of personal responsibility, professional integrity, comfort with uncertainty, an appreciation for the difference between authority and power, open-mindedness, and a nonintimidating milieu.

Educational activities often take the form of case-based ethics rounds, lectures, panel discussions, debates, role modeling, and development of pamphlets. Obviously, the format varies depending on the target audience. Sometimes the audience is the clinical professional staff, and at other times it is patients and their family members. Recent guidelines from the Joint Commission for the Accreditation of Health Care Organizations (JCAHO) promote mechanisms to educate patients about their rights to have advance directives and know about relevant institutional and state policies (Joint Commission on Accreditation Manual for Hospitals, 1993). Unfortunately, many of the educational materials that have been developed lack motivational appeal and merely focus on the logistics of completing advance directives.

The development of ethics education in the clinical setting poses numerous challenges. First, the culture of learning in most medical centers is case-based or patient-centered. Thus, educational activities often need to be tailored to specific cases and/or the clinical interests and needs of the clinicians. This culture often inhibits discussion of general ethical theories and principles, and yet such discussion may help provide a structure for thinking about new challenges. Second, effective teaching often occurs at the bedside. This requires having either consultants or clinicians with ethics training available during routine clinical teaching sessions. Third, many clinician-trainees consider ethics, humanistic medicine, and interactional skills less important than other aspects of clinical knowledge. Thus, attitudinal biases frequently interfere with clinician receptivity. Partial responses to this barrier include competent educators, education evaluations leading to refinement in teaching, and repeated role-modeling and support by clinician mentors.

Case Consultation

Clarification of goals is an important priority before the initiation of consultations and case review. In many health care institutions goals are formulated to identify morally sound solutions to ethical problems that arise in the medical context and to help resolve ethical dilemmas. Some ethics committees assume a more patient-centered role, such that the "interests of all parties, especially those of the incapacitated person, are adequately represented, and that the decision reached lies within the range of permissible alternatives" (President's Commission for the Study of Ethical Problems in Medicine and Biomedical Research, 1983). Despite efforts to define clearly the goals of consultative work, many questions remain. Papers by La Puma and Schneidermayer (1991) and by West and Gibson (1992) included in Part III discuss these questions in detail. Of paramount importance is whether cases are brought to the committee on a voluntary basis, or a committee reviews all cases of a certain type (e.g., withholding of artificial hydration and nutrition).

With the sharing of experience around the country, most American hospitals have adopted the time-honored tradition of voluntary consultations as the most appropriate format and as least antithetical to the medical culture (Lomax, Fraser, 1992). More recently, many policies for ethics committees specify inclusion of nonphysicians as members, and the opportunity for patients and family members to request ethics committee consultations. Patient knowledge of this resource, however, remains elusive. Even fewer committees as a matter of practice explicitly invite patients or their family members to participate in case discussions. Lack of patient involvement, however, procedurally undermines a common committee objective, the protection of patients.

The practical aspects of providing ethics consultations raises interesting questions: whether consultative recommendations should be advisory (optional) or mandatory, and whether the results of a consultation should be documented in the medical record or written and recorded elsewhere. In most institutions these questions have been resolved by having ethics consultations model clinical consultation services (Lomax, Fraser, 1992; Stadler, Morrissey, Williams-Rice, et al. 1994). Thus, consultations usually are advisory and written in the medical record, and ethics committees usually are called ethics advisory committees.

It has been argued, however, that the one *special* task of ethics committees is to exercise authority to postpone medical decisions it counsels against or to initiate judicial review of such decisions (Capron, 1984). A minor challenge for ethics committees is the additional question of what to do about advisory recommendations when consensus is lacking after case deliberation. When a range of ethically acceptable decisions exists, a committee's recommendations delineating one course of action may appear to foreclose other options due to clinicians' excessive deference to ethics committees. To prevent this, consultation notes may present conflicting opinions and rationales so that several options emerge as ethically defensible. Moreover, as consultative advice is advisory and potentially at variance with professionals' understanding of power and authority, negotiation and facilitation techniques and skills are useful for ethics consultants (West and Gibson, 1992).

The ethical analysis that occurs in case consultations usually reflects both inductive and deductive reasoning. Although members may be well-versed in distinct bioethical principles or methods of casuistic analysis, the nature of committee membership (involving multiple disciplines) and the orientation of discussion (being case-oriented) often foster analyses that combine approaches. In these discussions common principles such as respect for persons and autonomy, beneficence, nonmaleficence, and fairness are often considered. So too are the particularities of the case, experience with similar situations, the test of generalizability, the test of publicity (How would this read in tomorrow's newspaper?), legal constraints, and professional standards. When deliberations involve honest and explicit communication with critical questioning of assumptions, the end result is a rigorous process that represents the eclectic nature of contemporary ethical reasoning.

Hospital Policies

Health care institutions frequently involve ethics committees to assist with developing policies pertaining to withholding and withdrawing life-sustaining treatments (see the selections from Ruark and colleagues (1988), and Brennan (Brennan, 1988) included in Part III), medical record confidentiality, determination of mental incompetence, HIV testing and counseling, and advance care planning. Most committees quickly learn that subcommittee delegation fosters efficient progress. Many committees also learn that reviewing and critiquing other institutions' policies help prevent recreating the wheel.

Unfortunately, unforeseen challenges often await the implementation of policies. For example, even after do-not-resuscitate policies were implemented in hospitals, it became apparent that many physicians did not initiate communication about this until after the patient became mentally incapacitated, and thus the conversation involved family members (Bedell, Pelle, Maher, Cleary, 1986). Similarly, hospitals responded to the Patient Self-Determination Act's goal of educating patients about advance directives but were forced to consider the work demands of hospital personnel. As a result, many hospital policies about advance directives became administrative tools to ensure procedural compliance with JCAHO requirements. Empirical research identifying these and other challenges in clinical practice has enabled refinements in understanding of ethical problems and established the need for periodic review and modification of policies.

Policies from Nonclinical Settings

Professional organizations, individual scholars, and state and federal initiatives also have contributed to the formulation of policies relevant to the practice of bioethics. Selections from each of these sources are included in Part III. In many circumstances the purpose of such policies has been to facilitate decision making for mentally incapacitated patients and increase the likelihood that previously expressed wishes are honored, or, if prior wishes are unknown, that the best interests standard for surrogate decision making and reasonableness prevails (Braithwaite and Thomasma, 1986; American College of Physicians Ethics Committee, 1992; Omnibus Budget Reconciliation Act of 1990, 1990; Joint Commission on Accreditation Manual for Hospitals, 1993). Policies, especially legislative ones, are blunt instruments of change, and therefore can lack sufficient specificity to provide guidance in situations with additional clinical complexity. Using policies about advance directives as an example, the Patient Self-Determination Act (PSDA) was passed to promote awareness and respect for advance directives. The PSDA did not address the more important questions of how to talk to patients about their preferences for medical treatment in the face of mental incapacity, and how to assess the level of a patient's mental incapacity to know when to shift focus to an advance directive. The PSDA also did not address how to develop policies that are ethically and logistically feasible to facilitate decision making when a patient's wishes are not known and how to adjudicate apparent conflicts between prior preferences and current best interests.

Policy recommendations occasionally present competing ideas that lead to better understanding of bioethical issues. Unfortunately, different policies about the same issue in different settings may foster variability in practice based on the specifics of the accepted policy. Medical futility is a case in point. Some policies assert that physicians and nurses are not obligated to provide futile treatment (Council on Ethical and Judicial Affairs, American Medical Association, 1994). Others identify value elements and thus require patient involvement to avoid bias (Curtis, Park, Krone, et al., 1995). Other policies with futility judgments regard the use of physiologically futile interventions as falling outside the standards of professional behavior (Tomlinson and Brody, 1990). As these policies are discussed and evaluated, the concept of medical futility becomes more refined in ethical deliberations.

Different policy proposals also can lead to frustration among patients and educators in bioethics. This occurs, for example, with physician-assisted suicide. Competing policy recommendations from scholars and professional organizations about physician-assisted suicide have prevented consensus about decriminalizing or retaining the criminal status of this behavior. One group of scholars and clinicians has offered a policy that anchors physician involvement to reduction of suffering and compassion, and then offers suggestions to reduce the likelihood of abuse (Quill, Cassell, and Meier, 1992). By contrast, other policies pertaining to physician-assisted suicide argue against physician involvement in this activity due to potential future harms, such as diminution of respect and trust in the profession or service organization, insidious pressure for older and disabled persons to avail themselves of assisted suicide, and inequitable access to this service. The relative inertia within the medical profession about changing the status of physician-assisted suicide has led to patient frustration and the resultant consumer initiatives to decriminalize physician-assisted suicide in the states of Washington and Oregon. Frustration sometimes exists among educators in bioethics. An example is the American College of Physicians' policy about professional ethics. In one voice the College admonishes physicians to avoid conflicts of interest, but in another section discusses the physician's duty to render care *after* the relationship and its financial arrangements are secure (American College of Physicians' Ethics Committee, 1992). This potential inconsistency undermines the educational value of such a policy when taken in its entirety.

Quality Assurance

Like other activities in health care, ethics advisory committee activities and ethics-related policies can be evaluated for their effectiveness (Hoffmann, 1993). With regard to committee functions, empirical methods can be employed to characterize the scope and intensity of activities, assess effectiveness of educational programs, and identify which elements, approaches, or target audiences are associated with greater effectiveness. In addition, these types of research methods can characterize the relative contributions of different types of membership configurations, lines of authority, and chairmanship qualifications. To date there is limited information about these relationships and their ramifications. Similar types of questions are relevant to evaluating policies. Do they ensure consistent, ethically acceptable behaviors, augment education, or result in the desired outcomes?

Ethics consultations are another activity that might benefit from quality assurance. Currently, professional standards are lacking, quality control is questionable, credentialing of ethics consultants is a topic of debate, and questions exist as to the value and effectiveness of ethics consultations. Some critics charge that anyone can hang a shingle and call him- or herself an ethicist. In response to this gap in knowledge, the Agency for Health Care and Policy Research funded a conference in 1995 to promote a research agenda for quality assurance in ethics consultation.

If and when standards for ethics consultations develop, they should address the following areas of concern:

(1) the consultation discusses a course of action that is at variance with an institution's policy and does not advise the consultee of the conflict with the institution's policy
(2) the consultation fails to consider a central element or component of the clinical case
(3) the consultation discusses a course of action that is against the law without informing the consultee of the potential liability
(4) the consultant breaches patient confidentiality
(5) the consultant fails to inform the consultee of new major insights or a change in advice obtained from the full committee's review

(6) the consultation recommends a course of action that discriminates against a class of people by virtue of their age, gender, race, ethnicity, disability, or vulnerability. These possible behaviors raise questions of irresponsibility.

The challenge of quality assurance is to identify a way to reduce the likelihood of these events, promote quality service, and simultaneously not create a cumbersome monitoring system or meaningless activity that merely gives the appearance of promoting quality. In the absence of quality assurance efforts, the kinds of problems Bernard Lo details (Lo, 1987) can create obstacles to the functioning of ethics committees and consultants.

New and Future Challenges

Ethics committees have assumed a central role in the emergence of clinical ethics. In the future ethics committees will be forced to deal with concerns such as rationing and cost containment, the cultural diversity of patients, and the availability of new genetic information. Policies also will be needed to respond to the challenges of a changing system of health care delivery, diversification of the patient population, and technological advances that add to biological knowledge and may provide benefit to persons with appreciable concomitant risks of harm.

Managed Care and Rationing

Pressures to control health care costs and provide access to persons who are uninsured or underinsured, as well as the general sense that society is getting less than what it is paying for, are reshaping the delivery of health care in the United States. Managed care arrangements and rationing of treatments that provide marginal benefit or benefit only a few at great cost are two new issues confronting ethics committees.

Managed care will raise concerns as the old ethics of patient autonomy and fiduciary responsibility mix with business ethics and competing responsibilities. Physicians and nurses will seek guidance as they struggle over conflicts of interest and conscience. Without clear and explicit guidelines health providers will experience conflicts about whether their primary responsibility should be the best interests of the patient, the well-being of society, or the success of the health plan. Informed consent policies and practices will be challenged by business interests not to divulge information about the availability of services in other health care plans. Patients likely will seek support from ethics advisory committees either to protect their newly identified "rights," or to appeal policies that prevent access to beneficial treatments.

In response to emerging ethical problems, ethics committees will have to clarify their missions and goals. The greatest challenge that will confront ethics committees may be identifying and managing their own conflicting roles and advocacy responsibilities. Will ethics committees be able to protect the interests of patients and simultaneously help articulate and nurture business goals in health care institutions? Questions like this await ethics committees in the near future. It is hoped that ethics committees will serve as role models for health professionals by demonstrating how to protect patients and at the same time support institutional policies that have been developed with involvement of all stakeholders and that are fair, explicit, and accessible.

At the policy level, not only ethics committees, but also federal and state groups, professional associations, health care institutions, and scholars will attempt to develop policies that maximize health for society in general and are sensitive to fiscal constraints. Policies will attempt, for example, to distinguish basic from nonbasic health care, identify fair criteria and strategies for rationing, and develop fair mechanisms to develop and appeal policies. Explicit rationing policies will be tested and challenged by politics, a culture that embraces rescue medicine, and the mainstream societal preference to avoid difficult choices. Simultaneously, policy development will need to safeguard the integrity of the health care professions and patients' trust in health care providers. For a discussion of the various levels of clinical policy development see Part III, Section 2 of this anthology.

Cultural Diversity

Demographic changes in the composition of the country suggest a very different future American. In the near future, white, Anglo-Saxon protestants will be the minority in a polycultural society. Increasing numbers of patients will speak languages other than English and will have non-Western values. For example, the priority of individual autonomy is not embraced by all patients, and formalized informed consent practices may be offensive to others. See, for example, Carrese's and Rhodes's (1995) discussion of Navajo patients' responses to informed consent practices (in Part III, Section 4). Physicians and nurses will come to ethics committees seeking guidance about how to be "ethical" (per their understanding of ethical principles and ethics-related policies) and culturally sensitive at the same time. Committees will have to help providers to identify the underlying goals and values expressed in ethics-related policies and procedures, so that they can try to appeal to these fundamental goals in the context of another culture. At times it may seem like the integrity of the profession is challenged, and the role of the ethics committee may ultimately be to help physicians understand the true meaning of integrity. The role of ethics committees will be, first, to help identify strategies that support Western ideals while being sensitive and respectful of non-Western cultural beliefs; second, to help identify commonalities in values across cultures when strategies present cultural conflicts; and third, to identify the limits of acceptable practices to maintain the provider's professional integrity and personal moral beliefs. As Sherwin (1992) argues in Part III, Section 3, of this book, unequal power arrangements within health care institutions can perpetuate patterns of oppression that are unjust to nondominant social groups.

Ethics committees and institutional policies will struggle with cultural diversity. Issues such as advance care planning, intergenerational responsibility, personal responsibility for health, respect for persons, and the role of the community in decision making may become topics for ethics consultations and policy development. Cultural diversity and the resultant differences in meaning attributed to principles and ideas will help refine ethical analysis and ensure that it is not merely dominance of one cultural view over another.

Genetic Information

Advances in molecular biology occurring as a result of the project's genome goal of mapping human DNA will force the health care profession to confront issues about the ethical use of medical information. The ability to screen genetically for risks of conditions has just started to challenge ethics committees and hospital policies. Similar to the heart transplant issue in the early 1980s, new technological advances will have to be evaluated in terms of need, anticipated benefit, cost, and negative impact on other services. Future questions may focus on the value of knowing more about one's genetic make-up, problems of confidentiality when one family member's results implicate others, whether or not informed consent and genetic counseling accurately characterize the risks of learning genetic information, the relationship between probabilities for a population and the implications for an individual, and legitimate grounds for access to this knowledge in a health care system that is attempting to control health care costs. Empirical research will help identify the magnitude of anticipated and unanticipated consequences resulting from access to greater genetic knowledge.

Ethics committees will be asked to help develop policies that delineate access to genetic testing and the handling of confidential information. Health care workers likely will seek help from ethics committees when they perceive that patients want confirmation of their anticipated health. This pursuit of health-related knowledge is akin to the executive's desire for a yearly comprehensive health examination. Each type of behavior raises questions of whether patients and providers are acting responsibly. Health professionals also will struggle with parents who want to know the genetic predisposition of their fetus in order to decide whether or not to carry a pregnancy to term. The challenge for committees will be balancing respect for autonomous desires with both societal pressure to control health care costs and committee members' personal views. An additional challenge will be for ethics committees to nurture a medical culture that prevents wholesale use of medical technology simply because it is available. It is possible for ethics committees to help create a framework for handling the challenges of these new medical advances. Ethics committees and ethics-related policies can be agents for responding to future ethical challenge.

References

Alexander, S. "They decide who lives, who dies: medical miracle puts a moral burden on a small committee." *Life* 53:102ff, 1962.

American College of Physicians Ethics Committee. "American College of Physicians' Ethics Manual," 3d ed. *Annals of Internal Medicine* 117:947–960, 1992.

Barber v. Superior Court, 195 California Reporter 484, 486 (California Appellate 1983).

Bedell, S. E. W., Pelle, D., Maher, P. L., Cleary, P. D. "Do-not-resuscitate orders for critically ill patients in the hospital: How are they used and what is their impact?" *Journal of the American Medical Association* 256:233–237, 1986.

Braithwaite, S., Thomasma, D. C. "New guidelines for foregoing life-sustaining treatment for incompetent patients: an anti-cruelty policy." *Annals of Internal Medicine* 104:711–725, 1986.

Buchanan, A. E., Brock, D. W. *Deciding for Others: The Ethics of Surrogate Decision-making.* Cambridge, England: Cambridge University Press, 1989.

Capron, A. M. "Decision review: a problematic task." In: Cranford, R. E., Doudera, A. E., eds. *Institutional Ethics Committees and Health Care Decision Making.* Ann Arbor, MI: Health Administration Press, 1984.

Council on Ethical and Judicial Affairs, American Medical Association. "Guidelines for the appropriate use of do-not-resuscitate orders" *Journal of the American Medical Association* 265:1868–1871, 1991.

Cranford, R. E., Doudera, A. E. "The emergence of institutional ethics committees." In: Cranford, R. E., Doudera, A. E., eds. *Institutional Ethics Committees and Health Care Decision Making.* Ann Arbor, MI: Health Administration Press, 1984.

Curtis, R. C., Park, D. R., Krone, M. R., Pearlman, R. A. "Use of the medical futility rationale in do not attempt resuscitation orders." *Journal of the American Medical Association* 273:124–128, 1995.

Faden, R. R., Beauchamp, T. L., King N. M. P. *A History and Theory of Informed Consent.* New York, NY: Oxford Press, 1986.

Fletcher, J. C., Hoffmann, D. E. "Ethics committees: time to experiment with standards." *Annals of Internal Medicine* 120:335–338, 1994.

Fox, R. C., Swazey, J. P. *The Courage to Fail.* Chicago, IL: University of Chicago, 1974.

Hoffman, D. E. "Evaluating ethics committees: a view from the outside." *Milbank Quarterly* 71:677–701, 1993.

"*In re Quinlan*," 355 A.2d 647 (NJ 1976).

Infant Doe v. Baker, No. 482 S 140 (Indiana Supreme Court, May 27, 1982).

Joint Commission on Accreditation Manual for Hospitals. R1.1.1.3.2.1. Oak Brook Terrace, IL: Joint Commission on the Accreditation of Health Care Organizations, 1993.

Jonsen, A. R., Siegler, M., Winslade, W. J. *Clinical Ethics*, 3d ed. New York, N.Y.: Macmillan, 1992.

La Puma, J., Schneidermayer, D. L. Ethics consultation: skills, roles and training. *Annals of Internal Medicine* 114: 155–160, 1991.

Lomax, K. J., Fraser, J. E. "A survey of ethics advisory committees in the V. A. medical centers." Veterans' Administration National Center for Clinical Ethics, White River Junction, VT; 1992 (unpublished data).

Lusted, L. B. *Introduction to Medical Decision Making.* Springfield, IL: Charles C. Thomas, 1968.

"Nondiscrimination on the Basis of Handicap; Procedures and Guidelines relating to Health Care for Handicapped Infants; Final Rule," *49 Federal Register 1622, 1623* (January 16, 1984) (codified at 45 C. F. R. 84.55).

Omnibus Budget Reconciliation Act of 1990 (Western Supplement 1991). Pub. L. No. 101–508 4206, 4751.1990.

President's Commission for the Study of Ethical Problems in Medicine and Biomedical Research. *Deciding to Forego Life-Sustaining Treatment: Ethical, Medical and Legal Issues in Treatment Decisions.* Washington, D.C.: U.S. Government Printing Office, 1983.

Quill, T. E., Cassell, C. K., Meier, D. E. Care of the hopelessly ill: proposed clinical criteria for physician assisted suicide. *New England Journal of Medicine* 327:1380–1384, 1992.

Scribner, B. H. Ethical problems of using artificial organs to sustain life. Trans. *Amer Soc Artif Intern Organ* 10:209–212, 1964.

Singer, P. A., Pellegrino, E. D., Siegler, M. "Ethics committees and consultants." *Journal of Clinical Ethics* 1: 263–267, 1990.

Snaders, D., Dukeminier, J. "Medical advance and legal lag: hemodialysis and kidney transplantation." *University of California Law Association Law Review* 15:357–413, 1968.

Stadler, H. A., Morrissey, J. M., Williams-Rice, B., Tucker, J. E., Paige, J. A., McWilliams, J. E., Kay, D. "HEC consortium survey: current perspectives of physicians and nurses." *Hospital Ethics Committee Forum* 6:269–281, 1994.

Tomlinson, T., Brody, H. Futility and the ethics of resuscitation. *Journal of the American Medical Association* 264:1276–1280, 1990.

West, M. B., Gibson, J. M. "Facilitating medical ethics case review: what ethics committees can learn from mediation and facilitation techniques." *Cambridge Quarterly Healthcare Ethics* 1:63–74, 1992.

CLINICAL BIOETHICS

ৈ

Hospital Ethics Committees: Is There a Role?

Robert M. Veatch

Robert M. Veatch is a philosopher at the Kennedy Center for Ethics at Georgetown University and a senior associate at the Hastings Center. He has published extensively on topics in clinical ethics and the ethics of medical practitioners. In this article he considers four functions of ethics committees. He rules out an active decision-making role for ethics committees but endorses other functions such as developing and recommending ethics-related policies, advising and helping clarify ethically ambiguous cases, and confirming prognoses. In the course of assessing appropriate ethics committee functions, he illuminates concerns that ethics committees need to consider further.

On March 31, 1976, the New Jersey Supreme Court announced its decision in the case of Karen Quinlan. In addition to the personal impact of that decision on those involved in the case, the court's opinion had a significant impact on the broader public. The proposal to establish what Chief Justice Richard J. Hughes called a hospital "Ethics Committee" gave a major impetus to a new trend. Before the decision, there had been a few attempts to establish committees at the local hospital level to make, review, or advise in decisions regarding the care of the terminally ill, and since then the idea has been given substantial attention.

It is, therefore, an appropriate moment to ask a number of questions. . . .

. . . . should hospital ethics committees function primarily to review technical, medical facts, such as prognoses, or should they review the ethical and other value issues involved in the actual treatment-stopping decision once the prognosis has been determined?

Robert M. Veatch. "Hospital Ethics Committees: Is There A Role?" Abridged from *The Hasting Center Report*, Volume 7, 1977, pp. 22–25. Reprinted by permission.

Possible Tasks for Hospital Ethics Committees

Four general types of hospital committees can be identified: committees to review the ethical and other values involved in individual patient care decisions, committees to make larger ethical and policy decisions, committees for counseling, and prognosis committees.

1. Committees to review ethical and other values in individual patient care decisions   The committee originally proposed by Karen Teel and similar committees that have been proposed at other institutions are designed to review the appropriateness of decisions pertaining to the care of individual patients, in particular, determining when it is appropriate to stop treatment. Such a committee would take into account the patient's condition, but would move well beyond that to make decisions about whether treatment is appropriate, reasonable, or "ordinary."

According to many ethical traditions in medicine, a useless or gravely burdensome treatment is expendable. The tradition of Catholic moral theology defines such treatments as "extraordinary." Clearly, however, decisions about which treatments are expendable because they are unreasonable involve questions of ethics and other values. To say that a treatment is useless is to say that it will serve no appropriate or fitting purpose. It is an open question, for instance, whether a treatment which would sustain an individual's life in coma is useful or not. According to some ethical views that emphasize the duty to prolong life without asking questions about the quality of that life, such intervention may well be deemed useful. However, other, and in my view more plausible, ethical views emphasize that biological life *per se* should not be preserved unless other capacities and qualities are also present.

Deciding what counts as an expendable treatment or under what circumstances treatment should be discontinued once a prognosis has been determined is clearly a question of ethical and other value judgment[s]. If there is to be a committee at all to decide these questions, it should be a very broad one representing a range of ethical and other values. Some might argue that the committee should be made up of the ethically wisest people in the community, although selecting them would raise problems. However, individual patients who are competent have the right to refuse any medical treatment that is proposed for their own good. In the case of the incompetent patient, there is a recognized range of privacy and integrity for which the courts recognize familial discretion. Thus the question arises: why should there be any committee at all if the sole purpose is to review the wisdom of the decision? The conclusion seems inescapable that hospital committees have no appropriate role in actually making treatment-stopping decisions when the issue is one of whether the care is reasonable or unreasonable. They may still have counseling and other roles, to be considered below.

2. Committees to make larger ethical and policy decisions   Hospital committees may serve a second function, however. Questions arise that clearly involve ethical and other values, yet which in principle cannot be resolved by referring to the individual patient for the patient's own decision or, in the case of the incompetent, to the guardian and family. Institutional review boards for the protection of human subjects in biomedical research are an example of committees established to deal with this kind of question. Such committees must decide what information must be disclosed for a consent to be adequately informed for the research. In principle, one cannot ask the individual whether a particular risk should be disclosed without in the process disclosing that risk.

Another basic question faced by such institutional review boards is whether a hospital or other research facility should permit research even if the patient consents. Some hospitals might decide that research is sufficiently dangerous or useless that as a matter of ethical principle the research cannot be tolerated even with adequate consent.

A similar policy question is allocation of scarce hospital resources. In the 1960s when hemodialysis machines were scarce, committees were established at some hospitals to decide which patients would receive dialysis treatment. Those judgments involved medical criteria, but ethical judgments were central. Deciding which of two patients should receive a kidney machine when there is only one machine available cannot be left to the individual patient. Dialysis machines are no longer scarce, but there is a similar situation in neonatal intensive care units. Similarly a hospital might have a committee to make policy decisions about whether to build a new intensive care unit or to remodel the emergency room. Deciding whether obstetrics and abortion facilities or an alcoholism treatment unit should be established are other examples.

It seems reasonable that these policy-making committees should be broadly based, representing a wide range of ethical and sociological positions within the community or those responsible for the hospital. Different perspectives are important, since the committees are serving as agents for the broader community.

3. Counseling committees A third kind of committee might be called a counseling committee. It could be established to deal with specific terminally ill patients, but for the purpose of counseling and support rather than actual decision making. The hospital might have available an ongoing committee made up of a psychiatrist, a psychologist, a social worker, chaplain, and others with moral counseling skills. This committee might meet to discuss ongoing problems of the care of the terminally ill, but also make itself available for counseling when necessary.

Several existing committees, such as the Optimum Care Committee at the Massachusetts General Hospital, exist primarily to provide counsel (*New England Journal of Medicine*, 295 [August 12, 1976], 362–64). Many of the existing committees, however, see themselves as providing counsel not to the patient, but to the physician. Clearly, if one holds that the patient (or his agent in cases when he is incompetent) is the primary decision maker, it would be appropriate for the counseling committee to provide services for the patient instead of or in addition to the physician. For some patients such a committee might not be necessary, since moral counseling is likely to come from outside the hospital—from one's clergyman, family, or friends. Such a counseling committee would not be composed of representatives of a cross-section of ethical and sociological positions, but of individuals who have appropriate counseling skills.

Other functions related to counseling might also be appropriate. Although the committee should not have a role in making the actual decision to stop treatment, occasionally there may be cases where the decision made by a parent or other guardian is so questionable that the physician, nurse, or other hospital personnel are convinced that it should be reviewed. The morally and legally appropriate course is to bring the matter to court. If the court finds that the parental judgment is so unreasonable that it cannot be tolerated, it will appoint a new guardian for the purposes of authorizing the treatment. In such cases, however, the hospital staff member may want some guidance before deciding to initiate the court review. A hospital committee, especially one that was broadly representative of the community's moral sensitivities, could provide a sounding board for the health care professional who had such doubts. The committee could even initiate the court review proceedings itself. In such cases, however, the court, not the committee, would finally override the guardian's judgment.

4. Prognosis committees   The emphasis in the Quinlan opinion that the so-called "Ethics Committee" was in fact to confirm a prognosis has led to suggestions that such committees should really be called "Prognosis Committees." In January 1977 in New Jersey the Attorney General, the Health Commissioner, the head of the State Licensing Board, and several medical professional organizations jointly endorsed guidelines for prognosis committees called "Guidelines for Health Care Facilities to Implement Procedures Concerning the Care of Comatose Non-Cognitive Patients." The committee's purpose is to confirm the prognosis that no reasonable possibility exists of the patient's return to a cognitive, sapient state.

The guidelines propose that the committee include physicians trained in general surgery, medicine, neurosurgery or neurology, anesthesiology, pediatrics (if so indicated), and two additional physicians from outside the hospital staff. Such a committee should be made up of those with the relevant medical and other scientific skills for establishing the prognosis. The New Jersey guidelines provide for no lay committee members; but if lay people without such medical skills were on such a committee, their only function would be to ask questions and provide a modest public presence.

The New Jersey guidelines are recommendations that have no official weight. In fact, one of the main thrusts of the *Quinlan* opinion was to recognize that the consensus of the medical profession need not be binding on guardians or the state in approving guardian treatment refusals. By analogy one might question whether the consensus of the medical professional societies and other health-related professionals would be binding in recommendations about the establishment of a prognosis committee.

Second, the guidelines state that "the attending physician, guided by the committee's decision with the concurrence of the family, may then proceed with the appropriate course of action and, if indicated, shall personally withdraw life-support systems." In this recommendation the New Jersey guidelines clearly go beyond the *Quinlan* opinion. It is my understanding that this provision was added at the urging of nurses and others who might be ordered by physicians to actually stop the life-support apparatus.

Furthermore, the guidelines say that the attending physician *may* then proceed rather than that he *shall* proceed, leaving open the question of what would happen should such a physician decide against stopping the life-support apparatus. Presumably the physician would normally be the one who stops an ongoing treatment if the patient or the patient's agent so decides. Especially when a court has already reviewed the specific case or cases of the same type, however, the physician should not have the discretion in deciding whether to follow such instructions. He may, of course, feel morally obliged to withdraw from the case and normally would be permitted to do so provided a suitable replacement can be found to provide professional medical support. To say that the physician *may* then proceed, however, implies that he may also continue treatment which legally, since consent is lacking, has the quality of an assault and morally the quality of violating the patient's, the agent's, or the family's autonomy. It also forecloses the possibility that someone else might be the more appropriate person for the task. While nurses or other hospital personnel should never be forced to participate in the treatment stopping, there may be cases where they or others who are not directly connected with the hospital would be the more appropriate ones. In some circumstances the patient himself, the family, a clergy-man, or someone else in a special relationship with the patient may be more appropriate.

In spite of these reservations, the New Jersey guidelines are generally sound and the most concrete help available for a hospital in the process of establishing a committee. The commitment to prognosis review is clearly stated. The committee to review prognosis should be used whenever there is a difficult technical situation or concern that the individual physician's judgment needs review. As long as the committee does not mistakenly generalize its responsibilities and move into the area of approving or disapproving of the treatment decision arrived at by the patient or the patient's agent, the guidelines should be helpful.

There is one final problem, however. Deciding the prognosis of a patient may not be completely a technical question. We have become increasingly aware of a blurring between facts and values. When one is attempting to make a judgment of prognosis involving such vague terms as "reasonable hope," and "cognitive, sapient state," questions of value may impinge upon even the determination of prognosis. That may be one reason why a committee was established in the first place: to avoid depending exclusively on a single physician's evaluation of the prognosis. Those who advocate a prognosis committee should be aware of this difficulty. If a case were to be made for lay membership on a prognosis committee, this would provide one of the grounds.

These are just a few issues raised by proposals for hospital ethics committees to deal with decisions pertaining to the care of the terminally ill. Some of the proposals for hospital committees seem to me to be dangerous and misguided, for example, the use of a committee to approve or disapprove a treatment-stopping decision made by a patient or made by an agent for an incompetent patient. Other committee models make more sense. The committee made up of lay people to establish hospital policy or make resource allocation decisions, the counseling committee made up of those with counseling skills, and the prognosis committee made up of those with appropriate technical skills, are all reasonable ideas and could serve important functions. Hospital ethics committees are a new development, and it is still unclear which types will gain support and how they will evolve. The issues they pose are significant ones, and their resolution will merit further study.

The Inner Workings of an Ethics Committee
Latest Battle over Jehovah's Witnesses

Ruth Macklin

Ruth Macklin is a professor of ethics in the Department of Epidemiology and Social Medicine at Albert Einstein College of Medicine. She has contributed to the literature on many issues in clinical ethics and has been involved most recently in reproductive ethics. She served on the President's Advisory Committee on Human Radiation Experiments (1994–1995) and currently is a consultant to the Ethics Committee for the Department of Veteran Affairs. In this article she describes the evolution of a policy concerning consent for blood transfusion in Jehovah's Witnesses. The Ethics Committee's deliberations and discussions with noncommittee members resulted in several revisions to the section on pregnancy. The section on pregnancy became an explication of the competing principles and serves as a reminder that ethical analysis does not always lead to consensus about the most appropriate good course of action.

Is there anything new in the ongoing saga of Jehovah's Witness patients who seek to conform to the dictates of their religion, which prohibits transfusion of whole blood or blood products (including autologous transfusions, removal and replacement of the patient's own blood). . . .

. . . That issue is the right of a pregnant Jehovah's Witness to refuse a blood transfusion, resulting in the likelihood of her death and that of the fetus.* . . .

Policy Regarding Consent for Blood Transfusion in the Jehovah's Witness

Under New York State Public Health Law (Section 2805-d) an informed consent discussion should be conducted by the responsible physician with any patient about to undergo treatment. The patient should be told all the information that a reasonable person would consider material to the decision to accept treatment.

Ruth Macklin. "The Inner Workings of an Ethics Committee: Latest Battle over Jehovah's Witnesses." Abridged from *The Hastings Center Report*, Volume 18, 1988, pp. 15–20. Reprinted by permission.

*See for example, David A. Sacks and Richard A. Koppes, "Blood Transfusion and Jehovah's Witnesses: Medical and Legal Issues in Obstetrics and Gynecology," *American Journal of Obstetrics and Gynecology* 154:3 (1986), 483–86.

Information must be clearly and understandably presented in language the patient can reasonably be expected to understand. Information may not be withheld because of concern that disclosure could cause the patient to refuse treatment. The elements of the informed consent discussion should include:

a) The nature of the patient's illness
b) The nature and purposes of the proposed treatment, including:
   1. Risks or consequences
   2. Benefits
   3. Alternatives, including no treatment, and the risks of alternatives
c) The opportunity to question the proposed treatment

The Jehovah's Witness and Blood Transfusion Consent

A. Adult
   The risks, benefits, and alternatives, if any, to a proposed blood transfusion must be explained, as described above, to an adult Jehovah's Witness. Any adult patient who is not incapacitated has the right to refuse treatment no matter how detrimental such a refusal may be to his health.

Special Circumstances

1. Capacity

If there are reasonable grounds to doubt the capacity of the patient to understand the risks, or benefits of and alternatives to transfusion, psychiatric evaluation must be obtained. If the evaluation confirms the patient's capacity to understand, transfusion will *not* be administered.

If the patient is found to lack the capacity to make the decision to refuse transfusion, transfusion will be withheld only if there is clear and convincing evidence of the patient's wish to reject treatment, such as the following. . . .

a) If there is a document recently executed by the patient which directs unequivocally that transfusion should be withheld under all circumstances, or
b) If, prior to intervening incapacity during the hospitalization, the current chart documents the patient's unequivocal and consistent refusal to accept transfusion under any circumstances, or
c) If, in a patient who presents incapacitated, there is documentation in a prior hospital record within one year of an unequivocal and consistent refusal to accept transfusion under any circumstances.

Under any other circumstances, transfusion will be given.

2. Voluntariness

Any Jehovah's Witness who refuses transfusion will be offered an opportunity to discuss this refusal with a physician not directly involved in providing care, in order to ensure that the patient's decision is freely and voluntarily made. This physician should ordinarily be a psychiatrist unless the patient prefers otherwise.

3. Emergencies

In the event a Jehovah's Witness presents to the hospital with an immediate need for life-saving blood transfusion, transfusion will be given unless condition a, b, or c of Section 1 (Capacity) obtains.

In the event a life-threatening emergency requiring transfusion arises in the course of hospitalization, the same standard (Section 1, Capacity) will apply.

It is inappropriate to wait until a foreseeable emergency need for transfusion arises in order to avoid an informed consent discussion with a Jehovah's Witness. There is a positive obligation reasonably to anticipate the development of such an emergency need for transfusion.

B. Children

Parents have the right to consent to care for their dependent children; they do *not* have a coequal right to refuse care for their dependent children (Family Court Act Section 233). Parents do not have the right to deny minor children transfusions that are deemed medically necessary. In the event that a parent withholds consent for transfusion, the hospital administration must be contacted immediately and asked to seek a court order for transfusion. In the event that medical judgment holds any delay to be immediately life-threatening to the child or would produce irreversible harm, transfusion should be given.

For purposes of this policy a child is defined as anyone below the age of eighteen years. Emancipated minors will be treated as adults. (N.Y. State Public Health Law 2504 states: A minor parent or married minor may give consent. According to case law, a minor in the military may give consent; and a financially independent minor, living alone, may give consent.)

C. Pregnancy

In the case of a pregnant Jehovah's Witness's refusal of transfusion, policies relating to adult patients will apply before the third trimester. If the pregnancy has entered the third trimester, the State's interest in life requires the decision to be referred to the courts for adjudication. If in such a case medical judgment holds any delay to constitute an immediate threat to the pregnancy, transfusion should be given.

Competent adult patients have the right to refuse medical treatment. This right extends to pregnant women. However, some members of society assert that the fetus has "interests" or "rights" that compete with the rights of the mother to control her own body. In general, the rights of the mother are clearly acknowledged to take precedence in early pregnancy. As gestation advances, it becomes increasingly difficult for some members of society to ignore the "interests of the fetus." Because of the dilemma that arises out of these opposing interests, physicians have an obligation to disclose from the outset if, under specified circumstances, they would be unable to honor a patient's wishes.

Because society and the law have not resolved the conflict between fetal and maternal interests, the policy cannot establish clear guidelines for action where a clinician's interpretation of the interests of the fetus are in conflict with the wishes of the mother. The clinician and patient, with ethical consultation, must seek to resolve such conflicts within the context of the doctor-patient relationship and resort to other means for conflict resolution, including hospital administration, when necessary. Every physician has the right and the obligation to try to turn the care of such a patient over to another caregiver if the patient's wishes are incompatible with the physician's professional and ethical values. This course of action is ethically superior to the coercion of an unwilling patient.

Ethics Consultation: Skills, Roles, and Training

John La Puma and David L. Schiedermayer

John La Puma, the first author of this paper, is a general internist at the North Suburban Clinic in Elk Grove Village, Illinois, and a Chicago-based ethics consultant. In his role as consultant he helps physicians and managers develop programs in the area of managed health care. Dr. Schiedermayer is a general internist at the Medical College of Wisconsin. In addition to teaching ethics to medical students, residents, and faculty, he is a published poet. In the following article, these authors delineate the myriad of skills and roles for an ethics consultant. They emphasize that ethics consultants should be accountable for the process and outcome of their work. They also assert that clinical judgment, based on experience with patients and the natural history of diseases, is a prerequisite for effective ethics consulting. Thus they indirectly imply that the role of ethics consulting is primarily for clinician-ethicists. However, they recognize that nonclinicians could acquire the skills of an ethics consultant with years of clinical experience. This paper has been interpreted by some as suggesting that ethics consultants should be physician-ethicists.

What Legitimates Ethics Consultation?

Moral authority for ethics consultation arises from several sources. The primary justification for ethics consultation derives from the mandate to protect and foster shared decision making in the clinical setting.[1] Physicians should share health care decisions with well-informed patients who can understand their diagnoses, prognoses, and the various alternatives of proposed treatment and of nontreatment, and who can make decisions.[2] When an ethical problem arises, ethics consultation should be used to assure that issues are clarified so that decision making can be shared.

Ethics consultants' demonstrated ability to help resolve ethical dilemmas in patient care legitimates the use of ethics consultation. Ethics consultants have practical expertise in the clinical arena and are increasingly recognized as members of the health care team. The physician's need for analysis and advice in individual cases, the institution's need for counsel in patient-related policy issues, and the patient's need for an advocate further legitimate the use of ethics consultation. Courts and presidential commissions have recommended that clini-

John La Puma and David L. Schiedemayer. "Ethics Consultation: Skills, Roles, and Training." Abridged from *Annals of Internal Medicine*, Volume 114, 1991, pp. 155–160. Reprinted by permission.

cians seek appropriate assistance in making moral decisions.[3,4] The American College of Physicians and the American Medical Association have recognized that protecting and enhancing shared doctor-patient decision making is an ethical responsibility.[5,6] Physicians' concerns about liability and payers' concerns about the costs of care have fueled the search for special expertise.

Ethics consultants should be accountable for the process and outcome of their work. Having an institutional locus of accountability is reasonable, although the specific lines of authority and reporting relationship will differ according to each institution's structure and mission.[7] Vision and commitment are necessary to support the consultant in synergistic ventures with health care professionals specializing in other clinical areas.[8] A consultant may wish to report to or be sponsored by the medical staff executive committee, the department chairperson, the chief executive officer, the dean, or the board of trustees. Accountability keeps the consultant honest and humble and permits the consultant to work effectively within an institution. Finally, in the clinical model of ethics consultation, the consultant is accountable to his or her patients and their physicians.

Consultants should inform institutional ethics committees of relevant clinical activities. Ethics committees can use the consultant's knowledge of individual cases to reflect on larger trends and, when needed, suggest institutional policy; in addition, the committee may be able to provide the consultant with a multidisciplinary critique of his or her work.

Ethics Consultants and Ethics Committees

Ethics consultants are professionals with specialized training and experience that equip them to identify, analyze, and help resolve moral problems that arise in the care of individual patients. Consultants have the specific task of collecting disparate, but essential, aspects of a patient's medical course and personal history. The professional charge of gathering the relevant data, identifying opposing arguments and values, and restoring a central ethical focus to a case makes the consultant's role "ethical" in nature.[9] Assisting physicians in developing structured, coherent, and humane strategies for identifying, analyzing, and resolving ethical dilemmas is the clinical ethics consultant's special responsibility.[9]

Ethics consultants may choose to work with ethics committees (Table 1). The consultant is often the chairperson or co-chairperson of the committee and may go to the bedside, do the consultation, and report back to the committee at its regularly scheduled meeting. The consultant-chairperson may form a consulting subcommittee of several members, or the entire committee may meet to consider cases, either at the bedside or in a committee room. . . .

The Ethics Consultant's Clinical Skills

The consultant should be able to identify and analyze moral problems in a patient's care; use reasonable clinical ethical judgment in solving these problems; communicate effectively with health care professionals, patients, and families;

TABLE 1 Institutional Credibility, Sponsorship, and Relationships for Ethics
Consultants

Institutional credibility
  Clinical, practical, and ethical expertise
  Fellowship training in medical ethics
  Demonstrated patient advocacy
  Legal and professional acceptance
  Mastery of medical ethical information and patient-related policy issues

Institutional sponsorship
  Medical staff executive committee
  Department chairperson
  Chief executive officer
  Dean
  Board of trustees

Institutional relationships
  Chairperson of ethics committee
  Chairperson of consulting subcommittee
  Consultant on hospital policy
  Liaison with hospital legal office
  Educator of and advisor to various hospital committees, such as ethics, quality assurance,
    utilization review, and institutional review

negotiate and facilitate negotiations; and teach medical students, housestaff, and
attending physicians how to identify, analyze, and resolve similar problems in
similar cases (Table 2).

The ability to analyze and separate the ethical questions in a complex case
is among the most important of the ethics consultant's skills.[10] Data gathering
usually begins with an interview with and examination of the patient, followed
by a review of the medical record and hospital course and interviews with

TABLE 2 Skills and Roles for Ethics Consultants

Fundamental skills
  Identify and analyze clinical ethical problems
  Use and model reasonable clinical judgment
  Communicate with and educate team, patient, and family
  Negotiate and facilitate negotiations
  Teach and assist in problem resolution

Appropriate roles
  Professional colleague
  Patient advocate
  Case manager
  Negotiator
  Educator

physicians, nurses, family members, and others of importance to the patient. Through consultation, ethical issues are often identified and clarified: In one series, the consultant identified a mean of 3.0 issues per case and was "very important" or "somewhat important" in clarifying ethical issues in 94% of cases.[11] Considerable change in case management has been reported in 18 of 44 cases at county and Veterans Affairs hospitals,[12] 20 of 51 cases at university hospitals,[11] and 53 of 104 cases at community hospitals.

Clinical judgment, based on both long experience with many patients and familiarity with the natural histories of many diseases,[13,14] is difficult to acquire. Skill in clinical judgment underlies effective consultation, enabling the consultant to make the medical distinctions that are technically and morally relevant in each case. The consultant considers the care of a particular patient in a particular circumstance with a particular illness, as particularity is the hallmark of good medical practice.

Excellent interpersonal and communication skills are necessary for ethics consultants. Consultants can teach and model effective communication (listening, reflecting, encouraging discussion) and appropriate attitudes (respect, compassion, and courteousness). Ethics consultants use both verbal and nonverbal communication as diagnostic and therapeutic tools.[15]

The ethics consultant must be especially competent in helping to resolve interpersonal conflicts in patient care. Emotionally charged situations may be identified as "ethical dilemmas," but are more usually the result of miscommunication.[16] The consultant must be able to negotiate—at the bedside, in hospital conference rooms, and with administrators and third party payers. The consultant's expertise includes the ability to facilitate understanding, emphasize common interests instead of opposing positions, and remain tactful while suggesting a course of action. The consultant must consider the interests of patients, doctors, nurses, and administrators, because the clinical setting is a place of compromise. The consultant's ability to resolve cases in conflict hinges largely on mediation skills.[17]

Finally, the ethics consultant teaches medical students, housestaff, and attending physicians how to identify, analyze, and resolve ethical problems in similar cases.[18,19] Case process and case synthesis are inextricably integrated in ethics consultation: Both illustrate how ethical issues change over time. In addition, the consultant's written report may provide a detailed case analysis. Appended references of didactic and practical value allow requesting physicians to consider several views as they construct their own frameworks for decision making.

The Ethics Consultant's Roles

The consultant's roles may properly include those of professional colleague, educator, negotiator, advocate, and case manager (Table 2). The ethics consultant is a professional colleague. Rudd describes a professional colleague as "someone with whom to share the case's complexity and from whom discernible help will emerge."[20] The consultant's clinical judgment and ability to analyze ethical issues in individual cases identify the consultant as a professional colleague. The consultant should tailor the information, perspective, critique, or reassurance that he or she provides to help the requesting physician.[21] As Goldman and colleagues[22] note, the effective consultant communicates directly and nonthreateningly with the requesting physician.

Teaching ethical decision making to physicians is a central goal of ethics consultation.[23] The ethics consultant recognizes the requesting physician's ability and experience in analyzing and managing ethical dilemmas and provides effective, individualized instruction. The consultant then emphasizes principles that may apply to similar future cases.

The role of negotiator requires effective interpersonal and communication skills. The consultant can try to be a consensus-builder, but reasonable persons may disagree about the decisions made in a particular case.[24] The consultant acts as a rational, clear-headed participant who seeks to help disagreeing parties come to morally permissible conclusions. More often than not, disagreeing parties can agree on a practical solution, although their reasons for agreeing will be different.[25] The role of negotiator may properly include using persuasion, because ethics consultants have a professional obligation to effect morally permissible outcomes.

When a patient's situation mandates it, the consultant must be a patient advocate. The ethics consultant's primary duty is to the patient, but he or she also has duties to the requesting physician to be timely, clear, and specific.[18] Dual loyalty can be risky for the consultant, especially if he or she opposes the wishes or actions of family members, legal proxies, or physicians. When a patient's interests seem threatened by planned treatment, financial constraints, legal proceedings, or an unreliable proxy, the consultant's obligation may extend to confronting the family or physician, appealing economic constraints, and pursuing legal appeals.[26–28] Such actions may be difficult and time-consuming, but when harm to a patient seems imminent, consultants should try to prevent it.

The ethics consultant will seldom be required to manage a patient's case, even when a patient, family, or physician requests it. The attending physician should retain decision-making responsibility and authority, using the consultant's ongoing involvement as needed.[29] Ethics consultants should be prepared to help manage difficult cases when a patient's medical interests are threatened or when a patient, family, or professional colleague requires the consultant's skills in case management.

Ethics consultants can anticipate some pressure to assume other roles in the clinical setting. These roles properly belong to others, however, and should be referred to persons with the needed expertise. Ethics consultants may be asked to act as a case conscience (this role belongs to all physicians managing the case); case counsel (this role belongs to the legal office or the patient's attorney); case quality reviewer (this role belongs to hospital quality assurance); case psychoanalyst (this role belongs to a psychiatrist or psychologist); or case clergy (this role belongs to the hospital chaplain).

Difficulties for Ethics Consultants

Several general objections to ethics consultants have been raised.[30] Whether "objective" advice can be given by ethics "experts" and, if so, how this expertise is acquired are debated.[31,32] The long-term effects of ethics consultation in the hospital are unknown.[33] Trained in moral philosophy, not in decision making, philosopher-ethicists may lack clinical judgment. They may be aloof, unavailable, or uncomfortable in the clinical setting. Alternatively, a physician-ethicist may focus on problem solving and neglect important social, philosophical, or theologic aspects of a case.

A second objection is financial: Ethics consultants presently generate little or no revenue. Although consultants' revenue-generating potential may increase with use of the resource-based relative value scale (a weighting scale that increases compensation for cognitive work), whether ethics consultants ought to be paid as well as at what rate and by whom are unresolved questions of practical, political, and moral import.[34] As an institution-based service, like radiology or anesthesiology, consultants require costly malpractice coverage. If cost-savings criteria are used to evaluate ethics consultation, morality may become a charade for cost-cutting, to the patient's disadvantage.

Third, ethics consultants' risk for legal liability is unknown. We have previously suggested a standard of care for ethics consultants.[9] To our knowledge, however, an ethics consultant has not yet been sued. In 1986, charges were brought against an ethics committee in southern California; the suit was dismissed in 1990, but reportedly has dissuaded the committee from reconvening (Ross JW. Personal communication).

Fourth, questions remain about intrusion into the doctor-patient relationship. Who has the authority to request a consult? For whom does the consultant work? These questions are controversial. In our view, physicians may ask ethics consultants to speak with families, third-party payers, or patients; patients may speak with consultants directly.

The consultant should be able to answer requests from many quarters, but the primary physician engages and dismisses the consultant. In a clinical model of ethics consultation, the consultant works for both the physician and the patient. If a team member wants an ethics consultation, suggesting it first to the primary physician may promote an open dialogue and help to resolve the problem. If the suggestion is not taken, the team member can appeal the refusal to his or her supervisor. Uninvited consultants should not intercede in cases: Ethics consultants should not be moral policemen.

Finally, whether ethics consultants must be physicians or may also be nonphysicians is controversial. Nonphysicians may have the years of clinical experience necessary for the development of clinical judgment; if this is not the case, the clinical expertise of a physician colleague is required. More important than a medical degree is a consultant's ability to acquire and use the necessary skills and fulfill the appropriate roles of the ethics consultant. A professional who wishes to do ethics consultation should be trained in those skills and roles.

Training and Certification in Ethics Consultation

Training program curricula should provide the necessary skills for consultation practice. Ethics consultants need substantial patient care and hospital experience,[35] instruction in case law and legal processes,[36] practice in casuistic moral reasoning and ethical decision making,[37] and knowledge of medical humanism and humanistic behavior.[38-40] The experience of consulting with a skilled, well-trained mentor, reading carefully about the patient's medical and ethical presentation, and following the patient's case to its conclusion, constitutes a practical, established process of medical learning.

Who should train as an ethics consultant? Ideal candidates are clinicians who are expert in their own medical discipline and who have or wish to gain the skills and play the roles of the consultant.[41,42] Such candidates include physicians who are completing a primary care residency or who are the ethics committee chairperson or co-chairpersons.

To acquire the clinical skills of an ethics consultant, nonphysicians require several years of clinical experience and routine participation with medical teams in clinics, hospital rooms, and special care units. Training in different medical settings provides the necessary foundation for understanding the diversity and details of many medical illnesses and for developing clinical judgment. The complexity of the doctor-patient relationship; the individuality of patients' and families' preferences, goals, and interests; and the exigencies of hospitals, health care professionals, and third-party payers are best appreciated when observed firsthand.

To become ethics consultants, most nonphysicians and many physicians would require training in medical humanism, clinical psychology, medical sociology, and health law. Essential topics in medical humanism include integration of the qualities of integrity, respect, and compassion with bedside behavior; in clinical psychology, differentiation between organic and functional illnesses, recognition of differing doctor-patient relationships in different medical specialties, and determination of patient decision-making capacity; in medical sociology, comprehension of the special language, interrelationships, and hierarchies of hospital medicine, nursing, and medical social work; and, in health law, case and statutory law relevant to life-sustaining treatment, advance directives, and surrogate decision making.

Physicians who wish to become ethics consultants require training in moral reasoning and ethical decision making. Training must provide opportunities to reflect on and critique clinical ethical dilemmas, discover and discuss multidisciplinary perspectives, and learn and apply techniques of facilitation and negotiation. Continuing to hold primary clinical responsibilities during training is a direct, vital way of appreciating ethical dilemmas in patient care.

Whether clinical ethicists can or must have certification in a new medical field is controversial. Certification requires a defined body of useful clinical knowledge and an evaluation process that determines whether the candidate has mastered the knowledge and possesses a specified level of clinical competency. The American Board of Internal Medicine criteria for a new discipline include a significant scientific base and clearcut relation to internal medicine or its subspecialties; a recognition of the discipline in the medical, academic, and scientific communities; the potential for a significant number of practitioners in a well-defined practice; a requirement for formal training with prescribed standards; and improved patient care.[43] Ethics consultants, particularly those who are physicians, have begun to meet several of these criteria (for example, an identifiable base of scientific knowledge and improved clinical practice). Practical, political, and professional questions remain, however, about the incorporation of nonphysician ethics consultants (currently, the majority of ethics consultants) into a field of expertise in medicine.

Conclusion

The ethics consultant's role will continue to evolve. We favor a clinical model of ethics consultation, the process and outcome of which require continued study. Empiric data and critical review are necessary to evaluate the utility and limitations of consultation. An important question is whether patients, families, and physicians find ethics consultation to be beneficial. The issue of specialty certification in ethics consultation also requires further consideration and debate.

The consultant teaches the analytic, interpersonal, and communication skills that physicians need to solve ethical problems. The consultant assists in the decision-making process as a negotiator or advocate when the physician, the patient, or the family requires such assistance. Finally, the consultant is a clinical colleague with specialized training and experience who is available for consultation. Consultants who are competent in clinical ethics and who can use their skills and knowledge to assist patients and physicians at the bedside should be trained and available to assist patients, families, and physicians.

References

1. President's Commission for the Study of Ethical Problems in Medicine and Biomedical and Behavioral Research. *Making Health Care Decisions: The Ethical and Legal Implications of Informed Consent in the Patient-Practitioner Relationship.* Washington, DC. U.S. Government Printing Office; 1982.
2. Jonsen AR, Siegler M, Winslade WJ. *Clinical Ethics: A Practical Approach to Ethical Decisions in Clinical Medicine.* 2d ed. New York: Macmillan; 1986.

3. The National Commission for the Protection of Human Subjects of Biomedical and Behavioral Research. *The Belmont Report: Ethical Principles and Guidelines for the Protection of Human Subjects of Research*. Washington, DC: U.S. Government Printing Office; 1978:DHEW pub no (OS) 78-0012, 78-0013, 78-0014.

4. *President's Commission for the Study of Ethical Problems in Medicine and Biomedical and Behavioral Research*. Washington, DC: U.S. Government Printing Office; 1983.

5. Council on Ethical and Judicial Affairs of the American Medical Association. *Current Opinions*. Chicago: American Medical Association; 1989.

6. Ethics Committee, American College of Physicians. American College of Physicians ethics manual Part I. History: the patient; other physicians. *Ann Intern Med* 1989;111:245–52.

7. La Puma J. Clinical ethics, mission and vision: practical wisdom in health care. *Hospital and Health Services Admin*. 1990;35:321–6.

8. La Puma J. Researching for-profit research, the obligations of hospital ethicists. *Clin Res*. 1989;37:569–73.

9. La Puma J, Toulmin SE. Ethics consultants and ethics committees. *Arch Intern Med*. 1989;149:1109–12.

10. Rothenberg LS. Clinical ethicists and hospital ethics consultants: the nature of the "clinical" role In: Fletcher JC, Quist N, Jonsen AR, eds. *Ethics Consultation in Health Care*. Ann Arbor, Michigan: Health Administration Press; 1989:19–35.

11. La Puma J, Stocking CB, Silverstein MD, DiMartini A, Siegler M. An ethics consultation service in a teaching hospital: utilization and evaluation. *JAMA*. 1988;260:808–11.

12. Perkins HS, Saathoff BS. Impact of medical ethics consultations on physicians: an exploratory study. *Am J Med*. 1988;85:761–5.

13. Jonsen AR. Do no harm. *Ann Intern Med*. 1978;88:827–32.

14. Tumulty PA. What is a clinician and what does he do? *N Engl J Med*. 1970;283:20–4.

15. Cassell EJ. *Talking With Patients*. v. 1 and 2. Cambridge, Massachusetts: MIT Press; 1985.

16. Waitzkin H. Doctor-patient communication, clinical implications of social scientific research. *JAMA*. 1984;252:2441–6.

17. Drane JF. Hiring a hospital ethicist. In: Fletcher JC, Quist N, Jonsen AR. *Ethics Consultation in Health Care*. Ann Arbor, Michigan: Health Administration Press; 1989:117–33.

18. Self DJ, Lynn-Loftus GT. A model for teaching ethics in a family practice residency. *J Fam Pract*. 1983;16:355–9.

19. Barnard D. Residency ethics teaching: a critique of current trends. *Arch Intern Med*. 1988;148:1836–8.

20. Rudd P. Problems in consultation medicine: the generalist's reply. *J Gen Intern Med*. 1988;3:592–5.

21. Merli GJ, Weitz HW. The medical consultant. *Med Clin North Am*. 1987;71:353–5.

22. Goldman L, Lee T, Rudd P. Ten commandments for effective consultations. *Arch Intern Med*. 1983;143:1753–5.

23. Culver CM, Clouser KD, Gert B, et al. Basic curricular goals in medical ethics. *N Engl J Med*. 1985;312:253–6.

24. Moreno J. What means this consensus? Ethics committees and philosophic tradition. *The Journal of Clinical Ethics.* 1990;1:38–43.
25. Toulmin SE. The tyranny of principles. *Hastings Cent Rep.* 1981;11:31–9.
26. La Puma J, Schiedermayer DL, Toulmin SE, Miles SH, McAtee J. The standard of care: a case report and ethical analysis. *Ann Intern Med.* 1988;108:121–4.
27. La Puma J, Cassel CK, Humphrey H. Ethics, economics, and endocarditis: the physician's role in resource allocation. *Arch Intern Med.* 1988;148:1809–11.
28. Schiedermayer DL, La Puma J, Miles SH. Ethics consultations masking economic dilemmas in patient care. *Arch Intern Med.* 1989;149:1303–5.
29. La Puma J, Schiedermayer DL. Outpatient clinical ethics. *J Gen Intern Med.* 1989;4:413–9.
30. Nielsen K. On being skeptical about applied ethics. In: Ackerman TF, Graber GC, Reynolds CH, eds. *Clinical Medical Ethics: Exploration and Assessment.* New York: University Press of America; 1987;95–116.
31. Phillips DF. Physicians, journalists, ethicists, explore their adversarial, interdependent relationship. *JAMA.* 1988;260:751–7.
32. Perkins H. Teaching medical ethics during residency. *Academic Medicine.* 1989;64:262–6.
33. Siegler M, Singer PA. Clinical ethics consultation: Godsend or "God squad" *Am J Med.* 1988;85:759–60.
34. Purtilo RB. Ethics consultation in the hospital. *N Engl J Med.* 1984;311:983–6.
35. Siegler M. Cautionary advice for humanists. *Hastings Cent Rep.* 1981;11:19–20.
36. Burt R. *Taking Care of Strangers: the Rule of Law in Doctor-Patient Relations.* New York: Free Press; 1979.
37. Jonsen AR, Toulmin S. *The Abuse of Casuistry: A History of Moral Reasoning.* Berkeley: University of California Press; 1988.
38. American Board of Internal Medicine Subcommittee on Evaluation of Humanistic Qualities of the Internist. Evaluation of humanistic qualities in the internist. *Ann Intern Med.* 1983;99:720–4.
39. Arnold RM, Povar G, Howell J. The humanities, humanistic behavior and the humane physician: a cautionary note. *Ann Intern Med.* 1987;106:313–8.
40. The American Board of Internal Medical Subcommittee on Humanistic Qualities. *A Guide to the Awareness and Evaluation of Humanistic Qualities in the Internist.* Portland: American Board of Internal Medicine; 1990.
41. Siegler M, Pellegrino EJ, Singer PA. Clinical medical ethics. *J Clin Eth.* 1990;1:5–9.
42. Perkins H. Clinical ethics fellowships. *SGIM Newsletter.* 1989;12:6.
43. American Board of Internal Medicine. *Criteria for the Definition of New Medical Areas.* Portland: American Board of Internal Medicine; 1984.

Facilitating Medical Ethics Case Review

What Ethics Committees Can Learn from Mediation and Facilitation Techniques

Mary Beth West and Joan McIver Gibson

Mary Beth West is an attorney with the U.S. State Department in Washington, D. C. Joan Gibson is the director of the Health Sciences Ethics Program at the University of New Mexico. The program involves the schools of medicine, nursing, pharmacy, and allied health. They received a grant from the National Institute for Dispute Resolution in Washington, D. C., to assess how ethics committees could benefit from facilitation and mediation techniques. In the accompanying article they discuss how several methods of alternative dispute resolution (shuttle facilitation, mediation, and large-group facilitation) can facilitate ethics case consultations as well as other internal committee processes.

Case Consultation Models and Dispute Resolution Processes

Parallels can be drawn between case consultation models and three facilitated processes—shuttle facilitation, mediation, and large-group facilitation. This section explores those parallels.

Case Consultation and Shuttle Facilitation

In some healthcare institutions, medical ethics issues may be addressed without getting the interested parties together in a meeting. For example, a social worker, physician, chaplain, or another [ethics] committee member may meet with parties individually and resolve the issue before it gets to the committee. Alternatively, the [entire] committee may meet with the physician, while a committee member may talk individually with the family, patient, surrogate, or other party. In another format, the committee may designate one or more committee members as "liaisons" to meet with each party individually as a prelude to a meeting in which the committee develops advice outside the presence of the parties.

These models bear some similarities to shuttle facilitation—the process in

---

Mary Beth West and Joan McIver Gibson. "Facilitating Medical Ethics Case Review: What Ethics Committees Can Learn from Mediation and Facilitation Techniques." Abridged from *Cambridge Quarterly Healthcare Ethics*, Volume 1, 1992, pp. 64–74. Reprinted with the permission of Cambridge University Press.

which a facilitator works toward resolution through separate meetings with the parties. A shuttle facilitator meets individually with each party to explore underlying interests and needs. Options for resolution and eventual consensus are also developed as the facilitator shuttles between or among the parties. One major distinction between shuttle facilitation and the types of ethics committee consultation models described above, however, is that ethics committees do not necessarily base their strategies on the underlying assumption that they are neutral facilitators. Nor do they attempt to balance the power between or among the participants. For example, committees may meet with one party without meeting with the other, or may invite one party to the committee meeting, while meeting with the other only outside the framework of the committee. To the extent that a committee sees its function as helping parties work toward a resolution of issues, the lack of balance and neutrality, or the parties' perception of lack of balance and neutrality, may make it more difficult for the committee to fulfill that function.

Case Consultation and Mediation

Where committees bring together parties with a subset of two or three committee members, case consultation may resemble a mediation or small group facilitation. Whether this type of consultation in fact exhibits the characteristics of mediation or facilitation, however, depends on how the committee members perceive their roles in the case consultation. To the extent that the committee members are without independent interests and views concerning the issues, and to the extent that they see their roles as helping the parties work toward resolution, their actions may resemble those of a neutral mediator or facilitator. Because committees often view their roles as educational, however, one or more committee members in case review may have independent views or expertise to offer. Where committee members are "interested" participants, it may be difficult for those members to act as facilitators. Even "interested" participants can act as facilitators, however, where they perceive their roles as neutral and use their expertise to help the parties explore interests and solutions rather than to advocate particular ideas or resolutions.

The role of facilitator in small-group case consultation is to create an atmosphere of trust in which the parties are able to express and explore their underlying interests and needs, identify solutions, and work toward consensus. Some committees appear to view their roles as encompassing some but not all of these elements. For example, some committees see themselves as a resource to help parties explore ideas, but not to help them work toward consensus on a particular solution or plan. The functions of such committees may resemble mediation, without the steps of agenda setting and reaching resolution, and follow-up.

The extent to which small-group case consultation resembles mediation or facilitated settlement may also depend on the nature of the parties. If one party is a medical professional and the other is a patient or family member, the patient or family member may view himself or herself as an "outsider" and may view the committee and the medical professional as essentially one entity. In that case, the situation may appear as "4 or 5 on 1" rather than as a more balanced mediation or facilitation involving facilitators and two or more parties. Because the committee members are not perceived as neutral, it becomes significantly more difficult for the committee to fulfill a facilitation role. A committee that wishes to fulfill the role of facilitator must consider ways to minimize power imbalances among parties.

Case Consultation and Large-Group Facilitation

Where committees bring together parties and a number of committee members who may have positions or views to offer concerning the matter at issue, the process more closely resembles large-group mediation or facilitation. In a case involving differences between a physician and a patient's family concerning withdrawal of life support, for example, the physician, individual members of the patient's family, and various committee members (such as the chaplain, an ethicist, and a neurologist) may each have positions or interests in the resolution. While the chaplain, ethicist, and other medical personnel are not "parties" in the true sense, one or more of them may have views he or she feels should be recognized and taken into account in the discussion. An ethics committee meeting that brings together all these players faces some of the same challenges as a large-group facilitation of a public policy issue.

Facilitators in large-group meetings face significant challenges. They must create an atmosphere of trust in which the parties can explore their underlying interests and needs, in which the parties and other participants in the group are heard and understood, and in which parties are able to explore options for resolution within the framework of the applicable interests and needs. Ethics committees face similar challenges but with important differences. Large-group facilitations are often led by one or two neutral facilitators, whose sole responsibilities are to nurture the atmosphere of trust and to move the participants through the steps necessary to reach consensus. In the ethics committee setting, on the other hand, the person running the meeting may be one of the participants with a position or interest rather than a designated neutral facilitator. Even if the person running the meeting does not have an interest in the outcome, he or she may not have been trained in facilitation techniques. This adds to the difficulty in moving the process through the steps necessary to reach the committee's goal.

Recommendations for Ethics Committees in Case Consultation

Understanding the relationship among committee role, source(s) of power, and process is a prerequisite for successful case consultation. Even committees with defined roles have given little thought to how process assists case consultation.

In doing so, committees should focus on three primary stages of consultation. These are intake, the consultation itself, and follow-up.

Intake

Intake is critical. This stage offers the opportunity to diagnose the issue and determine the most effective process or method for its resolution. In addition, many cases are resolved at this stage. Hospital chaplains, social workers, physicians, and others who are members of ethics committees reported that they are able to resolve issues at this stage, often using shuttle facilitation techniques without involving the committee.

Little attention has been given to intake as an integral and constitutive function of ethics committee process. Although some committees have designated a person to call meetings, others could not describe a "normal" method by which issues arrive before and are presented to the committee. Even in committees using a designated process to convene meetings, the person exercising that function often fails to consider the best process for handling specific types of cases.

The intake stage can play an important diagnostic role. In the dispute resolution context, courts throughout the country[1] are setting up multidoor programs designed to offer a variety of opportunities for resolution, depending on the nature of the dispute and the parties. A careful intake process staffed by a person trained in techniques for diagnosis and resolution of problems could help committees identify interested parties, identify the interests and nature of the problem, and set up a case consultation structure and process designed most effectively to address those issues requiring committee attention. Careful intake also offers the potential of resolving some issues without the need for committee involvement.

We recommend that each ethics committee designate one member as its intake specialist. That member should in most cases be a hospital employee or someone who is readily available in the institution on short notice. The intake specialist should receive training in techniques for diagnosis and resolution of problems and in dispute resolution processes. Although formal training in diagnosis of bioethics conflicts/issues has not yet been developed, training in general facilitation and mediation techniques would be helpful. The process used by such intake specialists would likely involve the following stages, which closely resemble those designed by the trainers of the American Bar Association for referrals in multidoor courthouse programs: identification of interested parties; introduction, making each party comfortable, and establishing rapport; gathering information and maintaining an open, sensitive climate; problem clarification and summary; review of possible processes for addressing the issue; and selection of the option.[2]

Once the intake specialist has identified the interested parties, he or she can meet with them together or separately to determine the outlines of the issue and to determine which committee process would be most appropriate. In this preliminary process, some disputes and dilemmas will, no doubt, be resolved.

Case Consultation

Models for case consultation processes should vary, depending on the committee's perceived role in its institution, the nature of the issue, and the parties involved. Several critical elements are involved. These include, first, matters of form: the place the consultation is held, the number of people involved, the relationships of those people to the issue, whether both parties attend, and whether or not one or more members are present as neutral facilitators. Second are elements of process. Here the committee needs to determine how best to design the consultation to meet its goals. If the goal is to assist the parties in reaching consensus on a solution, for example, perhaps the process should incorporate the basic stages of mediation.

Committees should develop form and process guidelines that reflect their views of their roles in case consultation. This section outlines several models. Additional work is necessary to refine these models and to develop intake and consultation processes specifically designed for ethics committees. The ideal appears to involve design of several forms and processes that can be used flexibly by each committee, depending on the nature of the issue, the parties involved, and the goals for that consultation.

Issue resolution   For committees who see their roles as attempting to facilitate resolution, the process should be designed to most closely resemble a mediation or facilitated settlement. This model would call for one or two members of the committee trained as a neutral facilitator(s) to meet with the parties. Keeping in mind the persons necessary for resolution, the group should be as small as possible; the meeting could involve only the parties and the facilitator or could also involve a few other committee members. Alternatively, other committee members with views or interests could be brought in as "experts" to assist the parties at the appropriate time in the process.

The facilitator(s) should be flexible in designing and carrying out the process but should basically structure it along the lines of the mediation stages: introduction and explanation of the process, information gathering and issue identification, agenda setting and reaching resolution, and agreement. The facilitator(s) may meet with parties separately in caucus and should be willing to bring in others with views or expertise that will be helpful to the parties in considering the issues. The facilitator(s) should also be flexible in helping the parties design interim solutions or steps where final resolution is not attainable.

For example, assume that the family of a comatose patient takes the position that life-support treatment should be terminated immediately. The doctor, on the other hand, may insist that more information is needed before making that kind of decision. Delving beneath the outcome sought by the family, the participants might find such a position based on the anger, frustration, and pain that comes from dealing with what the family perceives as an uncaring, unresponsive institution rather than from a basic wish to let the patient die. The family's underlying interest may be in ending a situation that is unbearable for the family members. On the other hand, in advocating delay, the physician may be looking not so much for more information but rather for emotional and legal support. The doctor's underlying interest may be to avoid legal liability or to be faithful to a moral commitment to sustain a patient's life. In this situation, where the patient's family members feel that their concerns have not been heard and responded to by the physicians and hospital staff, the facilitator(s) might help the family and hospital design a method for future communication that must be implemented before the family is ready to consider the more basic treatment issues.

Issue exploration   Committees who see their roles as helping the parties explore issues, but not necessarily as assisting them in reaching resolution, may structure the process somewhat differently. However, it would still be helpful to have a trained member of the committee act as a neutral facilitator. The committee, however, may meet in a larger group and may meet with both parties together or with the parties separately. The committee should start with an introduction and explanation of the process and should then attempt to gather information and help the parties identify and explore the issues. Committee members and the facilitator(s) may also assist the participants in determining potential solutions but would not see their role as attempting to help the parties reach consensus on a solution.

Education   Finally, committees who see their primary roles as education of the parties may use yet a different process. Those committees may choose to meet in large session, including all the committee members (and possible outsiders) who have views to offer. Such committees may meet with the parties, either at the same time or separately, or may choose to meet without the parties, either at the same time or separately, or may choose to meet without the parties. In the latter case, the committee's views or advice would be transmitted to the parties by one or more committee members. Involvement of a person trained as a facilitator would be helpful where the committee meets with one or more of the parties. Where the committee does not, facilitation training is less critical.

Where the committee sees its role as educational and simply offers its advice and views to one or both parties, the parties still must reach consensus to proceed. In some cases, provision of information alone may pave the way for resolution. In others, however, the parties may need further assistance. Such assistance could be provided by a trained intake specialist or by one of the committee members trained in communication and facilitation.

Follow-up

Few of the committees surveyed follow up on case consultations. Occasionally a report is made at the next full meeting of the committee. Only rarely do committees formally follow up with the parties to determine what action was taken or to offer further assistance. Chaplains or social workers may occasionally perform this function informally.

We recommend that the intake specialist formally follow up with participants after case consultations. The purpose of the follow-up would be twofold. First, it would provide information to the committee concerning the outcome of the case consultation. Second, it would make further assistance available to the parties should they need such assistance to reach consensus or should additional issues arise after the formal case consultation.

Conclusion

. . . Facilitation and mediation techniques *can* be helpful in case review consultations as well as in other internal committee processes. *How* those techniques can best assist committees depends on an understanding of each committee's role in its institution, the applicable source(s) of committee power, the types of cases typically coming before the committee, and the committee's goals in consultation. Processes currently in use by ethics committees resemble certain forms of facilitation, such as shuttle facilitation, mediation, and large-group facilitation. The ideal format might encompass a more flexible approach designed to reflect and respond to the variety of issues, parties, and institutional roles that a single committee may confront.

We recommend that committees review and analyze the processes they use, their level of success with case consultations, and the cause and effect relationship between the two. As the initial step, committees should consider training one or more of their members in facilitation and communication techniques. Using these newly trained members, committees should then review and appropriately revise the structure and techniques used in case consultation, paying special attention to the roles and activities of intake and follow-up. Based on our preliminary research, it is clear that these stages play a key role in individual consultations as well as in committees' overall relationships to their institutions. It is also clear that when preliminary intake and postconsultation follow-up are undertaken, it is only in a most abbreviated fashion. Finally, it will be important for committees periodically to review and evaluate the success of revised procedures in responding to their needs and goals.

References

1. National Institute of Justice. Toward the multi-door courthouse—dispute resolution intake and referral. Washington, D.C.: NIJ Reports; 1986(Jul); SNI 198.
2. See above. National Institute of Justice, 1986.

Behind Closed Doors
Promises and Pitfalls of Ethics Committees

Bernard Lo

Bernard Lo is a physician (internal medicine)-ethicist at the University of California-San Francisco Medical School. He received fellowship training in ethics at the University of California-San Francisco while in the Robert Wood Johnson Clinical Scholars Program. He has contributed to the clinical ethics literature with articles invoking different methodologies, including ethical analysis, anthropological observation, survey research, and quantitative health services research. In the following article he primarily discusses the threats to optimal ethics committee function. Examples include imprecise goals, restricted access (who can request a consultation, who can attend a meeting, who can review the results of the discussion), and "groupthink." At the conclusion the author specifies several useful criteria for evaluating both the process by which ethics committees review cases and the results of their deliberations.

Hospital ethics committees have been hailed as providing a promising way to resolve ethical dilemmas in patient care. Although ethics committees may have various tasks, such as confirming prognoses, educating care givers, or developing hospital policies, their most innovative role is making recommendations in individual cases.[1-5] This role has been supported by the President's Commission for the Study of Ethical Problems in Medicine and Biomedical and Behavioral Research, the American Medical Association, and the American Hospital Association. Strictly speaking, such recommendations are not binding, but they undoubtedly carry great weight, especially if they are cogently justified.[6] It is predicted that most ethics committees will make recommendations in particular cases[3] and that the courts will respect them.[3]

Ethics committees may offer an attractive alternative to the courts.[3-5] The judicial system may be too slow for clinical decisions.[7,8] Moreover, the adversarial judicial process may polarize physicians, patients, and families,[9] whereas ethics committees may reconcile divergent views. The 1986 New York State Task

Bernard Lo. "Behind Closed Doors: Promises and Pitfalls of Ethics Committees." Reprinted from *The New England Journal of Medicine*, Volume 317, 1987, pp. 46–50. Reprinted by permission of *The New England Journal of Medicine*. Copyright © 1987, Massachusetts Medical Society.

Supported in part by a grant (1 P50 MH42459-01) from the National Institute of Mental Health and a grant from the Commonwealth Foundation.

Force on Life and the Law encouraged resolving patient care dilemmas at the hospital level, rather than turning to the courts, and suggested that ethics committees might mediate such disagreements.[10]

Although I support ethics committees, several questions trouble me. First, are these committees ethical? The goals and procedures of some committees may conflict with established ethical principles. Second, is agreement by committees always desirable? Group dynamics may lead to flawed information, reasoning, or recommendations. Third, are these committees effective? Like other medical innovations, they need to be rigorously evaluated.

Goals and Procedures of Ethics Committees

The very name suggests that ethics committees base their recommendations on ethical principles and rational deliberation, rather than on mere custom, political power, or self-interest. A consensus on medical decision making has emerged in the medical literature, court decisions, and reports of the President's Commission.[1,7,8,11,12] According to this consensus, competent patients should give informed consent or refusal to the recommendations of physicians. Care givers need not accede to patient requests for treatments, however, if there are no medical indications. In cases in which patients are incompetent, decisions should be based on their previously expressed preferences or, if such preferences are unclear or unknown, on their best interests. The goals of some ethics committees, however, may conflict with these ethical guidelines. Goals vary substantially among committees.[1-3,13-15] Some do not have explicit goals. One committee has said, "We have never formally stated in writing the exact purpose or purposes of our committee but have decided to proceed in an informal manner. . . . We felt that to formalize our objectives might be counterproductive to the work of our committee."[14] But as ethics committees mature, and especially as they wish to serve as alternatives to the courts, they need to define their goals more clearly. Some so-called ethics committees have as goals confirming prognoses, providing emotional support for care givers, or reducing legal liability for physicians or hospitals.[1-3,13-15] One hospital administrator has even suggested that the ethics committee be used as a public relations "tool" for justifying unpopular decisions to discontinue unprofitable services.[16] Although committees on quality assurance, staff support, risk management, or public relations are important, there is little reason for patients, their surrogates, or the public to accept their recommendations about patient care.

After clarifying goals, committees can establish procedures. Ethics committees must decide who can refer cases or attend meetings. Many committees limit participation by patients and families. According to a 1982 survey, only 25 percent of ethics committees that reviewed cases allowed patients to bring cases to the committee. Only 19 percent of committees allowed patients to attend meetings, whereas 44 percent allowed family members to do so.[17] Limiting access to committee proceedings may seem desirable. It may be sound political strategy to overcome initial resistance to the ethics committee within the hospital. For example, attending physicians may fear that their authority will be undermined if patients, families, or nurses can ask the committee to review cases. Restricting access may also facilitate frank discussions by care givers and committee members about sensitive topics. In addition, discussions with other health professionals may help physicians to clarify their thinking before they talk to patients or families.

Restricted discussions, however, may not be accepted by patients, families, and society. Patients or surrogates who disagree with physicians are unlikely to regard the committee as impartial if they may not convene the committee or present their views directly, whereas physicians may do so. Disagreements that reach ethics committees usually involve important personal issues—even questions of life and death. In such vital decisions, patients and their proxies are not likely to accept recommendations by a committee whose members they have not met or that seems to meet behind closed doors.

The composition of ethics committees may not reassure patients that their wishes and interests are represented. Typically, most members of ethics committees are physicians, who may assess the importance of medical problems or the risks and benefits of treatment differently from patients.[18,19] Patients or surrogates who disagree with the committee's recommendations may say that the composition of the committee was biased against them.

Some committees meet with patients or family members who take the initiative and request meetings. But people who need the most help in expressing their preferences or interests may be the least likely to request a meeting. They may be cognitively impaired or unable to navigate the medical system, or there may be cultural, language, or educational barriers. Hence, it is desirable for the committee to take steps to inform patients, as well as care givers, of its work. Such information is particularly important if the committee can review a case without the consent of the parties. Mandatory review has been recommended, for example, when withholding life-sustaining treatment from neonates or from incompetent adults without surrogates is being considered.[20] A pamphlet about the committee might be distributed when patients are admitted. Patients or surrogates who are concerned that committee discussions or recommendations may invade their privacy can then express those concerns in advance. Before the committee discusses a case, it should inform patients or surrogates and invite them to participate in the deliberations.

Most ethics committees also restrict the access of nurses. The 1982 survey found that only 31 percent of committees allowed nurses to present cases, and only 50 percent allowed nurses to attend meetings.[17] But it may be advisable to increase the access of nurses. Nurses have close contact with patients and families and may take the role of patient advocates.[21] They may raise previously overlooked issues, contribute new information, or express the questions and viewpoints of patients and families. Disagreements by nurses with physicians' orders often indicate a need to reconsider decisions.[22]

Because ethics committees are touted as an alternative to the courts, it may be useful to compare their safeguards with those in legal procedures.[23] The legal system notifies parties of the proceedings, allows them to give evidence, and ensures representation for patients. If the patient is incompetent, the court may appoint a guardian ad litem to represent the interests of the patient or to argue for continuing treatment. Moreover, parties are notified of the decision and the reasons for it, so that the decision can be reviewed or appealed. Ethics committees that make recommendations may not need safeguards that are as elaborate as those in a legal system that makes binding decisions. But for ethics committees to be accepted as a quicker and less acrimonious alternative to the courts, they must be perceived to be as fair as the courts.

In order for ethics committees to assist in decision making, their recommendations and the reasons for them must be known by all parties. In addition to communicating with the patient or surrogate and the attending physician, a representative of the committee might write a note in the medical record, so that nurses, consultants, and physicians understand the committee's recommendation and reasoning. Ethics committees, however, may seem reluctant to allow their recommendations to be reviewed. Some committees do not note their recommendations and reasoning in the medical record. In addition, articles about ethics committees discuss how to reduce the liability of individual committee members by keeping records from being "discoverable"—that is, from being subpoenaed in civil suits.[20,24] Such apparent secrecy may evoke the suspicion that the committee is more concerned with protecting physicians, the hospital, or itself than with helping patients.

Pitfalls of Committee Discussions

Pressures on ethics committees to reach agreement may lead to recommendations that are ethically questionable. Agreement or even consensus does not confer infallibility. For example, in the 1960s, hospital committees selected patients with chronic renal failure for treatment with life-prolonging dialysis machines, which were limited in number. When it was disclosed that criteria of social worth were implicitly applied, these committee decisions were criticized as being unfair and discriminatory.[25]

In some circumstances, committees may impair rather than improve decision making. Political scientists and psychologists have shown that committees may inadvertently pressure members to reach consensus, avoid controversial issues, underestimate risks and objections, or fail to consider alternatives or to search for additional information.[26,27] In other words, committees may not serve their intended function of considering diverse viewpoints and arguments. Such undesirable qualities of committee discussions, which have been called "groupthink," may lead to grave errors in judgment.

Ethics committees may fall victim to groupthink. First, these committees may reach consensus too easily, by not adequately considering patients' preferences. Despite the ideal of informed consent, patients are often not involved in decisions about their care.[28-30] Second, committees may accept secondhand information uncritically. Physicians appreciate that medical consultants should take new histories, examine patients, and review x-ray films and scans.[31,32] Similarly, an ethics committee should scrutinize information about the medical situation and the patient's preferences. Conclusions and inferences, rather than primary data, may be presented. For instance, patients may be described as "terminal" or "hopelessly ill," or it may be reported that an incompetent patient would not want "heroic care." Since such phrases are ambiguous and potentially misleading, committees should require and, if necessary, seek out more specific information. Third, ethics committees may overlook imaginative means of resolving disagreements. Disputes over patient care are not always caused by conflicts of ethical principles or obligations. They may also result from misunderstandings, stress, or lack of attention to the details of care.[22] Despite stalemates over conflicting ethical principles or duties, agreements on particular recommendations for patient care may be possible.[33]

Ethics committees should appreciate that they work under conditions that predispose them to groupthink. A rapid recommendation may be needed despite uncertain information and conflicting values and interests. Such clinical urgency may press the committee to reach agreement. The committee may feel attacked by various groups: attending physicians who fear that their power is being usurped, nurses who think that they are given unreasonable orders, administrators who wish to control costs, or risk managers who want to avoid legal difficulties. If committee chairpeople are forceful leaders who control discussions, they may unintentionally discourage frank debate and disagreement. Tendencies toward groupthink may be reinforced if access to the committee is limited.

Ethics committees that recognize the dangers of groupthink can take steps to avoid them. First, committees can guard against premature agreement. The chairperson may explicitly ask that doubts and objections be expressed or may appoint members to make the case against the majority. Second, committees can scrutinize any secondhand information they receive. To understand the patient's preferences, the committee might talk with the patient or proxy directly, invite the patient or surrogate to participate in some discussions, or assign a committee member to act as a patient advocate. Third, the committee can look for innovative ways to settle disputes. Improved communication may resolve disagreements. Families, nurses, or house staff may accept the attending physician's decisions after they hear the reasons for it and have an opportunity to ask questions. Alternatively, a compromise may be negotiated.[34] For example, a patient who threatens to sign out of a cardiac care unit may agree to further treatment if he or she is given more control over the timing of the administration of medications and nursing care and if one physician and one nurse take responsibility for answering his or her questions.

Evaluating Ethics Committees

Ultimately, the question of whether ethics committees are useful is an empirical one. Before consulting ethics committees can be considered to be a standard decision-making procedure rather than a promising innovation, they need to be evaluated. Because enthusiastic anecdotes about innovations may not be confirmed in controlled trials, pleas have been made to evaluate new technological procedures, such as angioplasty, before they are accepted and put into wide use.[35] Institutional innovations should also be evaluated, even if they seem to be obviously beneficial. For instance, hospices were expected to provide more humane and less expensive care for patients with terminal illnesses. Controlled studies, however, suggest that hospice care may not differ substantially from current conventional care and may be more expensive.[36-38]

As in any evaluation, deciding on clinically meaningful outcomes and designing unbiased studies require thought and planning. I suggest several criteria for evaluating both the process by which ethics committees review cases and the results of their deliberations. First, patients and their surrogates should have access to the ethics committees. Specifically, they should be able to ask the committees to review their cases and to meet with the committees if they desire. Second, recommendations by the committee and the reasons for them should be available to the parties in each case. Generally, a note in the medical record would be required. Third, recommendations by ethics committees and actual decisions by attending physicians should be consistent with ethical and legal guidelines. The gold standard should be the widespread ethical consensus that has emerged on many issues.[39] Evaluations might focus on whether ethics committees reduce discrepancies between this consensus and actual decisions by physicians. For instance, studies indicate that care givers often fail to discuss management options with patients or the surrogates of incompetent patients.[28-30] Ethics committees should recommend such discussions when appropriate. If their recommendations have an effect on care givers, fewer decisions will be made without such discussions with patients or their surrogates. Committees should also increase informed refusals of care by patients. Moreover, committees should decrease decisions based on ambiguous or uncorroborated secondhand information about the indications for treatment or about patient preferences. Fourth, parties in disagreements should be satisfied with the process of review and with the recommendations of the ethics committee. Although the degree of satisfaction of care givers with ethics consultations has been studied,[40] it is also important to determine the reactions of patients or their surrogates. Finally, ethics committees that make recommendations should have their own internal systems of review, to ensure that the suggested criteria are met.

In summary, the promise that ethics committees will resolve dilemmas about patient care and avoid legal disputes needs to be examined critically. If recommendations by ethics committees are to be accepted by patients, families, society, and the courts, the wishes and interests of patients must be represented and ethical guidelines must be followed. Committees can take active steps to reduce the risk of groupthink. Empirical studies may indicate what kinds of committees improve decisions relating to patient care and in which clinical circumstances.

References

1. President's Commission for the Study of Ethical Problems in Medicine and Biomedical and Behavioral Research. Deciding to forego life-sustaining treatment: a report on the ethical, medical, and legal issues in treatment decisions. Washington, D.C.: Government Printing Office, 1983.
2. Cranford RE, Doudera AE, eds. Institutional ethics committees and health care decision making. Ann Arbor, Mich.: Health Administration Press, 1984.
3. Bayley SC, Cranford RE. Ethics committees: what we have learned. In: Friedman E, ed. Making choices: ethics issues for health care professionals. Chicago: American Hospital Publishing, 1986:193–9.
4. Lynn J. Roles and functions of institutional ethics committees: the President's Commission's view. In: Cranford RE, Doudera AE, eds. Institutional ethics committees and health care decision making. Ann Arbor, Mich.: Health Administration Press, 1984:22–30.
5. Committee on Ethics and Medical-Legal Affairs. Institutional ethics committee's [sic]: roles, responsibilities, and benefits for physicians. Minn Med 1985; 68:607–12.
6. Siegler M. Ethics committees: decisions by bureaucracy. Hastings Cent Rep 1986; 16(3):22–4.
7. Lo B, Dornbrand L. The case of Claire Conroy: Will administrative review safeguard incompetent patients? Ann Intern Med 1986; 104:869–73.
8. Lo B. The Bartling case: protecting patients from harm while respecting their wishes. J Am Geriatr Soc 1986; 34:44–8.
9. Burt RA. Taking care of strangers: the rule of law in doctor-patient relations. New York: Free Press, 1979.
10. New York State Task Force on Life and the Law. Do not resuscitate orders: the proposed legislation and report of the New York State Task Force on Life and the Law, April 1986.
11. Wanzer SH, Adelstein SJ, Cranford RE, et al. The physician's responsibility towards hopelessly ill patients. N Engl J Med 1984; 310:955–9.
12. Lo B, Jonsen AR. Clinical decisions to limit treatment. Ann Intern Med 1980; 93:764–8.
13. Levine C. Questions and (some very tentative) answers about hospital ethics committees. Hastings Cent Rep 1984; 14(3):9–12.
14. Kushner T, Gibson JM. Institutional ethics committees speak for themselves. In: Cranford RE, Doudera AE, eds. Institutional ethics committees and health care decision making. Ann Arbor, Mich.: Health Administration Press, 1984:96–105.
15. Fost N, Cranford RE. Hospital ethics committees: administrative aspects. JAMA 1985; 253:2687–92.
16. Summers JW. Closing unprofitable services: ethical issues and management responses. Hosp Health Serv Adm 1985; 30:8–28.

17. Youngner SJ, Jackson DL, Coulton C, Juknialis BW, Smith E. A national survey of hospital ethics committees. Crit Care Med 1983; 11:902–5.
18. Friedin RB, Goldman L, Cecil RR. Patient–physician concordance in problem identification in the primary care setting. Ann Intern Med 1980; 93:490–3.
19. McNeil BJ, Weichselbaum R, Pauker SG. Fallacy of the five-year survival in lung cancer. N Engl J Med 1978; 299:1397–401.
20. Winslow GR. From loyalty to advocacy: a new metaphor for nursing. Hastings Cent Rep 1984; 14(3):32–40.
21. Robertson JA. Ethics committees in hospitals: alternative structures and responsibilities. Conn Med 1984;48:441–4.
22. Lo B. The death of Clarence Herbert: withdrawing care is not murder. Ann Intern Med 1984; 101:248–51.
23. Baron C. The case for the courts. J Am Geriatr Soc 1984; 32:734–8.
24. Cranford RE, Hester FA, Ashley BZ. Institutional ethics committees: issues of confidentiality and immunity. Law Med Health Care 1985,13:52–60.
25. Fox RC, Swazey JP, eds. The courage to fail: a social view of organ transplants and dialysis. Chicago: University of Chicago Press, 1974:240–79.
26. Janis IL, Mann L. Decision-making: a psychological analysis of conflict, choice, and commitment. New York: Free Press, 1977.
27. George A. Towards a more soundly based foreign policy. In: Commission on the Organization of the Government for the Conduct of Foreign Policy, appendix B. Washington, D.C., Government Printing Office, 1975.
28. Lidz CW, Meisel A, Osterweis M, Holden JL, Marx JH, Munetz MR. Barriers to informed consent. Ann Intern Med 1983; 99:539–43.
29. Bedell SE, Pelle D, Maher PL, Cleary P. Do-not-resuscitate orders for critically ill patients in the hospital: How are they used and what is their impact? JAMA 1986; 256:233–7.
30. Goldman L, Lee T, Rudd P. Ten commandments for effective clinicians. Arch Intern Med 1983; 143:1753–5.
31. Lo B, Saika G, Strull W, Thomas E, Showstack J. 'Do not resuscitate' decisions: a prospective study at three teaching hospitals. Arch Intern Med 1985; 145:1115–7.
32. Tumulty PA. The effective clinician: his methods and approach to diagnosis and care. Philadelphia: W.B. Saunders, 1973:45–8.
33. Beauchamp TL, Childress J. Principles of biomedical ethics. 2nd ed. New York: Oxford University Press, 1983.
34. Steinbrook R, Lo B. The case of Elizabeth Bouvia: Starvation, suicide, or problem patient? Arch Intern Med 1986; 146:161–4.
35. Mock MB, Reeder GS, Schaff HV, et al. Percutaneous transluminal coronary angioplasty versus coronary artery bypass: Isn't it time for a randomized trial? N Engl J Med 1985; 312:916–9.
36. Kane RL, Wales J, Bernstein L, Leibowitz A, Kaplan S. A randomised controlled trial of hospice care. Lancet 1984; 1:890–4.
37. Kane RL, Bernstein L, Wales J, Rothenberg R. Hospice effectiveness in controlling pain. JAMA 1985; 253:2683–6.
38. Birnbaum HG, Kidder D. What does hospice cost? Am J Public Health 1984; 74:689–97.
39. Jonsen AR. A concord in medical ethics. Ann Intern Med 1983; 99:261–4.
40. Perkins HS, Saathoff BS. How do ethics consultations benefit clinicians? Clin Res 1986, 34:831A. abstract.

Questions for Discussion
Part III, Section 1

1. According to Veatch, what are the benefits of including people with diverse professional and educational backgrounds on an ethics committee? Why is it important to have community representation on an ethics committee?

2. Did the ethics committee which developed the policy (discussed by Macklin) regarding blood transfusion among Jehovah's Witness patients do an adequate job of dealing with ethical concerns?

3. How do La Puma and Schiedermayer describe the education, training, and experience that are essential for someone who functions as an ethics consultant?

4. Do West and Gibson regard facilitation and mediation as parts of ethical analysis, complementary skills to be used in the dissemination of opinions, or both, depending on the circumstances?

5. Lo maintains that ethics committees should be rigorously evaluated. How would you evaluate the usefulness of ethics committees by means of quantitative and qualitative research methods?

SECTION 2

CLINICAL POLICY DEVELOPMENT
એ

Part 1340—Child Abuse and Neglect Prevention and Treatment

*Office of Human Development Services,
Health and Human Services*

In the following federal regulation pertaining to child abuse and neglect prevention and treatment, the Office of Human Development Services of Health and Human Services sets forth rules that enter the arena of decision making in the pediatric intensive care unit. These regulations, often referred to as the Baby Doe rules, preclude the withholding or withdrawal of artificial hydration and nutrition from newborns with severe disabilities and impaired quality of life. These rules are meant to prevent discrimination on the basis of disability and allow for hotlines to report clinician behaviors that appear to be outside these standards. These regulations may be compared in spirit, language, and effect with the American Disabilities Act.

Subpart A—General Provisions
§1340.1 Purpose and Scope

(a) This part implements the Child Abuse Prevention and Treatment Act ("Act"). As authorized by the Act, the National Center on Child Abuse and Neglect seeks to assist agencies and organizations at the national, State and community levels in their efforts to improve and expand child abuse and neglect prevention and treatment activities.

Office of Human Development Services, Health and Human Services, "Child Abuse and Neglect Prevention and Treatment," Part 1340, *Code of Federal Regulations* 45. Abridged from the October 1, 1993 version.

(b) The National Center on Child Abuse and Neglect seeks to meet these goals through:

(1) Conducting activities directly (by the Center);

(2) Making grants to States to improve and expand their child abuse and neglect prevention and treatment programs;

(3) Making grants to and entering into contracts for: Research, demonstration and service improvement programs and projects, and training, technical assistance and informational activities; and

(4) Coordinating Federal activities related to child abuse and neglect. This part establishes the standards and procedures for conducting the grant funded activities and contract and coordination activities.

(c) Requirements related to child abuse and neglect applicable to programs assisted under title IV-B of the Social Security Act are implemented by regulation at 45 CFR parts 1355 and 1357.

(d) Federal financial assistance is not available under the Act for the construction of facilities.

§1340.2 Definitions

For the purposes of this part; . . .

Child abuse and neglect means the physical or mental injury, sexual abuse or exploitation, negligent treatment, or maltreatment of a child under the age of eighteen, or the age specified by the child protection law of the State, by a person including any employee of a residential facility or any staff person providing out of home care who is responsible for the child's welfare under circumstances indicating harm or threatened harm to the child's health or welfare. The term encompasses both acts and omissions on the part of a responsible person.

(1) The term *sexual abuse* includes the following activities under circumstances which indicate that the child's health or welfare is harmed or threatened with harm: The employment, use, persuasion, inducement, enticement, or coercion of any child to engage in, or having a child assist any other person to engage in, any sexually explicit conduct (or any simulation of such conduct) for the purpose of producing any visual depiction of such conduct; or the rape, molestation, prostitution, or other form of sexual exploitation of children, or incest with children. With respect to the definition of sexual abuse, the term "child" or "children" means any individual who has not attained the age of eighteen.

(2)(i) "Negligent treatment or maltreatment" includes failure to provide adequate food, clothing, shelter, or medical care.

(ii) Nothing in this part should be construed as requiring or prohibiting a finding of negligent treatment or maltreatment when a parent practicing his or her religious beliefs does not, for that reason alone, provide medical treatment for a child; provided, however, that if such a finding is prohibited, the prohibition shall not limit the administrative or judicial authority of the State to ensure that medical services are provided to the child when his health requires it.

(3) *Threatened harm to a child's health or welfare* means a substantial risk of harm to the child's health or welfare.

(4) *A person responsible for a child's welfare* includes the child's parent, guardian, foster parent, an employee of a public or private residential home or facility or other person legally responsible under State law for the child's welfare in a residential setting, or any staff person providing out of home care. For purposes of this definition, out-of-home care means child day care, i.e., family day care, group day care, and center-based day care; and, at State option, any other settings in which children are provided care. . . .

Subpart B—Grants to States

§1340.10 Purpose of This Subpart

This subpart sets forth the requirements and procedures States must meet in order to receive grants to develop, strengthen, and carry out State child abuse and neglect prevention and treatment programs under section 107 of the Act. . . .

§1340.14 Eligibility Requirements

In order for a State to qualify for an award under this subpart, the State must meet the requirements of §1340.15 and satisfy each of the following requirements:

(a) State must satisfy each of the requirements in section 107(b) of the Act.

(b) *Definition of Child Abuse and Neglect.* Wherever the requirements below use the term "Child Abuse and Neglect" the State must define that term in accordance with §1340.2. However, it is not necessary to adopt language identical to that used in §1340.2, as long as the definition used in the State is the same in substance.

(c) *Reporting.* The State must provide by statute that specified persons must report and by statute or administrative procedure that all other persons are permitted to report known and suspected instances of child abuse and neglect to a child protective agency or other properly constituted authority.

(d) *Investigations.* The State must provide for the prompt initiation of an appropriate investigation by a child protective agency or other properly constituted authority to substantiate the accuracy of all reports of known or suspected child abuse or neglect. This investigation may include the use of reporting hotlines, contact with central registers, field investigations and interviews, home visits, consultation with other agencies, medical examinations, psychological and social evaluations, and reviews by multidisciplinary teams.

(e) *Institutional child abuse and neglect.* The State must have a statute or administrative procedure requiring that when a report of known or suspected child abuse or neglect involves the acts or omissions of the agency, institution, or facility to which the report would ordinarily be made, a different properly constituted authority must receive and investigate the report and take appropriate protective and corrective action.

(f) *Emergency services.* If an investigation of a report reveals that the reported child or any other child under the same care is in need of immediate protection, the State must provide emergency services to protect the child's health and welfare. These services may include emergency caretaker or homemaker services; emergency shelter care or medical services; review by a multidisciplinary team; and, if appropriate, criminal or civil court action to protect the child, to help the parents or guardians in their responsibilities and, if necessary, to remove the child from a dangerous situation.

(g) *Guardian ad litem.* In every case involving an abused or neglected child which results in a judicial proceeding, the State must insure the appointment of a guardian ad litem or other individual whom the State recognizes as fulfilling the same functions as a guardian ad litem, to represent and protect the rights and best interests of the child. This requirement may be satisfied: (1) By a statute mandating the appointments; (2) by a statute permitting the appointments, accompanied by a statement from the Governor that the appointments are made in every case; (3) in the absence of a specific statute, by a formal opinion of the Attorney General that the appointments are permitted, accompanied by a Governor's statement that the appointments are made in every case; or (4) by the State's Uniform Court Rule mandating appointments in every case. However, the guardian *ad litem* shall not be the attorney responsible for presenting the evidence alleging child abuse or neglect.

(h) *Prevention and treatment services.* The State must demonstrate that it has throughout the State procedures and services [that] deal with child abuse and neglect cases. These procedures and services include the determination of social service and medical needs and the provision of needed social and medical services. . . .

§1340.15 Services and Treatment for Disabled Infants

(a) *Purpose.* The regulations in this section implement certain provisions of the Act, including section 107(b)(10) governing the protection and care of disabled infants with life-threatening conditions.

(b) *Definitions.* (1) The term "medical neglect" means the failure to provide adequate medical care in the context of the definitions of "child abuse and neglect" in section 113 of the Act and §1340.2(d) of this part. The term "medical neglect" includes, but is not limited to, the withholding of medically indicated treatment from a disabled infant with a life-threatening condition.

(2) The term "withholding of medically indicated treatment" means the failure to respond to the infant's life-threatening conditions by providing treatment (including appropriate nutrition, hydration, and medication) which, in the treating physician's (or physicians') reasonable medical judgment, will be most likely to be effective in ameliorating or correcting all such conditions, except that the term does not include the failure to provide treatment (other than appropriate nutrition, hydration, or medication) to an infant when, in the treating physician's (or physicians') reasonable medical judgment any of the following circumstances apply:

(i) The infant is chronically and irreversibly comatose:

(ii) The provision of such treatment would merely prolong dying, not be effective in ameliorating or correcting all of the infant's life-threatening conditions, or otherwise be futile in terms of the survival of the infant; or

(iii) The provision of such treatment would be virtually futile in terms of the survival of the infant and the treatment itself under such circumstances would be inhumane.

(3) Following are definitions of terms used in paragraph (b)(2) of this section:

(i) The term "infant" means an infant less than one year of age. The reference to less than one year of age shall not be construed to imply that treatment should be changed or discontinued when an infant reaches one year of age, or to affect or limit any existing protections available under State laws regarding medical neglect of children over one year of age. In addition to their applicability to infants less than one year of age, the standards set forth in paragraph (b)(2) of this section should be consulted thoroughly in the evaluation of any issue of medical neglect involving an infant older than one year of age who has been continuously hospitalized since birth, who was born extremely prematurely, or who has a long-term disability.

(ii) The term "reasonable medical judgment" means a medical judgment that would be made by a reasonably prudent physician, knowledgeable about the case and the treatment possibilities with respect to the medical conditions involved.

(c) *Eligibility requirements.* (1) In addition to the other eligibility requirements set forth in this part, to qualify for a basic State grant under section 107(b) of the Act, a State must have programs, procedures, or both, in place within the State's child protective service system for the purpose of responding to the reporting of medical neglect, including instances of withholding of medically indicated treatment from disabled infants with life-threatening conditions.

(2) These programs and/or procedures must provide for:

(i) Coordination and consultation with individuals designated by and within appropriate health care facilities;

(ii) Prompt notification by individuals designated by and within appropriate health care facilities of cases of suspected medical neglect (including instances of the withholding of medically indicated treatment from disabled infants with life-threatening conditions); and

(iii) The authority, under State law, for the State child protective service system to pursue any legal remedies, including the authority to initiate legal proceedings in a court of competent jurisdiction, as may be necessary to prevent the withholding of medically indicated treatment from disabled infants with life-threatening conditions.

(3) The programs and/or procedures must specify that the child protective services system will promptly contact each health care facility to obtain the name, title, and telephone number of the individual(s) designated by such facility for the purpose of the coordination, consultation, and notification activities identified in paragraph (c)(2) of this section, and will at least annually recontact each health care facility to obtain any changes in the designations.

(4) These programs and/or procedures must be in writing and must conform

with the requirements of section 107(b) of the Act and §1340.14 of this part. In connection with the requirement of conformity with the requirements of section 107(b) of the Act and §1340.14 of this part, the programs and/or procedures must specify the procedures the child protective services system will follow to obtain, in a manner consistent with State law:

(i) Access to medical records and/or other pertinent information when such access is necessary to assure an appropriate investigation of a report of medical neglect (including instances of withholding of medically indicated treatment from disabled infants with life-threatening conditions); and

(ii) A court order for an independent medical examination of the infant, or otherwise effect such an examination in accordance with processes established under State law, when necessary to assure an appropriate resolution of a report of medical neglect (including instances of withholding of medically indicated treatment from disabled infants with life-threatening conditions). . . .

APPENDIX TO PART 1340
INTERPRETATIVE GUIDELINES REGARDING
45 CFR 1340.15
SERVICES AND TREATMENT FOR DISABLED
INFANTS

1. In general: The statutory definition of "withholding of medically indicated treatment." . . . This definition has several main features. First, it establishes the basic principle that all disabled infants with life-threatening conditions must be given medically indicated treatment, defined in terms of action to respond to the infant's life-threatening conditions by providing treatment (including appropriate nutrition, hydration or medication) which, in the treating physician's (or physicians') reasonable medical judgment, will be most likely to be effective in ameliorating or correcting all such conditions.

Second, the statutory definition spells out three circumstances under which treatment is not considered "medically indicated." These are when, in the treating physician's (or physicians') reasonable medical judgment:

- The infant is chronically and irreversibly comatose:
- The provision of such treatment would merely prolong dying, not be effective in ameilorating or correcting all of the infant's life-threatening conditions, or otherwise be futile in terms of survival of the infant; or
- The provision of such treatment would be virtually futile in terms of survival of the infant and the treatment itself under such circumstances would be inhumane.

The third key feature of the statutory definition is that even when one of these three circumstances is present, and thus the failure to provide treatment is not a "withholding of medically indicated treatment," the infant must nonetheless be provided with appropriate nutrition, hydration, and medication.

Fourth, the definition's focus on the potential effectiveness of treatment in ameliorating or correcting life-threatening conditions makes clear that it does not sanction decisions based on subjective opinions about the future "quality of life" of a retarded or disabled person.

The fifth main feature of the statutory definition is that its operation turns substantially on the "reasonable medical judgment" of the treating physician or physicians. The term "reasonable medical judgment" is defined in §1340.15(b)(3)(ii) of the final rule, as it was in the Conference Committee Report on the Act, as a medical judgment that would be made by a reasonably prudent physician, knowledgeable about the case and the treatment possibilities with respect to the medical conditions involved.

The Department's interpretations of key terms in the statutory definition are fully consistent with these basic principles reflected in the definition. The discussion that follows is organized under headings that generally correspond to the proposed clarifying definitions that appeared in the proposed rule but were not adopted in the final rule. The discussion also attempts to analyze and respond to significant comments received by the Department.

2. The term "life-threatening condition."   Clause (b)(3)(ii) of the proposed rule proposed a definition of the term "life-threatening condition." This term is used in the statutory definition in the following context:

[T]he term "withholding of medically indicated treatment" means the failure to respond to the infant's *life-threatening conditions* by providing treatment (including appropriate nutrition, hydration, and medication) which, in the treating physician's or physicians' reasonable medical judgment, will be most likely to be effective in ameliorating or correcting all such conditions [, except that] . . . [Emphasis supplied].

It appears to the Department that the applicability of the statutory definition might be uncertain to some people in cases where a condition may not, strictly speaking, by itself be life-threatening, but where the condition significantly increases the risk of the onset of complications that may threaten the life of the infant. If medically indicated treatment is available for such a condition, the failure to provide it may result in the onset of complications that, by the time the condition becomes life-threatening in the strictest sense, will eliminate or reduce the potential effectiveness of any treatment. Such a result cannot, in the Department's view, be squared with the Congressional intent.

Thus, the Department interprets the term "life-threatening condition" to include a condition that, in the treating physician's or physicians' reasonable medical judgment, significantly increases the risk of the onset of complications that may threaten the life of the infant.

In response to comments that the proposed rule's definition was potentially overinclusive by covering any condition that one could argue "may" become life-threatening, the Department notes that the statutory standard of "the treating physician's or physicians' reasonable medical judgment" is incorporated in the Department's interpretation, and is fully applicable.

Other commenters suggested that this interpretation would bring under the scope of the definition many irreversible conditions for which no corrective treatment is available. This is certainly not the intent. The Department's interpretation implies nothing about whether, or what, treatment should be provided. It simply makes clear that the criteria set forth in the statutory definition for evaluating whether, or what, treatment should be provided are applicable. That is just the start, not the end, of the analysis. The analysis then takes fully into account the reasonable medical judgment regarding potential effectiveness of possible treatments, and the like.

Other comments were that it is unnecessary to state any interpretation because reasonable medical judgment commonly deems the conditions described as life-threatening and responds accordingly. HHS agrees that this is common practice followed under reasonable medical judgment, just as all the standards incorporated in the statutory definition reflect common practice followed under reasonable medical judgment. For the reasons stated above, however, the Department believes it is useful to say so in these interpretative guidelines.

3. The term "treatment" in the context of adequate evaluation.   Clause (b)(3)(ii) of the proposed rule proposed a definition of the term "treatment." Two separate concepts were dealt with in clause (A) and (B), respectively, of the proposed rule. Both of these clauses were designed to ensure that the Congressional intent regarding the issues to be considered under the analysis set forth in the statutory definition is fully effectuated. Like the guidance regarding "life-threatening condition," discussed above, the Department's interpretations go to the applicability of the statutory analysis, not its result.

The Department believes that Congress intended that the standard of following reasonable medical judgment regarding the potential effectiveness of possible courses of action should apply to issues regarding adequate medical evaluation, just as it does to issues regarding adequate medical intervention. This is apparent Congressional intent because Congress adopted, in the Conference Report's definition of "reasonable medical judgment," the standard of adequate knowledge about the case and the treatment possibilities with respect to the medical condition involved.

Having adequate knowledge about the case and the treatment possibilities involved is, in effect, step one of the process, because that is the basis on which "reasonable medical judgment" will operate to make recommendations regarding medical intervention. Thus, part of the process to determine what treatment, if any, "will be most likely to be effective in ameliorating or correcting" all life-threatening conditions is for the treating physician or physicians to make sure they have adequate information about the condition and adequate knowledge about treatment possibilities with respect to the condition involved. The standard for determining the adequacy of the information and knowledge is the same as the basic standard of the statutory definition: reasonable medical judgment. A reasonably prudent physician faced with a particular condition about which he or she needs additional information and knowledge of treatment possibilities would take steps to gain more information and knowledge by, quite simply, seeking further evaluation by, or consultation with, a physician or physicians whose expertise is appropriate to the condition(s) involved or further evaluation at a facility with specialized capabilities regarding the conditions(s) involved.

Thus, the Department interprets the term "treatment" to include (but not be limited to) any further evaluation by, or consultation with, a physician or physicians whose expertise is appropriate to the condition(s) involved or further evaluation at a facility with specialized capabilities regarding the condition(s) involved that, in the treating physician's or physicians' reasonable medical judgment, is needed to assure that decisions regarding medical intervention are based on adequate knowledge about the case and the treatment possibilities with respect to the medical conditions involved.

This reflects the Department's interpretation that failure to respond to an infant's life-threatening conditions by obtaining any further evaluations or consultations that, in the treating physician's reasonable medical judgment, are necessary to assure that decisions regarding medical intervention are based on adequate knowledge about the case and the treatment possibilities involved constitutes a "withholding of medically indicated treatment." Thus, if parents refuse to consent to such a recommendation that is based on the treating physician's reasonable medical judgment that, for example, further evaluation by a specialist is necessary to permit reasonable medical judgments to be made regarding medical intervention, this would be a matter for appropriate action by the child protective services system.

In response to comments regarding the related provision in the proposed rule, this interpretative guideline makes quite clear that this interpretation does not deviate from the basic principle of reliance on reasonable medical judgment to determine the extent of the evaluation necessary in the particular case. Commenters expressed concerns that the provision in the proposed rule would intimidate physicians to seek transfer of seriously ill infants to tertiary level facilities much more often than necessary, potentially resulting in diversion of the limited capacities of these facilities away from those with real needs for the specialized care, unnecessary separation of infants from their parents when equally beneficial treatment could have been provided at the community or regional hospital, inappropriate deferral of therapy while time-consuming arrangements can be affected, and other counterproductive ramifications. The Department intended no intimidation, prescription or similar influence on reasonable medical judgment, but rather, intended only to affirm that it is the Department's interpretation that the reasonable medical judgment standard applies to issues of medical evaluation, as well as issues of medical intervention.

4. The term "treatment" in the context of multiple treatments. Clause (b)(3)(iii)(B) of the proposed rule was designed to clarify that, in evaluating the potential effectiveness of a particular medical treatment or surgical procedure that can only be reasonably evaluated in the context of a complete potential treatment plan, the "treatment" to be evaluated under the standards of the statutory definition includes the multiple medical treatments and/or surgical procedures over a period of time that are designed to ameliorate or correct a life-threatening condition or conditions. Some commenters stated that it could be construed to require the carrying out of a long process of medical treatments or surgical procedures regardless of the lack of success of those done first. No such meaning is intended.

The intent is simply to characterize that which must be evaluated under the standards of the statutory definition, not to imply anything about the results of the evaluation. If parents refuse consent for a particular medical treatment or surgical procedure that by itself may not correct or ameliorate all life-threatening conditions, but is recommended as part of a total plan that involves multiple medical treatments and/or surgical procedures over a period of time that, in the treating physician's reasonable medical judgment, will be most likely to be effective in ameliorating or correcting all such conditions, that would be a matter for appropriate action by the child protective services system.

On the other hand, if, in the treating physician's reasonable medical judgment, the total plan will, for example, be virtually futile and inhumane, within the meaning of the statutory term, then there is no "withholding of medically indicated treatment." Similarly, if a treatment plan is commenced on the basis of a reasonable medical judgment that there is a good chance that it will be effective, but due to a lack of success, unfavorable complications, or other factors, it becomes the treating physician's reasonable medical judgment that further treatment in accord with the prospective treatment plan, or alternative treatment, would be futile, then the failure to provide that treatment would not constitute a "withholding of medically indicated treatment." This analysis does not divert from the reasonable medical judgment standard of the statutory definition; it simply makes clear the Department's interpretation that the failure to evaluate the potential effectiveness of a treatment plan as a whole would be inconsistent with the legislative intent.

Thus, the Department interprets the term "treatment" to include (but not be limited to) multiple medical treatments and/or surgical procedures over a period of time that are designed to ameliorate or correct a life-threatening condition or conditions.

5. The term "merely prolong dying."   Clause (b)(3)(v) of the proposed rule proposed a definition of the term "merely prolong dying," which appears in the statutory definition. The proposed rule's provision stated that this term "refers to situations where death is imminent and treatment will do no more than postpone the act of dying."

Many commenters argued that the incorporation of the word "imminent," and its connotation of immediacy, appeared to deviate from the Congressional intent, as developed in the course of the lengthy legislative negotiations, that reasonable medical judgments can and do result in nontreatment decisions regarding some conditions for which treatment will do no more than temporarily postpone a death that will occur in the near future, but not necessarily within days. The six principal sponsors of the compromise amendment also strongly urged deletion of the word "imminent."

The Department's use of the term "imminent" in the proposed rule was not intended to convey a meaning not fully consonant with the statute. Rather, the Department intended that the word "imminent" would be applied in the context of the condition involved, and in such a context, it would not be understood to specify a particular number of days. As noted in the preamble to the proposed rule, this clarification was proposed to make clear that the "merely prolong dying" clause of the statutory definition would not be applicable to situations where treatment will not totally correct a medical condition but will give a patient many years of life. The Department continues to hold to this view.

To eliminate the type of misunderstanding evidenced in the comments, and to assure consistency with the statutory definition, the word "imminent" is not being adopted for purposes of these interpretative guidelines.

The Department interprets the term "merely prolong dying" as referring to situations where the prognosis is for death and, in the treating physician's (or physicians') reasonable medical judgment, further or alternative treatment would not alter the prognosis in an extension of time that would not render the treatment futile.

Thus, the Department continues to interpret Congressional intent as not permitting the "merely prolong dying" provision to apply where many years of life will result from the provision of treatment, or where the prognosis is not for death in the near future, but rather the more distant future. The Department also wants to make clear it does not intend the connotations many commenters associated with the word "imminent." In addition, contrary to the impression some commenters appeared to have regarding the proposed rule, the Department's interpretation is that reasonable medical judgments will be formed on the basis of knowledge about the condition(s) involved, the degree of inevitability of death, the probable effect of any potential treatments, the projected time period within which death will probably occur, and other pertinent factors.

6. The term "not be effective in ameliorating or correcting all of the infant's life-threatening conditions" in the context of a future life-threatening condition. Clause (b)(3)(vi) of the proposed rule proposed a definition of the term "not be effective in ameliorating or correcting all the infant's life-threatening conditions" used in the statutory definition of "withholding of medically indicated treatment."

The basic point made by the use of this term in the statutory definition was explained in the Conference Committee Report:

Under the definition, if a disabled infant suffers more than one life-threatening condition and, in the treating physician's or physicians' reasonable medical judgment, there is no effective treatment for one of those conditions, then the infant is not covered by the terms of the amendment (except with respect to appropriate nutrition, hydration, and medication) concerning the withholding of medically indicated treatment. H. Conf. Rep. No. 1038, 98th Cong., 2d Sess. 41 (1984).

This clause of the proposed rule dealt with the application of this concept in two contexts: First, when the nontreatable condition will not become life-threatening in the near future, and second, when humaneness makes palliative treatment medically indicated.

With respect to the context of a future life-threatening condition, it is the Department's interpretation that the term "not be effective in ameliorating or correcting all of the infant's life-threatening conditions" does not permit the withholding of treatment on the grounds that one or more of the infant's life-threatening conditions, although not life-threatening in the near future, will become life-threatening in the more distant future.

This clarification can be restated in the terms of the Conference Committee Report excerpt, quoted just above, with the italicized words indicating the clarification, as follows: Under the definition, if a disabled infant suffers from more than one life-threatening condition and, in the treating physician's or physicians' reasonable medical judgment, there is no effective treatment for one of these conditions *that threatens the life of the infant in the near future,* then the infant is not covered by the terms of the amendment (except with respect to appropriate nutrition, hydration, and medication) concerning the withholding of medically indicated treatment; *but if the nontreatable condition will not become life-threatening until the more distant future, the infant is covered by the terms of the amendment.*

Thus, this interpretative guideline is simply a corollary to the Department's interpretation of "merely prolong dying," stated above, and is based on the same understanding of Congressional intent, indicated above, that if a condition will not become life-threatening until the more distant future, it should not be the basis for withholding treatment.

Also for the same reasons explained above, the word "imminent" that appeared in the proposed definition is not adopted for purposes of this interpretative guideline. The Department makes no effort to draw an exact line to separate "near future" from "more distant future." As noted above in connection with the term "merely prolong dying," the statutory definition provides that it is for reasonable medical judgment, applied to the specific condition and circumstances involved, to determine whether the prognosis of death, because of its nearness in time, is such that treatment would not be medically indicated.

7. The term "not be effective in ameliorating or correcting all life-threatening conditions" in the context of palliative treatment.   Clause (b)(3)(iv)(B) of the proposed rule proposed to define the term "not be effective in ameliorating or correcting all life-threatening conditions" in the context where the issue is not life-saving treatment, but rather palliative treatment to make a condition more tolerable. An example of this situation is where an infant has more than one life-threatening condition, at least one of which is not treatable and will cause death in the near future. Palliative treatment is available, however, that will, in the treating physician's reasonable medical judgment, relieve severe pain associated with one of the conditions. If it is the treating physician's reasonable medical judgment that this palliative treatment will ameliorate the infant's *overall* condition, taking all individual conditions into account, even though it would not ameliorate or correct *each* condition, then this palliative treatment is medically indicated. Simply put, in the context of ameliorative treatment that will make a condition more tolerable, the term "not be effective in ameliorating or correcting *all* life-threatening conditions" should not be construed as meaning *each and every* condition, but rather as referring to the infant's *overall* condition.

HHS believes Congress did not intend to exclude humane treatment of this kind from the scope of "medically indicated treatment." The Conference Committee Report specifically recognized that "It is appropriate for a physician, in the exercise of reasonable medical judgment, to consider that factor [humaneness] in selecting among effective treatments." H. Conf. Rep. No. 1038, 98th Cong., 2d Sess. 41 (1984). In addition, the articulation in the statutory definition of circumstances in which treatment need not be provided specifically states that "appropriate nutrition, hydration, and medication" must nonetheless be provided. The inclusion in this proviso of medication, one (but not the only) potential palliative treatment to relieve severe pain, corroborates the Department's interpretation that such palliative treatment that will ameliorate the infant's overall condition, and that in the exercise of reasonable medical judgment is humane and medically indicated, was not intended by Congress to be outside the scope of the statutory definition.

Thus, it is the Department's interpretation that the term "not be effective in ameliorating or correcting all of the infant's life-threatening conditions" does not permit the withholding of ameliorative treatment that, in the treating physician's or physicians' reasonable medical judgment, will make a condition more tolerable, such as providing palliative treatment to relieve severe pain, even if the overall prognosis, taking all conditions into account, is that the infant will not survive.

A number of commenters expressed concerns about some of the examples contained in the preamble of the proposed rule that discussed the proposed definition relating to this point, and stated that, depending on medical complications, exact prognosis, relationships to other conditions, and other factors, the treatment suggested in the examples might not necessarily be the treatment that reasonable medical judgment would decide would be most likely to be effective. In response to these comments, specific diagnostic examples have not been included in this discussion, and this interpretative guideline makes clear that the "reasonable medical judgment" standard applies on this point as well.

Other commenters argued that an interpretative guideline on this point is unnecessary because reasonable medical judgment would commonly provide ameliorative or palliative treatment in the circumstances described. The Depart-

322   Child Abuse and Neglect Prevention and Treatment

ment agrees that such treatment is common in the exercise of reasonable medical judgment, but believes it useful, for the reasons stated, to provide this interpretative guidance.

8. The term "virtually futile."   Clause (b)(3)(vii) of the proposed rule proposed a definition of the term "virtually futile" contained in the statutory definition. The context of this term in the statutory definition is:

[T]he term "withholding of medically indicated treatment" . . . does not include the failure to provide treatment (other than appropriate nutrition, hydration, or medication) to an infant when, in the treating physician's or physicians' reasonable medical judgment . . . the provision of such treatment would be *virtually futile* in terms of the survival of the infant and the treatment itself under such circumstances would be inhumane. Section 3(3)(C) of the Act (emphasis supplied).

The Department interprets the term "virtually futile" to mean that the treatment is highly unlikely to prevent death in the near future.

This interpretation is similar to those offered in connection with "merely prolong dying" and "not be effective in ameliorating or correcting all life-threatening conditions" in the context of a future life-threatening condition, with the addition of a characterization of likelihood that corresponds to the statutory word "virtually." For the reasons explained in the discussion of "merely prolong dying," the word "imminent" that was used in the proposed rule has not been adopted for purposes of this interpretative guideline.

Some commenters expressed concern regarding the words "highly unlikely," on the grounds that such certitude is often medically impossible. Other commenters urged that a distinction should be made between generally utilized treatments and experimental treatments. The Department does not believe any special clarifications are needed to respond to these comments. The basic standard of reasonable medical judgment applies to the term "virtually futile." The Department's interpretation does not suggest an impossible or unrealistic standard of certitude for any medical judgment. Rather, the standard adopted in the law is that there be a "reasonable medical judgment." Similarly, reasonable medical judgment is the standard for evaluating potential treatment possibilities on the basis of the actual circumstances of the case. HHS does not believe it would be helpful to try to establish distinctions based on characterizations of the degree of general usage, extent of validated efficacy data, or other similar factors. The factors considered in the exercise of reasonable medical judgment, including any factors relating to human subjects experimentation standards, are not disturbed.

9. The term "the treatment itself under such circumstances would be inhumane."   Clause (b)(3)(viii) of the proposed rule proposed a definition of the term "the treatment itself under such circumstances would be inhumane," that appears in the statutory definition. The context of this term in the statutory definition is that it is not a "withholding of medically indicated treatment" to withhold treatment (other than appropriate nutrition, hydration, or medication) when, in the treating physician's reasonable medical judgment, "the provision of such treatment would be virtually futile in terms of the survival of the infant and the treatment itself under such circumstances would be inhumane." §3(3)(C) of the Act.

The Department interprets the term "the treatment itself under such circumstances would be inhumane" to mean the treatment itself involves significant medical contraindications and/or significant pain and suffering for the infant that clearly outweigh the very slight potential benefit of the treatment for an infant highly unlikely to survive. (The Department further notes that the use of the term "inhumane" in this context is not intended to suggest that consideration of the humaneness of a particular treatment is not legitimate in any other context; rather, it is recognized that it is appropriate for a physician, in the exercise of reasonable medical judgment, to consider that factor in selecting among effective treatments.)

Other clauses of the statutory definition focus on the expected *result* of the possible treatment. This provision of the statutory definition adds a consideration relating to the *process* of possible treatment. It recognizes that in the exercise of reasonable medical judgment, there are situations where, although there is some slight chance that the treatment will be beneficial to the patient (the potential treatment is considered *virtually* futile, rather than futile), the potential benefit is so outweighed by negative factors relating to the process of the treatment itself that, under the circumstances, it would be inhumane to subject the patient to the treatment.

The Department's interpretation is designed to suggest the factors that should be taken into account in this difficult balance. A number of commenters argued that the interpretation should permit, as part of the evaluation of whether treatment would be inhumane, consideration of the infant's future "quality of life."

The Department strongly believes such an interpretation would be inconsistent with the statute. The statute specifies that the provision applies only where the treatment would be "virtually futile in terms of the survival of the infant," and the "treatment *itself* under such circumstances would be inhumane." (Emphasis supplied.) The balance is clearly to be between the very slight chance that treatment will allow the infant to survive and the negative factors relating to the process of the treatment. These are the circumstances under which reasonable medical judgment could decide that the treatment itself would be inhumane. . . .

The Patient Self-Determination Act and the Future of Advance Directives

*Peter J. Greco, Kevin A. Schulman, Risa Lavizzo-Mourey,
and John Hansen-Flaschen*

Peter Greco and Kevin Schulman were fellows in general internal medicine at the University of Pennsylvania when this paper was written. They were mentored by Risa Lavizzo-Mourey in geriatric medicine and John Hansen-Flaschen in critical care medicine. They summarize the components of the Patient Self-Determination Act, discuss limitations in the law, and provide advice about advance care planning. They consider (1) physicians not being required to discuss advance directives, and (2) the designation of inpatient settings for these discussions as two principal limitations to the Act. They recommend that clinicians and institutions go beyond the requirements of the Act with outpatient discussions, encouraging discussions with other forms of planning for the future (e.g., wills), public education, policy development for decision making in the absence of advance directives, and evaluative research.

On 5 November 1990, President Bush signed the Patient Self-Determination Act (1). This law was designed to increase patient involvement in decisions regarding life-sustaining treatment by ensuring that advance directives for health care are available to physicians at the time medical decisions are being made and that patients who have not prepared such documents are aware of their legal right to do so. Sponsors of the legislation hope that this proactive approach will not only ensure that existing directives are respected by health care providers but will also encourage many more persons to prepare these documents.

This legislation was passed in the wake of the *Cruzan* case (2), which had renewed national interest in the use of advance directives to avoid unwanted medical interventions. However, the first living will statutes were enacted 15 years ago, and most of these statutes have been in place for more than 5 years (3). Even though this means of expressing treatment preferences has been widely publicized in recent years, only 8% to 15% of American adults have prepared a living will (4–6). Similarly, only 4% of acute care hospitals routinely inquire about the existence of advance directives at the time of admission (7). Consequently, written advance directives still play only an occasional role in decisions to withhold or withdraw life-sustaining treatment (8–12).

Peter J. Greco, Kevin A. Schulman, Risa Lavizzo-Mourey, and John Hansen-Flaschen. "The Patient Self-Determination Act and the Future of Advance Directives." Abridged from *Annals of Internal Medicine*, Volume 115, 1991, pp. 639–643. Reprinted by permission.

Although few Americans have expressed their treatment preferences in writing, decisions to withhold or withdraw treatment are common in the United States (13–17). Approximately 80% of deaths in this country occur in acute care hospitals or chronic care facilities (18,19), and 70% of deaths in the hospital are preceded by a decision to limit medical treatment (13–17). Without advance directives, such decisions must be made by family members and physicians who often do not know what type of care the individual would have wanted under the circumstances (20). . . .

The New Law

As a condition of Medicare and Medicaid payment, the Patient Self-Determination Act requires health care providers in hospitals, skilled nursing facilities, and other health care settings to 1) develop written policies concerning advance directives; 2) ask all new patients whether they have prepared an advance directive and include this information in the patient's chart; 3) give patients written materials regarding the facility's policies on advance directives and the patient's right (under applicable state law) to prepare such documents; and 4) educate staff and the community about advance directives. These requirements are to take effect on 1 December 1991.

Health care providers must begin to prepare for the implementation of this new law. As a first step, facilities and organizations should develop institutional policies concerning advance directives and decisions to withhold or withdraw life-sustaining treatment. These policies should be detailed enough to address the following issues: 1) the philosophy of the institution regarding the discontinuation of life-sustaining treatment; 2) any specific limitations the institution might place on the implementation of advance directives; 3) the delegation of responsibility for discussing advance directives with patients; and 4) the development of mechanisms for ensuring that advance directives are incorporated into the medical record.

Health care institutions must also prepare written materials that explain these policies to patients and their families in language that is simple and clear. For example, a facility opposed to the withdrawal of nutrition and hydration from permanently unconscious patients would prepare a brochure for distribution to the public that describes its policies in the following manner: "This institution provides life-saving food and water to all patients who have not explicitly rejected this treatment in a living will." Disclosure of these policies well in advance of their application is intended to avoid future misunderstandings or conflicts; such disclosure may also allow patients to choose health care facilities with treatment policies more consistent with their personal beliefs.

Under the provisions of the new law, each state must develop written materials describing the state's legislation and case law concerning advance directives. While awaiting these materials, health care institutions should seek the advice of legal counsel in developing their policies. This will be of particular importance in developing policies on the withholding or the withdrawal of artificial nutrition and hydration from patients who are not terminally ill; many living will statutes apply only to terminal illness or prohibit the withholding or withdrawal of tube feeding, or both.

Limitations of the New Law

The Patient Self-Determination Act represents a fundamental change in the approach to advance directives in the United States. Enactment of this legislation is an acknowledgment that a purely voluntary approach to the promotion of advance directives has been unsuccessful. The approach outlined in the legislation, however, has certain limitations. First, the law does not specify that physicians must discuss advance directives with patients; this task could be delegated to an admissions clerk (21). Second, the law relies on inpatient facilities to perform a function that many believe should take place primarily in the outpatient setting. Third, with the exception of the provision of the law that applies to health maintenance organizations, the law does little to encourage the preparation of advance directives before the need for hospitalization or long-term care arises. Fourth, patients who most need to discuss their treatment preferences—those who are acutely ill and immediately in need of life-sustaining interventions—may be unable to do so because of their illness. Similarly, by the time a person is admitted to a skilled nursing facility it may be impossible to carry out a discussion of treatment preferences because of his or her cognitive impairment. Finally, although the law requires health care institutions and the federal government to engage in public education, this provision of the law is not supported by any specific funding.

Additional Steps

Because of these limitations, additional initiatives by institutions and policymakers will be necessary if advance directives are to have a greater effect on treatment decisions in health care. These efforts can be undertaken at the local level by hospitals and at the state and federal levels by legislatures or professional societies. We propose several approaches that are complementary to the Patient Self-Determination Act in promoting the preparation of advance directives.

1. Encourage outpatient discussions of advance directives. . . .
2. Encourage all health insurers to provide enrollees with information about advance directives. . . .
3. Encourage discussion of advance directives during preparation of traditional wills or durable powers of attorney. . . .
4. Educate the public about advance directives. . . .

Decision Making in the Absence of Advance Directives

Even the most comprehensive educational program cannot ensure that advance directives are prepared and periodically updated by all American adults. Moreover, situations inevitably arise in which advance directives exist but are difficult to interpret or apply. When the patient's wishes are not known, surrogate decision makers are advised to make treatment decisions by considering the patient's "best interests," as defined by "objective, societally shared criteria" (22). In determining the patient's best interests one must weigh the potential benefits and burdens of treatment, including such factors as the relief of suffering, the quality and extent of life sustained, and the effect of the decision on the patient's loved ones. As stated by the President's Commission for the Study of Ethical Problems in Medicine and Biomedical and Behavioral Research, "When a patient's likely decision is unknown . . . a surrogate decisionmaker should use the best interests standard and choose a course that will promote the patient's well-being as it would probably be conceived by a reasonable person in the patient's circumstances" (22).

One societal standard that is often decisive in these deliberations is a strong presumption in favor of preserving life, regardless of the prognosis for recovery. Thus, in many instances, the absence of an advance directive results in an implicit decision to institute or continue any life-sustaining treatment that is physiologically efficacious.

There is growing evidence, however, that most people would not want chronic life-sustaining treatment if they became terminally ill or permanently unconscious. A recent CBS-New York Times poll reported that 85% of people would not want to be kept alive by a feeding tube if they were "in a coma with no brain activity" (23). Another poll found that 82% of respondents were very willing (70%) or somewhat willing (12%) to have a "life-support system" disconnected if they became permanently unconscious (5). A study of outpatients and members of the general public in Boston found that approximately 80% did not want life-sustaining treatment (such as cardiopulmonary resuscitation, mechanical ventilation, or artificial nutrition) if permanently unconscious or if demented and terminally ill (24). A survey of community-dwelling elderly found that 86% would not want cardiopulmonary resuscitation or mechanical ventilation if terminally ill (25). Finally, a study of nursing home residents found that only 16% would want tube feeding if permanently unconscious, and only 20% would want cardiopulmonary resuscitation if terminally ill (26). Thus, the presumption in favor of preserving life by whatever means necessary conflicts with most people's wishes in cases of terminal illness or permanent loss of cognitive function.

One way to resolve this conflict would be for health care facilities to develop formal treatment guidelines that are based on the consensus of the surrounding community and the institution's staff (27). These guidelines would be specific to certain clinical conditions (such as persistent vegetative state) and treatments (such as cardiopulmonary resuscitation and artificial nutrition and hydration). In the absence of a written or verbal advance directive, patients would receive only those treatments that would be desired by most persons in the surrounding community. Within a given community, each facility could have different treatment guidelines (27) based, for example, on religious affiliation or on the particular patient population served. These policies would, of course, have to be consistent with relevant state law and legal precedent.

Under this proposal, an institution could conceivably implement a policy of not providing artificial nutrition and hydration to permanently unconscious patients unless such treatment had specifically been requested in an advance directive. Would this type of policy be feasible? The protests surrounding the removal of Nancy Cruzan's feeding tube demonstrate that some people in this country strongly oppose withholding or withdrawing such treatment under any circumstances; these individuals would, of course, vigorously oppose such a policy. This strong opposition, however, would make it very likely that these individuals would make their preferences for such treatment known—particularly if neglecting to do so would result in not receiving the desired treatment. Thus, publication of these explicit treatment guidelines would act as an incentive for the preparation of advance directives by the minority that did not agree with a particular guideline. . . .

Conclusions

The Patient Self-Determination Act is a major step toward ensuring that individuals' treatment preferences are respected when they lose decisional capacity. This law will help ensure that patients' existing advance directives are made available to health care providers and will increase the public's awareness of their right to prepare such documents. An evaluation program will be required to determine whether the law is successful in achieving its goals. Outcomes of interest in such an evaluation would include 1) the relative effectiveness of different ways of presenting information to patients about advance directives; 2) the stability over time of the preferences obtained from patients through routinized discussions; 3) successful solutions to the particular difficulties faced in the long-term care setting (such as the determination of patients' capacity to participate in such discussions); and 4) documentation of the role that advance directives play in actual treatment decisions.

Institutions and policymakers may choose to go beyond the requirements of the legislation and actively promote the preparation of advance directives. We have outlined several ways in which this can be accomplished. We have also outlined an approach with which to create guidelines for treatment decisions when a patient's preferences are unknown. Under this approach, decision makers would apply the preferences of the local community in deciding whether or not to provide particular treatments in certain well-defined situations. This approach depends on the existence of a community consensus regarding certain treatments, such as artificial nutrition and hydration in case of permanent unconsciousness. This assumption can be tested by a large public opinion survey with stratification according to age, religious affiliation, socioeconomic status, and other variables. For many conditions there may be no such consensus; in these situations, there would be no guidelines.

The Patient Self-Determination Act reaffirms that patients have a right to make their treatment preferences known and for those preferences to be respected. The Congress has now compelled the medical community and the public to begin to confront these difficult issues.

References

1. Omnibus Budget Reconciliation Act of 1990. Public law no. 101–508.
2. Cruzan v. Director, Missouri Department of Health. 110 S. Ct. 2841 (1990).
3. Society for the Right to Die. Handbook of living will laws. New York: Society for the Right to Die; 1987:5.
4. President's Commission for the Study of Ethical Problems in Medicine and Biomedical and Behavioral Research. Making health care decisions: a report on the ethical and legal implications of informed consent in the patient-practitioner relationship. Washington, DC: U.S. Government Printing Office; 1982:217–61.
5. Steiber SR. Right to die: public balks at deciding for others. Hospitals. 1987;61:72.
6. [Anonymous.] Most MDs favor withdrawal of life support—survey. *American Medical News*. 1988 Jun 3.
7. McCrary SV, Botkin JR. Hospital policy on advance directives: do institutions ask patients about living wills? JAMA 1989;262:2411–4.
8. Smedira NG, Evans BH, Grais LS, Cohen NH, Lo B. Cooke M, et al. Withholding and withdrawal of life support from the critically ill. New Engl J Med. 1990;322:309–15.
9. Lo B, Saika G, Strull W, Thomas E, Showstack J. "Do not resuscitate" decisions. A prospective study at three teaching hospitals. Arch Intern Med. 1985;145:1115–7.
10. Stolman CJ, Gregory JJ, Dunn D, Ripley B. Evaluation of the do not resuscitate orders at a community hospital. Arch Intern Med. 1989;149:1851–6.
11. Youngner SJ, Lewandowski W, McClish DK, Juknialis BW, Coulton C, Bartlett ET. "Do not resuscitate" orders: incidence and implications in a medical intensive care unit. JAMA. 1985;253:54–7.
12. Brennan TA. Ethics committees and decisions to limit care: the experience at the Massachusetts General Hospital. JAMA. 1988;260:803–7.
13. Bedell SE, Pelle D, Maher PL, Cleary PD. Do-not-resuscitate orders for critically ill patients in the hospital: how are they used and what is their impact? JAMA. 1986;256:233–7.
14. Lipton HL. Do-not-resuscitate decisions in a community hospital. Incidence, implications, and outcomes. JAMA. 1986;256:1164–9.
15. Levy MR, Lambe ME, Shear CL. Do-not-resuscitate orders in a county hospital. West J Med. 1984;140:111–3.
16. Jonsson PV, McNamee M, Campion EW. The "Do not resuscitate" order. A profile of its changing use. Arch Intern Med. 1988;148:2373–5.
17. Taffet GE, Teasdale TA, Luchi RJ. In-hospital cardiopulmonary resuscitation. JAMA. 1988;260:2069–72.
18. Sager MA, Easterling DV, Kindig DA, Anderson OW. Changes in the location of death after passage of medicare's prospective payment system. N Engl J Med. 1989;320:433–9.
19. President's Commission for the Study of Ethical Problems in Medicine and

Biomedical and Behavioral Research. Deciding to forego life-sustaining treatment: a report on the ethical, medical, and legal issues in treatment decisions. Washington, DC: U.S. Government Printing Office; 1983:17–8.

20. Uhlmann RF, Pearlman RA, Cain KC. Physicians' and spouses' predictions of elderly patients' resuscitation preferences. J Gerontol. 1988;43:M115–21.

21. Capron AM. The patient self-determination act: not now. *Hastings Center Report.* 1990;20:35–6.

22. President's Commission for the Study of Ethical Problems in Medicine and Biomedical and Behavioral Research. Deciding to forego life-sustaining treatment: a report on the ethical, medical, and legal issues in treatment decisions. Washington, DC: U.S. Government Printing Office; 1983:132–6.

23. [Anonymous]. Right to die: the public's view. The New York Times. 1990 Jun 26:sect A;18(col 2).

24. Emmanuel LL, Barry MJ, Stoeckle JD, Ettelson LM, Emmanuel EJ. Advance directives for medical care—a case for greater use. N Engl J Med. 1991; 324:889–95.

25. Gamble ER, McDonald PJ, Lichstein PR. Knowledge, attitudes, and behavior of elderly persons regarding living wills. Arch Intern Med. 1991;151:277–80.

26. Danis M, Southerland LI, Garrett JM, Smith JL, Hielema F, Pickard CG, et al. A prospective study of advance directives for life-sustaining care. N Engl J Med. 1991;324:882–8.

27. Emanuel EJ. A communal vision of care for incompetent patients. Hasting Cent Rep. 1987;17:15–20.

Deciding to Forego Life-Sustaining Treatment

*President's Commission for the Study of Ethical Problems in Medicine
and Biomedical and Behavioral Research*

The President's Commission for the Study of Ethical Problems in Medicine and Biomedical and Behavioral Research completed this report in 1983. It continues to be one of the strongest of the many reports prepared by the Commission. In the following selection several traditional moral distinctions are reviewed and clarified. These include the distinction between acting and omitting; between failing to initiate therapy and stopping therapy; between giving a pain-relieving medication with the unintended consequence of hastening death versus giving a drug to hasten death; and between ordinary and extraordinary as a reason for accepting or declining a treatment.

Reexamining the Role of Traditional Moral Distinctions

Most patients make their decisions about the alternative courses available to them in light of such factors as how many days or months the treatment might add to their lives, the nature of that life (for example, whether treatment will allow or interfere with their pursuit of important goals, such as completing projects and taking leave of loved ones), the degree of suffering involved, and the costs (financial and otherwise) to themselves and others. The relative weight, if any, to be given to each consideration must ultimately be determined by the competent patient.

Other bases are sometimes suggested for judging whether life-and-death decisions about medical care are acceptable or unacceptable beyond making sure that the results of the decisions are justified in the patient's view by their expected good. These bases are traditionally presented in the form of opposing categories. Although the categories—causing death by acting versus by omitting to act; withholding versus withdrawing treatment; the intended versus the unintended but foreseeable consequences of a choice; and ordinary versus extraordinary treatment—do reflect factors that can be important in assessing the moral and legal acceptability of decisions to forego life-sustaining treatment, they are inherently unclear. Worse, their invocation is often so

Abridged from the President's Commission for the Study of Ethical Problems in Medicine and Biomedical and Behavioral Research, *Deciding to Forego Life-Sustaining Treatment.* Washington, D.C.: U.S. Government Printing Office, 1983, pp. 60–90.

mechanical that it neither illuminates an actual case nor provides an ethically persuasive argument.

In considering these distinctions, which are discussed in detail in the remainder of this chapter, the Commission reached the following conclusions, which are particularly relevant to assessing the role of such distinctions in public policies that preclude patients and providers from choosing certain options.

- The distinction between acting and omitting to act provides a useful rule-of-thumb by separating cases that probably deserve more scrutiny from those that are likely not to need it. Although not all decisions to omit treatment and allow death to occur are acceptable, such a choice, when made by a patient or surrogate, is usually morally acceptable and in compliance with the law on homicide; conversely, active steps to end life, such as by administering a poison, are likely to be serious moral and legal wrongs. Nonetheless, the mere difference between acts and omissions—which is often hard to draw in any case—never by itself determines what is morally acceptable. Rather, the acceptability of particular actions or omissions turns on other morally significant considerations, such as the balance of harms and benefits likely to be achieved, the duties owed by others to a dying person, the risks imposed on others in acting or refraining, and the certainty of outcome.

- The distinction between failing to initiate and stopping therapy—that is, withholding versus withdrawing treatment—is not itself of moral importance. A justification that is adequate for not commencing a treatment is also sufficient for ceasing it. Moreover, erecting a higher requirement for cessation might unjustifiably discourage vigorous initial attempts to treat seriously ill patients that sometimes succeed.

- A distinction is sometimes drawn between giving a pain-relieving medication that will probably have the unintended consequence of hastening a patient's death and giving a poison in order to relieve a patient's suffering by killing the patient. The first is generally acceptable while the latter is against the law. Actions that lead to death must be justified by benefits to the patient that are expected to exceed the negative consequences and ordinarily must be within the person's socially accepted authority. In the case of physicians and nurses, this authority encompasses the use of means, such as pain-relieving medication, that can cure illnesses or relieve suffering but not the use of means, such as weapons or poisons, whose sole effect is viewed as killing a patient.

- Whether care is "ordinary" or "extraordinary" should not determine whether a patient must accept or may decline it. The terms have come to be used in conflicting and confusing ways, reflecting variously such aspects as the usualness, complexity, invasiveness, artificiality, expense, or availability of care. If used in their historic sense, however—to signify whether the burdens a treatment imposes on a patient are or are not disproportionate to its benefits—the terms denote useful concepts. To avoid misunderstanding, public discussion should focus on the underlying reasons for or against a therapy rather than on a simple categorization as "ordinary" or "extraordinary." . . .

The Moral Significance of the Difference [between actions and omissions]   Actual instances of actions leading to death, especially outside the medical context, are more likely to be seriously morally wrong than are omissions that lead to death, which, in the medical context, are most often morally justified. Usually, one or more of several factors make fatal actions worse than fatal omissions:

(1) The motives of an agent who acts to cause death are usually worse (for example, self-interest or malice) than those of someone who omits to act and lets another die.

(2) A person who is barred from acting to cause another's death is usually thereby placed at no personal risk of harm; whereas, especially outside the medical context, if a person were forced to intercede to save another's life (instead of standing by and omitting to act), he or she would often be put at substantial risk.

(3) The nature and duration of future life denied to a person whose life is ended by another's act is usually much greater than that denied to a dying person whose death comes slightly more quickly due to an omission of treatment.

(4) A person, especially a patient, may still have some possibility of surviving if one omits to act, while survival is more often foreclosed by actions that lead to death.

Each of these factors—or several in combination—can make a significant moral difference in the evaluation of any particular instance of acting and omitting to act. Together they help explain why most actions leading to death are correctly considered morally worse than most omissions leading to death. Moreover, the greater stringency of the legal duties to refrain from killing than to intervene to save life reinforces people's view of which conduct is worse morally.

However, the distinction between omissions leading to death and acts leading to death is not a reliable guide to their moral evaluation. In the case of medical treatment, the first and third factors are not likely to provide grounds for a distinction: family members and health professionals could be equally merciful in their intention—either in acting or omitting—and life may end immediately for some patients after treatment is withdrawn. Likewise, the second factor—based on the usual rule that people have fairly limited duties to save others with whom they stand in no special relation—does not apply in the medical context. Health professionals have a special role-related duty to use their skills, insofar as possible, on behalf of their patients, and this duty removes any distinction between acts and omissions.

Only the final factor—turning the possibility of death into a certainty—can apply as much in medical settings as elsewhere. Indeed, this factor has particular relevance here since the element of uncertainty—whether a patient really will die if treatment is ceased—is sometimes unavoidable in the medical setting. A valid distinction may therefore arise between an act causing certain death (for example, a poisoning) and an omission that hastens or risks death (such as not amputating a gangrenous limb). But sometimes death is as certain following withdrawal of a treatment as following a particular action that is reliably expected to lead to death.

Consequently, merely determining whether what was done involved a fatal act or omission does not establish whether it was morally acceptable. Some actions that lead to death can be acceptable: very dangerous but potentially beneficial surgery or the use of hazardous doses of morphine for severe pain are examples. Some omissions that lead to death are very serious wrongs: deliberately failing to treat an ordinary patient's bacterial pneumonia or ignoring a bleeding patient's pleas for help would be totally unacceptable conduct for that patient's physician.

Not only are there difficult cases to classify as acts or omissions and difficulties in placing moral significance on the distinction, but making the distinction also presupposes an unsound conception of responsibility, namely (1) that human action is an intervention in the existing course of nature, (2) that not acting is not intervening, and (3) that people are responsible only for their interventions (or, at least, are much more responsible for deliberate interventions than for deliberate omissions). The weaknesses of this position include the ambiguous meaning of "intervention" when someone takes an action as part of a plan of nonintervention (such as writing orders not to resuscitate), the inability to define clearly the "course of nature," and the indefensibility of not holding someone responsible for states of affairs that the person could have prevented.

In sum, then, actions that lead to death are likely to be serious wrongs, while many omissions in the medical context are quite acceptable. Yet this is not a fixed moral assessment based on the mere descriptive difference between acts and omissions, but a generalization from experience that rests on such factors as whether the decision reflects the pursuit of the patient's ends and values, whether the health care providers have fulfilled their duties, and whether the risk of death has been appropriately considered.

The Cause of Death   Sometimes acts that lead to death seem to be more seriously wrong than omissions that likewise lead to death because the cause of death in the first instance is seen to be the act while the cause of death in an omission is regarded as the underlying disease. For example, were a physician deliberately to inject a patient with a lethal poison, the physician's action would be the cause of the patient's death. On the other hand, if an otherwise dying patient is not resuscitated in the event of cardiac arrest, or if a pneumonia or kidney failure goes untreated, the underlying disease process is said to be the cause of death. Since people ordinarily feel responsible for their own acts but not for another person's disease, this is a very comforting formulation.

The difference in this common account of causation does not actually explain the different moral assessment—rather, the account of causation *reflects* an underlying assessment of what is right or wrong under the circumstances. Commonly, many factors play some causal role in a person's death. When "the cause" of a patient's death is singled out—for example, to be entered on a death certificate—the decision to designate one or more factors as "the cause(s)" depends upon the normative question at issue. Although the process begins with an empirical inquiry to identify the factors that were actually connected with a particular patient's death, both the process of narrowing to those factors that were "substantial" causes and that of deciding which ones should be held legally or morally responsible for the death involve value judgments. In some situations, although one person's action is unquestionably a factual cause of another's death, holding the person responsible for the death is unfair because the death could not reasonably have been foreseen or because the person was under no obligation to prevent the death.

Beyond selecting "the cause" of death from among the many factors empirically determined to have causally contributed to a patient's death, both the legal and the moral inquiry presuppose that some kinds of causal roles in a death are wrong, and then ask whether any person played any of those roles. Therefore, a determination of causation ordinarily must presuppose, and cannot itself justify, the sorts of decisions that ought to be permissible. For example, in a death following nontreatment, designating the disease as the cause not only asserts that a fatal disease process was present but also communicates acceptance of the physician's behavior in foregoing treatment. Conversely, if an otherwise healthy patient who desired treatment died from untreated pneumonia, the physician's failure to treat would be considered to have caused the patient's death. Although pneumonia is among the factual causes of death, one way of stating the physician's responsibility for the death is to identify the physician's omission of his or her duty to treat as the cause of death. As this example shows, the action/omission distinction does not always correspond to the usual understanding of whether the physician or the disease is the cause of death, and so the attribution of what caused a death cannot make acts morally different from omissions.

In addition, the physician's behavior is among the factual causes of a patient's death both in acting and in omitting to act. This is clear enough if a physician were to give a lethal injection—the patient would not have died at that time and in that way if the physician had not given the injection. But exactly the same is true of a physician's omission of treatment: had a physician not refrained from resuscitating or from treating a pneumonia or a kidney failure, a patient would not have died at that time and in that way. In either case, a different choice by the physician would have led to the patient living longer. To refrain from treating is justifiable in some cases—for example, if the patient does not want the treatment, is suffering, and will die very soon whatever is done. But the justification rests on these other reasons, rather than on not classifying a physician's omission as a cause of the patient's death. Thus, calling the disease the cause of death can be misleading but does reflect a sound point: that a physician who omits treatment in such a case is not morally or legally blameworthy.

The Role of the Distinction in Public Policy   The moral and legal prohibition against acting to take the life of another human being is deeply rooted in Western society and serves the laudable and extremely important value of protecting and preserving human life. Although health care professionals and families want to do the best they can for patients, both in respecting patients' self-determination and promoting their well-being, they face troubling conflicts when doing so would involve them in conduct that might be considered as the taking of another's life.

Yet in health care, and especially with critically or terminally ill patients, it is common to make decisions that one knows risk shortening patients' lives and that sometimes turn out to do so. As a result, there is a strong motivation to interpret the actions decided upon and carried out, especially if by people other than the patient, as something other than acts of killing. Thus, the concerned parties very much want these to be regarded as cases of "allowing to die" (rather than "killing"), of "not prolonging the dying process" (instead of "hastening death"), or of "failing to stop a disease from causing death" (rather than "someone's action was the cause of death"). Consequently, these distinctions, while often conceptually unclear and of dubious moral importance in themselves, are useful in facilitating acceptance of sound decisions that would otherwise meet unwarranted resistance. They help people involved to understand, in ways acceptable to them, their proper roles in implementing decisions to forego life-sustaining treatment.

Law, as a principal instrument of public policy in this area, has sought an accommodation that adequately protects human life while not resulting in officious overtreatment of dying patients. The present general legal prohibition against deliberate, active killing, reinforced by a strong social and professional presumption in favor of sustaining life, serves as a public affirmation of the high value accorded to each human life. The law, and public policy in general, has not interpreted the termination of life-sustaining treatment, even when it requires active steps such as turning off a respirator, as falling under this general prohibition. For competent patients, the principle of self-determination is understood to include a right to refuse life-sustaining treatment, and to place a duty on providers and others to respect that right. Providers, in turn, are protected from liability when they act to aid a patient in carrying out that right. Active steps to terminate life-sustaining interventions may be permitted, indeed required, by the patient's authority to forego therapy even when such steps lead to death. With adequate procedural safeguards, this right can be extended to incompetent patients through surrogates.

Although there are some cases in which the acting-omitting distinction is difficult to make and although its moral importance originates in other considerations, the commonly accepted prohibition of active killing helps to produce the correct decision in the great majority of cases. Furthermore, weakening the legal prohibition to allow a deliberate taking of life in extreme circumstances would risk allowing wholly unjustified taking of life in less extreme circumstances. Such a risk would be warranted only if there were substantial evidence of serious harms to be relieved by a weakened legal protection of life, which the Commission does not find to be the case. Thus the Commission concludes that the current interpretation of the legal prohibition of active killing should be sustained. . . .

Withholding Versus Withdrawing Treatment

A variation on the action/omission distinction sometimes troubles physicians who allow competent patients to refuse a life-sustaining treatment but who are uncomfortable about stopping a treatment that has already been started because doing so seems to them to constitute killing the patient. By contrast, not starting a therapy seems acceptable, supposedly because it involves an omission rather than an action.

Although the nature of the distinction between withholding and withdrawing seems clear enough initially, cases that obscure it abound. If a patient is on a respirator, disconnecting would count as stopping. But if the patient is on a respirator and the power fails, does failing to use a manual bellows mechanism count as "stopping" a therapy (artificial respiration) or "not starting" a therapy (manually generated respiration)? Many therapies in medicine require repeated applications of an intervention. Does failing to continue to reapply the intervention count as "stopping" (the series of treatments) or as "not starting" (the next element in the series)? Even when a clear distinction can be drawn between withdrawing and withholding, insofar as the distinction is merely an instance of the acting-omitting distinction it lacks moral significance.

Other considerations may be involved here, however. Even though health care professionals may not be obligated to initiate a therapy with a particular patient, its initiation may create expectations on the part of the patient and others. In some instances these expectations may lead the health care provider to feel obliged not to stop a therapy that initially could have been foregone. (Similarly, a physician, who is under no obligation to accept any particular person as a patient, may not abandon a patient once a physician-patient relationship has been established.)

This observation does not actually argue that stopping a treatment is in itself any more serious than not starting it. What it claims is that *if* additional obligations to treat have arisen from any expectations created once a treatment has been initiated, then stopping, because it breaches those obligations, is worse than not starting. The expectations, and the resultant obligation to continue, create whatever moral difference arises. The definition of the professional-patient relationship and the creation of expectations that care will be continued occur in complex ways—from professional codes, patterns of practice, legal decisions, and physician-patient communications. A particular physician faced with stopping or not starting therapy with a particular patient may have to accept a relationship and expectations that are at least partly givens.

Discussions between a physician and competent patient, however, allow redefinition of their relationship and alteration of their expectations and thus of any resulting obligations. For example, a physician and patient could agree to a time-limited trial of a particular intervention, with an understanding that unless the therapy achieved certain goals it should be stopped. Moreover, these relationships and expectations, with their resultant obligations, need not be treated as fixed when public policy is being made but can be redefined where appropriate. Of course, most withdrawals of treatment involve explicit decisions while withholdings are commonly implicit and not clearly discussed (although, in conformity with the Commission's recommendations, they should be discussed, except in emergency situations). Although this may make the withdrawal of treatment more anguishing, or even more likely to precipitate external review, it does not make it morally different.

Adopting the opposite view—that treatment, once started, cannot be stopped, or that stopping requires much greater justification than not starting—is likely to have serious adverse consequences. Treatment might be continued for longer than is optimal for the patient, even to the point where it is causing positive harm with little or no compensating benefit. An even more troubling wrong occurs when a treatment that might save life or improve health is not started because the health care personnel are afraid that they will find it very difficult to stop the treatment if, as is fairly likely, it proves to be of little benefit and greatly burdens the patient. The Commission received testimony, for example, that sometimes the view that a therapy that has been started could not be stopped had unduly raised the threshold for initiating some forms of vigorous therapy for newborns. In cases of extremely low birth weight or severe spina bifida, for example, highly aggressive treatment may significantly benefit a small proportion of the infants treated while it prolongs the survival of a great number of newborns for whom treatment turns out to be futile. Fear of being unable to stop treatment in the latter cases—no matter how compelling the reason to stop—can lead to failure to treat the entire group, including the few infants who would have benefited.

Ironically, if there is any call to draw a moral distinction between withholding and withdrawing, it generally cuts the opposite way from the usual formulation: greater justification ought to be required to withhold than to withdraw treatment. Whether a particular treatment will have positive effects is often highly uncertain before the therapy has been tried. If a trial of therapy makes clear that it is not helpful to the patient, this is actual evidence (rather than mere surmise) to support stopping because the therapeutic benefit that earlier was a possibility has been found to be clearly unobtainable.

Behind the withholding/withdrawing distinction lies the more general acting/omitting distinction in one of its least defensible forms. Given that the Commission considers as unwarranted the view that steps leading to death are always more serious when they involve an act rather than an omission, it also rejects the view that stopping a treatment ("an act") is morally more serious than not starting it ("an omission") could be.

Little if any legal significance attaches to the distinction between withholding and withdrawing. Nothing in law—certainly not in the context of the doctor-patient relationship—makes stopping treatment a more serious legal issue than not starting treatment. In fact, not starting treatment that *might* be in a patient's interests is more likely to be held a civil or criminal wrong than stopping the same treatment when it has proved unavailing.

As is the case with the distinction between acting and omitting, many other factors of moral importance may differentiate the appropriateness of a particular decision not to start from one to stop. Yet whatever considerations justify not starting should justify stopping as well. Thus the Commission concludes that neither law nor public policy should mark a difference in moral seriousness between stopping and not starting treatment.

Intended Versus Unintended but Foreseeable Consequences

Since there are sound moral and policy reasons to prohibit such active steps as administering strychnine or using a gun to kill a terminally ill patient, the question arises as to whether physicians should be able to administer a symptom-relieving drug—such as a pain-killer—knowing that the drug may cause or accelerate the patient's death, even though death is not an outcome the physician seeks. The usual answer to this question—that the prohibition against active killing does not bar the use of appropriate medical treatment, such as morphine for pain—is often said to rest on a distinction between the goals physicians seek to achieve or the means they use, on the one hand, and the unintended but foreseeable consequences of their actions on the other.

One problem with assigning moral significance to the traditional distinction is that it is sometimes difficult to determine whether a particular aspect of a course of action ought to be considered to be intended, because it is an inseparable part of the "means" by which the course of action is achieved, or whether it is merely an unintended but foreseeable consequence. In medicine, and especially in the treatment of the critically or terminally ill, many of the courses that might be followed entail a significant risk, sometimes approaching a certainty, of shortening a patient's life. For example, in order to avoid additional suffering or disability, or perhaps to spare loved ones extreme financial or emotional costs, a patient may elect not to have a potentially life-extending operation. Risking earlier death might plausibly be construed as the intended means to these other ends, or as an unintended and "merely foreseeable" consequence. Since there seems to be no generally accepted, principled basis for making the distinction, there is substantial potential for unclear or contested determinations.

Even in cases in which the distinction is clear, however, health care professionals cannot use it to justify a failure to consider all the consequences of their choices. By choosing a course of action, a person knowingly brings about certain effects; other effects could have been caused by deciding differently. The law reflects this moral view and holds people to be equally responsible for all the reasonably foreseeable results of their actions and not just for those results that they acknowledge having intended to achieve. Nevertheless, although medication is commonly used to relieve the suffering of dying patients (even when it causes or risks causing death), physicians are not held to have violated the law. How can this failure to prosecute be explained, since it does not rest on an explicit waiver of the usual legal rule?

The explanation lies in the importance of defining physicians' responsibilities regarding these choices and of developing an accepted and well-regulated social role that allows the choices to be made with due care. The search for medical treatments that will benefit a patient often involves risk, sometimes great risk, for the patient: for example, some surgery still carries a sizable risk of mortality, as does much of cancer therapy. Furthermore, seeking to cure disease and to prolong life is only a part of the physician's traditional role in caring for patients; another important part is to comfort patients and relieve their suffering. Sometimes these goals conflict, and a physician and patient (or patient's surrogate) have the authority to decide which goal has priority. Medicine's role in relieving suffering is especially important when a patient is going to die soon, since the suffering of such a patient is not an unavoidable aspect of treatment that might restore health, as it might be for a patient with a curable condition.

Consequently, the use of pain-relieving medications is distinguished from the use of poisons, though both may result in death, and society places the former into the category of acceptable treatment while continuing the traditional prohibition against the latter. Indeed, in the Commission's view it is not only possible but desirable to draw this distinction. If physicians (and other health professionals) became the dispensers of "treatments" that could only be understood as deliberate killing of patients, patients' trust in them might be seriously undermined. And irreparable damage could be done to health care professionals' self-image and to their ability to devote themselves wholeheartedly to the often arduous task of treating gravely ill patients. Moreover, whether or not one believes there are some instances in which giving a poison might be morally permissible, the Commission considers that the obvious potential for abuse of a public, legal policy condoning such action argues strongly against it.

For the use of morphine or other pain-relieving medication that can lead to death to be socially and legally acceptable, physicians must act within the socially defined bounds of their role. This means that they are not only proceeding with the necessary agreement of the patient (or surrogate) and in a professionally skillful fashion (for example, by not taking a step that is riskier than necessary), but that there are sufficiently weighty reasons to run the risk of the patient dying. For example, were a person experiencing great pain from a condition that will be cured in a few days, use of morphine at doses that would probably lead to death by inducing respiratory depression would usually be unacceptable. On the other hand, for a patient in great pain—especially from a condition that has proved to be untreatable and that is expected to be rapidly fatal—morphine can be both morally and legally acceptable if pain relief cannot be achieved by less risky means.

This analysis rests on the special role of physicians and on particular professional norms of acceptability that have gained social sanction (such as the difference between morphine, which can relieve pain, and strychnine, which can only cause death). Part of acceptable behavior—from the medical as well as the ethical and legal standpoints—is for the physician to take into account all the foreseeable effects, not just the intended goals, in making recommendations and in administering treatment. The degree of care and judgment exercised by the physician should therefore be guided not only by the technical question of whether pain can be relieved but also by the broader question of whether care providers are certain enough of the facts in this case, including the patient's priorities and subjective experience, to risk death in order to relieve suffering. If this can be answered affirmatively, there is no moral or legal objection to using the kinds and amounts of drugs necessary to relieve the patient's pain.

The Commission concludes that the distinction between the decisionmakers' "intending" a patient's death and their "merely foreseeing" that death will occur does not help in separating unacceptable from acceptable actions that lead to death. But, as proved true of the distinctions already discussed, this does point to ethically and legally significant factors—here, the real and symbolic role traditionally assigned to physicians and other practitioners of the healing arts, who can be expected to have developed special sensitivity and skills regarding the judgments to be made, and who are an identifiable group that can be readily held accountable for serious error. Furthermore, the acceptable treatment options that carry a risk of death are limited to those within the special expertise of health care professionals.

The highly valued traditional professional role is not undermined when a physician, with due care, employs a measure—whether radical surgery or medication to relieve pain—that could lead to the patient's death but that is reasonably likely to cure or relieve pain. The relevant distinction, then, is not really that death is forbidden as a means to relieve suffering but is sometimes acceptable if it is merely a foreseeable consequence. Rather, the moral issue is whether or not the decisionmakers have considered the full range of foreseeable effects, have knowingly accepted whatever risk of death is entailed, and have found the risk to be justified in light of the paucity and undesirability of other options. . . .

The Meaning of the Distinction   "Extraordinary" treatment has an unfortunate array of alternative meanings, as became obvious in an exchange that took place at a Commission hearing concerning a Florida case involving the cessation of life-sustaining treatment at the request of a 76-year-old man dying of amyotrophic lateral sclerosis. The attending physician testified:

> I deal with respirators every day of my life. To me, this is not heroic. This is standard procedure. . . .

By contrast, the trial judge who had decided that the respirator could be withdrawn told the Commission:

> Certainly there is no question legally that putting a hole in a man's trachea and inserting a mechanical respirator is extraordinary life-preserving means. . . .

The most natural understanding of the ordinary/extraordinary distinction is as the difference between common and unusual care, with those terms understood as applying to a patient in a particular condition. This interprets the distinction in a literal, statistical sense and, no doubt, is what some of its users intend. Related, though different, is the idea that ordinary care is simple and that extraordinary care is complex, elaborate, or artificial, or that it employs elaborate technology and/or great efforts or expense. With either of these interpretations, for example, the use of antibiotics to fight a life-threatening infection would be considered ordinary treatment. On the statistical interpretation, a complex of resuscitation measures (including physical, chemical, and electrical means) might well be ordinary for a hospital patient, whereas on the technological interpretation, resuscitation would probably be considered extraordinary. Since both common/unusual and simple/complex exist on continuums with no precise dividing line, on either interpretation there will be borderline cases engendering disagreement about whether a particular treatment is ordinary or extraordinary.

A different understanding of the distinction, one that has its origins in moral theology, inquires into the usefulness and burdensomeness of a treatment. Here, too, disagreement persists about which outcomes are considered useful or burdensome. Without entering into the complexity of these debates, the Commission notes that any interpretation of the ordinary/extraordinary distinction in terms of usefulness and burdensomeness to an individual patient has an important advantage over the common/unusual or simple/complex interpretations in that judgments about usefulness and burdensomeness rest on morally important differences. . . . characterize treatments as being required or permissibly foregone. For example, the New Jersey Supreme Court in the *Quinlan* case recognized a distinction based on the possible benefit to the individual patient:

> One would have to think that the use of the same respirator or life support could be considered "ordinary" in the context of the possibly curable patient but "extraordinary" in the context of the forced sustaining by cardio-respiratory processes of an irreversibly doomed patient.

Likewise, the Massachusetts Supreme Judicial Court quoted an article in a medical journal concerning the proposition that ordinary treatment could become extraordinary when applied in the context of a patient for whom there is no hope:

> We should not use *extraordinary* means of prolonging life or its semblance when, after careful consideration, consultation and application of the most well conceived therapy it becomes apparent that there is no hope for the recovery of the patient. Recovery should not be defined simply as the ability to remain alive; it should mean life without intolerable suffering.

Even if the patient or a designated surrogate is held to be under no obligation to accept "extraordinary" care, there still remains the perplexing issue about what constitutes the dividing line between the two. The courts have most often faced the question of what constitutes "ordinary" care in cases when the respirator was the medical intervention at issue. Generally the courts have recognized, in the words of one judge, that "the act of turning off the respirator is the termination of an optional, extraordinary medical procedure which will allow nature to take its course."

For many, the harder questions lie in less dramatic interventions, including the use of artificial feeding and antibiotics. In one criminal case involving whether the defendant's robbery and assault killed his victim or whether she died because life-supporting treatments were later withdrawn after severe brain injury was confirmed, the court held that "heroic" (and unnecessary) measures included "infusion of drugs in order to reduce the pressure in the head when there was no obvious response to those measures of therapy." In another case, in which a patient's refusal of an amputation to prevent death from gangrene was overridden, antibiotics were described by the physician "as heroic measures, meaning quantities in highly unusual amounts risking iatrogenic disease in treating gangrene." Here the assessment, in addition to relying on "benefits," also seems to rely to some degree upon the risk and invasiveness of the intervention. One court did begin to get at the scope of the questions underlying the ordinary/extraordinary distinction. Faced with the question of treatment withdrawal for a permanently unconscious automobile accident victim, the Delaware Supreme Court asked what might constitute life-sustaining measures for a person who has been comatose for many months:

> Are "medicines" a part of such life-sustaining systems? If so, which medicines? Is food or nourishment a part of such life-sustaining systems? If so, to what extent? What extraordinary measures (or equipment) are a part of such systems? What measures (or equipment) are regarded by the medical profession as not extraordinary under the circumstances? What ordinary equipment is used? How is a respirator regarded in this context?

The Moral Significance of the Distinction   Because of the varied meanings of the distinction, whether or not it has moral significance depends upon the specific meaning assigned to it. The Commission believes there is no basis for holding that whether a treatment is common or unusual, or whether it is simple or complex, is in itself significant to a moral analysis of whether the treatment is warranted or obligatory. An unusual treatment may have a lower success rate than a common one; if so, it is the lower success rate rather than the unusualness of the procedure that is relevant to evaluating the therapy. Likewise, a complex, technological treatment may be costlier than a simple one, and this difference may be relevant to the desirability of the therapy. A patient may choose a complex therapy and shun a simple one, and the patient's choice is always relevant to the moral obligation to provide the therapy.

If the ordinary/extraordinary distinction is understood in terms of the usefulness and burdensomeness of a particular therapy, however, the distinction does have moral significance. When a treatment is deemed extraordinary because it is too burdensome for a particular patient, the individual (or a surrogate) may appropriately decide not to undertake it. The reasonableness of this is evident—a patient should not have to undergo life-prolonging treatment without consideration of the burdens that the treatment would impose. Of course, whether a treatment is warranted depends on its usefulness or benefits as well. Whether serious burdens of treatment (for example, the side effects of chemotherapy treatments for cancer) are worth enduring obviously depends on the expected benefits—how long the treatment will extend life, and under what conditions. Usefulness might be understood as mere extension of life, no matter what the conditions of that life. But so long as mere biological existence is not considered the *only* value, patients may want to take the nature of that additional life into account as well.

This line of reasoning suggests that extraordinary treatment is that which, in the patient's view, entails significantly greater burdens than benefits and is therefore undesirable and not obligatory, while ordinary treatment is that which, in the patient's view, produces greater benefits than burdens and is therefore reasonably desirable and undertaken. The claim, then, that the treatment is extraordinary is more of an expression of the conclusion than a justification for it.

The Role of the Distinction in Public Policy   Despite its long history of frequent use, the distinction between ordinary and extraordinary treatments has now become so confused that its continued use in the formulation of public policy is no longer desirable. Although those who share a common understanding of its meaning may still find it helpful in counseling situations, the Commission believes that it is better for those involved in the difficult task of establishing policies and guidelines in the area of treatment decisions to avoid employing these phrases. Clarity and understanding in this area will be enhanced if laws, judicial opinions, regulations, and medical policies speak instead in terms of the proportionate benefit and burdens of treatment as viewed by particular patients. With the reasoning thus clearly articulated, patients will be better able to understand the moral significance of the options and to choose accordingly. . . .

Natural Death Act

The State of California

The California Natural Death Act was passed in 1976. This Act became the precedent and template for other states interested in sanctioning living wills. The language of this first Living Will statute embodies the thinking of the time. This living will was intended for people with terminal illnesses and death anticipated imminently. It was meant to avoid unwanted life-sustaining treatment that would merely prolong the moment of death. More recent and generic advance directives and supplementary comments attached to Durable Power of Attorney for Health Care documents expand the scope of circumstances in which a mentally incapacitated person may forgo life-sustaining treatment.

*T*he people of the State of California do enact as follows:

Directive to Physicians

Directive made this ____ day of _____ (month, year).

    I _____ , being of sound mind, willfully, and voluntarily make known my desire that my life shall not be artificially prolonged under the circumstances set forth below, do hereby declare:

1. If at any time I should have an incurable injury, disease, or illness certified to be a terminal condition by two physicians, and where the application of life-sustaining procedures would serve only to artificially prolong the moment of my death and where my physician determines that my death is imminent whether or not life-sustaining procedures are utilized, I direct that such procedures be withheld or withdrawn, and that I be permitted to die naturally.

2. In the absence of my ability to give directions regarding the use of such life-sustaining procedures, it is my intention that this directive shall be honored by my family and physician(s) as the final expression of my legal right to refuse medical or surgical treatment and accept the consequences from such refusal.

3. If I have been diagnosed as pregnant and that diagnosis is known to my physician, this directive shall have no force or effect during the course of my pregnancy.

4. I have been diagnosed and notified at least 14 days ago as having a

---

Reprinted from "California Natural Death Act," from *California Health and Safety Code*, Part I, Division 7, Chapter 3.9, Section 7188. Approved by the Governor on the 30th of September, 1976.

terminal condition by _____ M.D., whose address is _____ and whose telephone number is _____.
I understand that if I have not filled in the physician's name and address, it shall be presumed that I did not have a terminal condition when I made out this directive.

5. This directive shall have no force or effect five years from the date filled in above.

6. I understand the full import of this directive and I am emotionally and mentally competent to make this directive.

   Signed _____
City, county and State of Residence _____
The declarant has been personally known to me and I believe him or her to be of sound mind.
Witness _____
Witness _____

When Others Must Choose

The New York State Task Force on Life and the Law

The New York State Task Force on Life and the Law was convened by Governor Mario Cuomo in 1984. The Task Force was charged with devising public policy recommendations on issues arising from medical and technological advances such as determination of death, withdrawal and withholding of life-sustaining treatment, organ transplantation, treatment of disabled newborns, and the new reproductive technologies. In 1992 the New York Task Force recommended that each health care facility establish a bioethics review committee or participate in a review committee that served more than one facility. In addition to recommending membership, functions, and procedures [e.g., patient or surrogate involvement], the Task Force recommended that three kinds of sensitive cases be reviewed even when conflicts do not arise. These include the following: (1) when a surrogate decides that life-sustaining treatment should be withdrawn or withheld from a patient who is neither terminally ill nor permanently unconscious; (2) when a decision is made to forego life-sustaining treatment for a patient without a surrogate; and (3) when an emancipated minor wishes to forego life-sustaining treatment. Interestingly, the Task Force recommended immunity for bioethics review Committee members working in good faith.

Establishing Bioethics Review Committees

The Task Force recommends that each health care facility should establish a bioethics review committee or participate in a review committee that serves more than one facility. . . .

In developing its recommendations, the Task Force also examined the role the courts might and should play in surrogate decisions. It concluded that the courts should always remain available as an alternative for those who do not want to participate in a facility-based process, and as a last resort for disputes or cases that cannot be resolved at the health care facility. The Task Force believes, however, that courts should not be the avenue of first resort, either as the sole alternative to address conflict or as the primary decision maker on behalf of all patients who are neither terminally ill nor permanently unconscious. The courts would be overwhelmed by this responsibility, and patients would be ill-served by the delays and demands of the judicial process. This approach would also intrude unnecessarily on the privacy of the family unit and relationships.

New York State Task Force on Life and the Law. Abridged from "When Others Must Choose" (New York State Task Force on Life and Law, March 1992).

Membership

The membership of the review committee should be diverse, in order to provide a range of experience and expertise and to ensure that a variety of perspectives inform committee deliberation. The composition of review committees will vary with the type and size of institution and the sorts of cases reviewed most often. The Task Force proposes that review committees should consist of at least five individuals; at many institutions, committees will be much larger.

Mandatory Members

Each review committee should include at least one physician; one registered nurse; one certified social worker or other person with training or expertise in providing psychosocial services to patients; one individual with training or expertise in bioethics, moral philosophy, or theology; and one lay community member unaffiliated with the facility. In long-term care facilities, at least one representative of the residents' council and one advocate for elderly or nursing home residents should participate on the committee. In addition, the Task Force encourages nursing home committees to include either a member of the bioethics review committee at an acute care hospital with which the nursing home is affiliated or to participate in a review committee that serves more than one nursing home.

Most committees will have more than one physician, representing different specialties and experience. The scientific and technical knowledge of physicians, as well as their clinical experience in caring for patients, is essential to committee deliberations. As the committee considers individual cases, it should begin by clarifying the medical facts, including the patient's diagnosis and prognosis, and treatment alternatives.

Nurses, like physicians, bring both clinical knowledge and experience with patients to committee discussion. Nurses spend extensive time with patients, caring for their personal and medical needs. Although nurses cannot serve on the committee when it considers a case involving one of their patients, this experience still informs their professional perspective. As suggested by a study of New York's DNR law, nurses may be more likely than many physicians to regard the promotion of patient rights as part of their professional mission.

Social workers and other persons with training or expertise in providing psychosocial services to patients also have a vital role in committee discussion, especially concerning the personal, social, and psychological dimensions of each case. They can help to clarify the preferences of patients and the roles and views of family members and others close to the patient. Information about social support and resources available to the patient and family may be critical in some cases.

Review committees should also include at least one individual with training or expertise in bioethics, moral philosophy, or moral theology. These individuals bring skill and experience in identifying ethical problems and analyzing critically the ethical claims and interests of all involved in the case. They can assist the committee to develop clear principles to guide decision making. Ethicists and chaplains may also be well versed in the literature on medical ethics and have experience applying ethical principles in the context of medical cases.

In many facilities, individuals with training or expertise in bioethics, philosophy, or theology will be members of the clergy. In addition to their contribution in evaluating ethical problems, clergypersons, including chaplains, may assist the committee to address religious issues that may be critical for some patients. A clergyperson can help identify the patient's religious values and ensure that the personal and religious views of all concerned are respected.

This responsibility must be approached with sensitivity to the religious and moral diversity likely to be encountered in health care facilities throughout New York State. A member of the clergy must be careful not to promote decisions based on his or her own religious convictions when these diverge from the patient's religious or moral outlook. Even if the patient and clergyperson share the same religious affiliation, their interpretations of that tradition may differ.

The Task Force recommends that review committees also include at least one community member who is not otherwise affiliated with the institution. These individuals should not participate as a "community representative" in the sense of promoting the interests of a group outside the institution, but rather should provide an independent perspective in advocating for patients. These individuals may notice practices and patterns that those affiliated with the facility might overlook or take for granted. They also add to the accountability and credibility of the committee. Their independence distances them from potential conflicts of interest, and enhances their freedom to take positions differing from those of facility administrators or others in a position of authority at the facility.

In acute care hospitals, the lay community member could be an individual who has recognized expertise or demonstrated interest in patient welfare or individual rights. . . .

In long-term care facilities, the lay community member should be an advocate for persons in long-term care or the elderly. This person could be a representative from the New York State Long-Term Care Ombudsman Program. The Ombudsman Program, administered by the New York State Office of the Aging, provides advocacy services for older residents of long-term care facilities. The program relies on trained volunteers as well as state staff to receive, investigate, and resolve complaints. The lay community member might also be a member of a not-for-profit organization that has as part of its mission advocacy for long-term care residents or the elderly, such as the Nursing Home Community Coalition or the state chapter of the American Association of Retired Persons.

The Task Force recognizes that the participation of lay community members raises potential problems. These individuals may be unfamiliar with the clinical setting in general and the facility in particular, making it difficult for them to understand and contribute to committee discussion. They also may be intimidated or ignored by other committee members. Some commentators have expressed concern that patient confidentiality might be compromised by the participation of an individual unaffiliated with the institution, especially one who might not be sensitive to legal requirements or professional standards of confidentiality. Some individuals might be more devoted to general social goals or a personal agenda than to the wishes and interests of individual patients. Finally, some committee members might feel that the participation of a community representative lessens their own responsibility as an advocate for the patient.

Despite these difficulties, the Task Force believes that the participation of lay community members who are not affiliated with the facility adds to committee deliberation and on balance makes an essential contribution. An individual unaffiliated with the institution can bring a critical independent perspective. The individual will also enhance the committee's accountability and public trust in the committee process.

In long-term care facilities, committees should also include at least one member of the residents' council. Required in all facilities by New York State Department of Health regulations, residents' councils are designed to provide a forum for resident participation in devising facility programs and policies. A member of the council can provide insight about treatment alternatives from the perspective of a patient at the facility. In addition, the resident can help to ensure that the patient's interests in each case are fully explored.

Additional Members

The participation of more than one individual from some of the above categories will generally enhance committee deliberation. Facilities can increase the expertise or perspectives available to the committee by inviting individuals affiliated with another health care facility or local institution such as a university to join the committee. Including individuals from another facility is especially important for nursing homes, which often have a more centralized administration than hospitals and may lack the independent viewpoints that coexist in many hospitals. The Task Force encourages committees in long-term care facilities to participate in a committee with another nursing home. When a single bioethics review committee serves more than one long-term care facility, the perspectives of members from different facilities are likely to enrich committee deliberation, and help guard against excessive deference to any one committee member or point of view. . . .

Procedures

Facilities should adopt a written policy governing committee functions, composition, and procedures. This policy should contain procedures for responding promptly to a request for a case consideration, informing appropriate persons of the case, and providing them with access to the committee. It should also specify the circumstances that would trigger the committee's participation or review.

The committee should inform the patient, when possible, the surrogate and involved family members, the attending physician, the facility, and other appropriate individuals of a pending case review, and provide information about the committee's procedures and function. These individuals should also be promptly informed of any decision or recommendation by the committee and should have the opportunity to present their concerns and views to the committee.

Patients and surrogates should also be allowed to bring a person with them to the meeting to assist them in understanding the issues discussed or in presenting their views. This person may be a family member, lawyer, member of the clergy, or simply a close friend. Especially for those who may be intimidated by the process, this is an important option.

While all persons connected with a case may present information to the review committee, health care professionals should not participate as committee members in a case that concerns them directly. For example, physicians caring for the patient whose case is under consideration should present their views to the committee in the same manner as individuals involved with the case, but should not otherwise participate in committee deliberations. This policy will facilitate frank discussion among committee members and enhance the fairness of committee review.

A quorum of the full committee should review surrogate decisions to withdraw or withhold life-sustaining treatment from a patient who is neither terminally ill nor permanently unconscious, or a decision to withhold or withdraw life-sustaining treatment from an emancipated minor or a patient without a surrogate. At a minimum, the proposed requirements for committee membership should be met: at least five members with the professional and other qualifications for committee composition should be present. A health care facility should identify the number of individuals that constitute a quorum of the committee. The presence of a quorum would help assure that cases are treated in a consistent manner and that principles or precedents reflected in the decisions are embraced by the review committee as a whole, not just by a few members. . . .

In general, facilities should maintain written records of committee decisions. The records will contribute to the continuity of the committee's activities, enabling the committee to examine its previous recommendations and to modify its decisions or procedures where appropriate. Maintaining records will also contribute to the committee's accountability.

Except for cases mentioned above when a quorum of the committee should always be present, committees should be allowed to delegate the review of cases to subcommittees. The full committee may be unable to consider every case, because of the frequency of decisions requiring review or the urgency of a particular case. Particularly in situations of conflict between family members or among members of the health care team, a subcommittee may be able to address the issues as well as a larger group and in a more timely way. Except for dispute mediation, which would not require any fixed number of individuals, at least three review committee members, including at least one physician, should participate in each case. Subcommittees should routinely report their activities to the review committee to maintain accountability and to allow the full committee to identify any patterns in subcommittee review that seem problematic.

Functions

Education and Policy Review

In addition to case consultation and review, bioethics review committees could undertake other responsibilities as authorized by the facilities they serve. Review committees could naturally fulfill other roles associated with ethics committees, such as education and policy development. In addition to their intrinsic importance, these activities generally strengthen the ability of committees to engage in case consultation and review. For facilities that already have ethics committees, those committees would probably provide the basis for or serve as the bioethics review committee.

Responding to Conflict or Requests for Consultation

. . . The Task Force recommends that review committees should be available for consultation and advice upon the request of persons involved with the case. In addition, it proposes that committees should seek to resolve cases whether a decision to provide treatment or a decision to withdraw or withhold treatment triggers the conflict. When disagreements arise between or among the physician or other health care professionals caring for the patient, family members, other persons on the surrogate list, or the facility, they should be brought to the committee. For example, the committee should consider any of the following cases:

- A physician objects to a surrogate's decision to discontinue life-sustaining treatment and refers the matter to a review committee rather than implement the decision or transfer the patient's care to another physician.
- A close family member (or other individual on the surrogate list) objects to a surrogate's decision to provide life-sustaining treatment for a dying patient.
- A parent objects to another parent's or guardian's decision to refuse life-sustaining treatment for a minor child, or a minor refuses life-sustaining treatment despite the objection of a parent or guardian.
- An attending physician and other health care professionals disagree about surgery for a patient who has no surrogate.

In these types of cases, the most appropriate role for the committee may be dispute mediation. The committee may be able to resolve a conflict by improving communication among those involved or exploring alternative courses of action. The committee should also identify disputes that arise because a proposed course of treatment conflicts with the substituted judgment and best interests standards or with the medical predicates for surrogate decisions.

Reviewing Sensitive Treatment Decisions

The Task Force believes that three kinds of cases are so sensitive that they should be reviewed routinely by a bioethics review committee, even in the absence of disagreement among those close to the patient and health care professionals: when a surrogate decides that life-sustaining treatment should be withdrawn or withheld for a patient who is neither terminally ill nor permanently unconscious; when a decision is made to forgo life-sustaining treatment for a patient without a surrogate; and when an emancipated minor wishes to forgo life-sustaining treatment. These types of cases present difficult treatment decisions for patients who are extremely vulnerable.

Under the Task Force's proposal, decisions by family members or other surrogates to forgo life-sustaining treatment for patients who are neither terminally ill nor permanently unconscious would not be authorized unless reviewed and approved by the committee or by a court. Committee review and approval would not change the fact that the surrogate and physician remain the decision makers, although it does establish a constraint on their authority. In essence, the committee should function in these sensitive cases to confirm that the decision-making standards have been met and that a surrogate's decision is made in good faith. For emancipated minors, the committee can serve as an advocate, assuring that health care professionals have explored the options for available care and informed the minor fully. For minors as well as surrogates, the committee can also determine whether the choice falls within a range of acceptable alternatives.

The review committee may enhance the surrogate's or minor's decision by seeking additional medical information, clarifying available alternatives, and raising issues that might have been overlooked in previous discussions. The committee should also issue a recommendation about the surrogate's or minor's decision, presenting a statement of the reasons for its recommendation. The statement may persuade the surrogate or minor to accept the committee's recommendation. The statement of reasons would also provide a basis for the surrogate, minor, or attending physician to respond to the committee or to challenge the committee's position. Surrogates, minors, or physicians acting on behalf of their patients can also bypass the committee altogether and seek judicial approval of the decision.

Extending Legal Protection

The Task Force proposes that individuals who serve on bioethics committees in good faith in accord with the proposed legislation should be protected from liability. It is appropriate to extend this legal protection. It is also essential to encourage individuals to serve on the committees. Given the authority vested in the committees, the potential for liability would be more real than when ethics committees perform a purely consultative role, as they do now. Fears of liability, if unaddressed, would not only discourage persons from participating on committees, but also would inhibit free and open discussion among committee members.

The Task Force proposes that individuals should be granted legal protection for actions taken in good faith as a member of or consultant to a review committee or as a participant in a review committee meeting. The protection proposed is broad but not unlimited; it would not encompass either activities outside the scope of committee duties or actions taken in deliberate disregard of the standards and requirements of the proposed legislation. For example, committee members who place the interests of the health care facility ahead of those of the patient whose case is considered would not be protected from liability.

This proposed protection from liability resembles protections afforded under New York law to participants in other health care committees that also function to improve patient care. For example, persons who participate in good faith in dispute mediation under the DNR law are protected from civil liability, criminal prosecution, and professional misconduct sanctions. Likewise, if a person's participation on a facility's quality assurance committee meets a good faith standard, New York law extends immunity from any action for civil damages or other relief as a result of the activity.

Maintaining Confidentiality

Confidentiality for committee deliberations is also crucial to foster committee activity and to protect the privacy of patients whose cases are reviewed. The Task Force recommends that internal committee discussions and records should remain confidential, except for the cases and circumstances specified below. As a general matter, neither the proceedings nor the records of the committee should be released by committee members, consultants, or others privy to such information, nor should the information be accessible to others for use in legal proceedings or government agency investigations. Under this standard, minutes, memoranda, or other written materials prepared for the committee would be kept confidential. Internal committee deliberations and views expressed at committee meetings would also remain private. This confidentiality should be accomplished in two ways. Committee members, consultants, and others with access to these materials and discussions should have a duty to maintain confidentiality. Also, persons external to the committee process, such as individuals who bring a legal action against a physician or the facility, generally should be unable to gain access to documents and discussions by means of subpoenas or other methods.

This confidentiality protection should be subject to two important exceptions. First, committee records and proceedings that address the withdrawal or withholding of life-sustaining treatment from a patient without a surrogate, an emancipated minor patient, or any patient who is neither terminally ill nor permanently unconscious, should be subject to review by the New York State Department of Health. The nature of these sensitive treatment decisions calls for greater oversight and openness about the decision-making process. Also, confidentiality protections should not prevent the patient, the surrogate, other persons on the surrogate list, or the parent or guardian of a minor patient from speaking about the committee proceedings to which they have access, if they choose to do so. For example, a spouse acting as the surrogate for her husband should not be constrained from describing the comments made by committee members during any part of a review committee meeting she attended.

Policies preserving the confidentiality of committee proceedings are also important to protect the privacy of patients. In order for the bioethics review committee to perform its function, committee members, consultants, and others must have access to relevant medical records and information. This access entails a duty to respect the patient's privacy and the confidentiality ordinarily accorded medical information. Any patient-specific information should be disclosed only to the extent strictly necessary to accomplish the purposes of the surrogate decision-making proposal or as otherwise provided by law. For example, the committee should be permitted to inform appropriate persons of a pending case, but should only give individuals the medical information necessary to foster decision making under the standards of the proposal. The patient's privacy should remain of utmost concern.

Health care facilities or the committees themselves should make special efforts to explain the confidentiality requirements to community members and long-term care residents who serve on the committees. These individuals, like others on the committee, should have a clear legal duty to respect the patient's privacy, but may not be familiar with the confidentiality that extends to medical information.

Mandating Committees

. . . The Task Force's proposal . . . requires facilities to establish review committees, . . . delineates the functions of the committees and sets minimum standards for their composition and process. Many of the proposed procedures are designed to make the committee process open and accessible. The committees would be required to function according to a written policy and to consider and respond to health care matters presented by patients, a person on the list of potential surrogates, health care providers, or an authorized state agency. They must also inform patients and those close to them that a matter is under consideration and tell them about the committee's function and procedures. Moreover, the proposed decision-making process, including the participation of committees, represents an alternative for patients and their family members. It would not prevent them from bypassing the committee altogether and seeking judicial intervention at any time. . . .

Recommendation

The Task Force recommends that each health care facility should establish one or more bioethics review committees or participate in a review committee that serves more than one facility. Each review committee should include at least one physician; one registered nurse; one certified social worker or other person with training or expertise in providing psychosocial services to patients; one individual with training or expertise in bioethics, moral philosophy, or theology; and one lay community member unaffiliated with the facility. In long-term care, the community member should be a representative of the Long-Term Care Ombudsman Program or of a not-for-profit organization that promotes the rights and interests of the elderly or nursing home residents as part of its mission. Review committees at long-term care facilities should also include at least one representative of the residents' council. Long-term care facilities should be encouraged, but not required, to include either a member of the bioethics review committee at the acute care hospital with which the facility is affiliated or representatives of more than one long-term care facility in a review committee serving more than one facility.

Facilities should adopt a written policy governing committee functions, composition, and procedures. This policy should include procedures for responding promptly to a request for case consideration and should permit persons connected with a case to present their views to the committee. The proceedings and records of the review committee should generally be kept confidential. All committee members have a duty to respect the confidentiality of patient information.

Review committees should be consulted in the event of conflict between and among health care professionals, family members, and others close to the patient or the facility. Committees should also review and be authorized to approve decisions to forgo life-sustaining treatment by emancipated minors and for patients who are neither terminally ill nor permanently unconscious, even in the absence of conflict. In both types of cases, review committees should determine whether the decision satisfies the standards for surrogate decisions and should issue a recommendation. Review committees should also review and be authorized to approve recommendations to forgo life-sustaining treatment for patients who do not have a family member or friend willing and able to serve as surrogate.

Ethical Issues Involved in the Growing AIDS Crisis

American Medical Association

The American Medical Association has been developing policy statements pertaining to ethical behavior since 1979. The Council on Ethical and Judicial Affairs has expanded the focus from professionalism to explicating ethical challenges facing the profession and providing recommendations derived from the ethical analyses. In this report, the Council believes that physicians may not ethically refuse to treat a patient whose condition is within the physician's competence solely because the patient is seropositive. The Council also states that physicians are ethically obligated to respect the rights of privacy and of confidentiality of AIDS patients and seropositive individuals. Guidelines for responding to situations in which seropositive individuals are endangering third parties are discussed. Guidelines about the question of continuing to practice medicine are presented for physicians with seropositivity or AIDS.

The council on Ethical and Judicial Affairs of the American Medical Association (AMA) recognizes the growing crisis created by the acquired immunodeficiency syndrome (AIDS) as a crucial health problem involving the physician's ethical responsibility to his patients and to society. The House of Delegates adopted Report YY (1987 Annual Meeting) of the Board of Trustees, which provides excellent guidance for a responsible public policy. As stated therein, AIDS patients are entitled to competent medical service with compassion and respect for human dignity and to the safeguard of their confidences within the constraints of the law. Those persons who are afflicted with the disease or who are seropositive have the right to be free from discrimination.

A physician may not ethically refuse to treat a patient whose condition is within the physician's current realm of competence solely because the patient is seropositive. The tradition of the AMA, since its organization in 1847, is that "when an epidemic prevails, a physician must continue his labors without regard to the risk to his own health." (See Principles of Medical Ethics, 1847, 1903, 1912, 1947, 1955.) That tradition must be maintained. A person who is afflicted

---

with AIDS needs competent, compassionate treatment. Neither those who have the disease nor those who have been infected with the virus should be subjected to discrimination based on fear or prejudice, least of all by members of the health care community. Physicians should respond to the best of their abilities in cases of emergency where first-aid treatment is essential, and physicians should not abandon patients whose care they have undertaken. (See Section 8.10 of *Current Opinions of the Council on Ethical and Judicial Affairs of the American Medical Association, 1986.*)

Principle VI of the 1980 Principles of Medical Ethics states: "A physician shall in the provision of appropriate patient care, except in emergencies, be free to choose whom to serve, with whom to associate and the environment in which to provide medical services." The Council has always interpreted this principle as not supporting illegal or invidious discrimination. (See Section 9.11 of *Current Opinions, 1986.*) Thus, it is the view of the Council that Principle VI does not permit categorical discrimination against a patient based solely on his or her seropositivity. A physician who is not able to provide the services required by persons with AIDS should make an appropriate referral to those physicians or facilities that are equipped to provide such services.

At its 1987 Annual Meeting, the House of Delegates adopted Substitute Resolution 18, which asked the Council on Ethical and Judicial Affairs to address "the patient confidentiality and ethical issues raised by known HIV antibody positive patients who refuse to inform their sexual partners or modify their behavior." Physicians have a responsibility to prevent the spread of contagious diseases, as well as an ethical obligation to recognize the rights to privacy and to confidentiality of the AIDS victim. These rights are absolute until they infringe in a material way on the safety of another person or persons. Those who are not infected with the virus are entitled to protection from transmission of the disease. Thus, the societal need for accurate information and public health surveillance must also be respected. As the Board of Trustees stated in Report YY, "A sound epidemiologic understanding of the potential impact of AIDS on society requires the reporting [on an anonymous or confidential basis to public health authorities] of those who are confirmed as testing positive for the antibody to the AIDS virus."

In those jurisdictions in which the reporting of individuals infected with the AIDS virus to public health authorities is not mandated, a physician who knows that a seropositive patient is endangering a third party faces a dilemma. The physician should attempt to persuade the infected individual to refrain from activities that might result in further transmission of the disease. When rational persuasion fails, authorities should be notified so that they can take appropriate measures to protect third parties. Ordinarily, this action will fulfill the physician's duty to warn third parties; in unusual circumstances, when all else fails, a physician may have a common-law duty to warn endangered third parties. However, notification of any third party, including public health authorities, without the consent of the patient may be precluded by statutes in certain states. Therefore, the Council reiterates and strongly endorses Recommendations 16 and 17 of Board Report YY. They are that:

Recommendation 16—Specific statutes must be drafted which, while protecting to the greatest extent possible the confidentiality of patient information, (a) provide a method for warning unsuspecting sexual partners, (b) protect physicians from liability for failure to warn the unsuspecting third party but, (c) establish clear standards for when a physician should inform the public health authorities, and (d) provide clear guidelines for public health authorities who need to trace the unsuspecting sexual partners of the infected person.

Recommendation 17—Given the risk of infection being transmitted sexually, and given the dire potential consequences of transmission, serious consideration should be given to sanctions, at least in circumstances where an unsuspecting sexual partner subsequently finds out about a partner's infection and brings a complaint to the attention of authorities. Pre-emptive sanctions are not being endorsed by this recommendation.

The civil rights and liberties of those who are infected with the AIDS virus, as well as those who are not, are entitled to protection. The ethical challenge to the medical profession is to maintain a judicious balance in this regard, including the issue of whether physicians who are infected with the human immunodeficiency virus must inform their patients or whether they may continue in patient care at all. The Council's new opinion on "Physicians and Infectious Diseases" is as follows: "A physician who knows that he or she has an infectious disease should not engage in any activity that creates a risk of transmission of the disease to others." In the context of the AIDS crisis, the application of the Council's opinion depends on the activity in which the physician wishes to engage.

The Council on Ethical and Judicial Affairs reiterates and reaffirms the AMA's strong belief that AIDS victims and those who are seropositive should not be treated unfairly or suffer from discrimination. However, in the special context of the provision of medical care, the Council believes that if a risk of transmission of an infectious disease from a physician to a patient exists, disclosure of that risk to patients is not enough; patients are entitled to expect that their physicians will not increase their exposure to the risk of contracting an infectious disease, even minimally. If no risk exists, disclosure of the physician's medical condition to his or her patients will serve no rational purpose; if a risk does exist, the physician should not engage in the activity. The Council recommends that the afflicted physician disclose his or her condition to colleagues who can assist in the individual assessment of whether the physician's medical condition or the proposed activity poses any risk to patients. There may be an occasion when a patient who is fully informed of the physician's condition and the risks that condition presents may choose to continue his or her care with the seropositive physician. Great care must be exercised to ensure that true informed consent is obtained.

Position of the American Academy of Neurology on Certain Aspects of the Care and Management of the Persistent Vegetative State Patient

Executive Board, American Academy of Neurology

The American Academy of Neurology's Quality Standards Subcommittee develops scientifically sound, literature-based practice guidelines to assist neurologists in the care of their patients. After a thorough review of the literature, the Subcommittee attempts to link the quality of the literature to the strength of their recommendations. In 1988, the American Academy of Neurology adopted a position on the care and management of patients in a persistent vegetative state. Besides reinforcing that artificial hydration and nutrition is a form of medical treatment, the Academy asserts that medical treatment provides no benefit to patients in a persistent vegetative state. The Academy statement reminds physicians that it often takes one to three months of complete unconsciousness before the condition can be reliably considered permanent.

I. The persistent vegetative state is a form of eyes-open permanent unconsciousness in which the patient has periods of wakefulness and physiological sleep/wake cycles, but at no time is the patient aware of him- or herself or the environment. Neurologically, being awake but unaware is the result of a functioning brainstem and the total loss of cerebral cortical functioning.

A. No voluntary action or behavior of any kind is present. Primitive reflexes and vegetative functions that may be present are either controlled by the brainstem or are so elemental that they require no brain regulation at all.

Although the persistent vegetative state patient is generally able to breathe spontaneously because of the intact brainstem, the capacity to chew and swallow in a normal manner is lost because these functions are voluntary, requiring intact cerebral hemispheres.

B. The primary basis for the diagnosis of persistent vegetative state is the careful and extended clinical observation of the patient, supported by laboratory studies. Persistent vegetative state patients will show no behavioral response whatsoever over an extended period of time. The diagnosis of permanent uncon-

---

Executive Board, American Academy of Neurology. "Position of the American Academy of Neurology on Certain Aspects of the Care and Managment of the Persistent Vegetative State Patient." Abridged from *Neurology*, Volume 39, 1989, pp. 125–126. Reprinted by permisssion.

sciousness can usually be made with a high degree of medical certainty in cases of hypoxic-ischemic encephalopathy after a period of 1 to 3 months.

C. Patients in a persistent vegetative state may continue to survive for a prolonged period of time ("prolonged survival") as long as the artificial provision of nutrition and fluids is continued. These patients are not "terminally ill."

D. Persistent vegetative state patients do not have the capacity to experience pain or suffering. Pain and suffering are attributes of consciousness requiring cerebral cortical functioning, and patients who are permanently and completely unconscious cannot experience these symptoms.

There are several independent bases for the neurological conclusion that persistent vegetative state patients do not experience pain or suffering.

First, direct clinical experience with these patients demonstrates that there is no behavioral indication of any awareness of pain or suffering.

Second, in all persistent vegetative state patients studied to date, postmortem examination reveals overwhelming bilateral damage to the cerebral hemispheres to a degree incompatible with consciousness or the capacity to experience pain or suffering.

Third, recent data utilizing positron emission tomography indicates that the metabolic rate for glucose in the cerebral cortex is greatly reduced in persistent vegetative state patients, to a degree incompatible with consciousness.

II. The artificial provision of nutrition and hydration is a form of medical treatment and may be discontinued in accordance with the principles and practices governing the withholding and withdrawal of other forms of medical treatment.

A. The Academy recognizes that the decision to discontinue the artificial provision of fluid and nutrition may have special symbolic and emotional significance for the parties involved and for society. Nevertheless, the decision to discontinue this type of treatment should be made in the same manner as other medical decisions, i.e., based on a careful evaluation of the patient's diagnosis and prognosis, the prospective benefits and burdens of the treatment, and the stated preferences of the patient and family.

B. The artificial provision of nutrition and hydration is analogous to other forms of life-sustaining treatment, such as the use of the respirator. When a patient is unconscious, both a respirator and an artificial feeding device serve to support or replace normal bodily functions that are compromised as a result of the patient's illness.

C. The administration of fluids and nutrition by medical means, such as a G-tube, is a medical procedure, rather than a nursing procedure, for several reasons.

1. First, the choice of this method of providing fluid and nutrients requires a careful medical judgment as to the relative advantages and disadvantages of this treatment. Second, the use of a G-tube is possible only by the creation of a stoma in the abdominal wall, which is unquestionably a medical or surgical procedure. Third, once the G-tube is in place, it must be carefully monitored by physicians, or other health care personnel working under the direction of physicians, to insure that complications do not arise. Fourth, a physician's judg-

ment is necessary to monitor the patient's tolerance of any response to the nutrients that are provided by means of the G-tube.

2. The fact that the placement of nutrients into the tube is itself a relatively simple process, and that the feeding does not require sophisticated mechanical equipment, does not mean that the provision of fluids and nutrition in this manner is a nursing rather than a medical procedure. Indeed, many forms of medical treatment, including, for example, chemotherapy or insulin treatments, involve a simple self-administration of prescription drugs by the patient. Yet such treatments are clearly medical and their initiation and monitoring require careful medical attention.

D. In caring for hopelessly ill and dying patients, physicians must often assess the level of medical treatment appropriate to the specific circumstances of each case.

1. The recognition of a patient's right to self-determination is central to the medical, ethical, and legal principles relevant to medical treatment decisions.

2. In conjunction with respecting a patient's right to self-determination, a physician must also attempt to promote the patient's well-being, either by relieving suffering or addressing or reversing a pathological process. Where medical treatment fails to promote a patient's well-being, there is no longer an ethical obligation to provide it.

3. Treatments that provide no benefit to the patient or the family may be discontinued. Medical treatment that offers some hope for recovery should be distinguished from treatment that merely prolongs or suspends the dying process without providing any possible cure. Medical treatment, including the medical provision of artificial nutrition and hydration, provides no benefit to patients in a persistent vegetative state, once the diagnosis has been established to a high degree of medical certainty.

III. When a patient has been reliably diagnosed as being in a persistent vegetative state, and when it is clear that the patient would not want further medical treatment, and the family agrees with the patient, all further medical treatment, including the artificial provision of nutrition and hydration, may be forgone.

A. The Academy believes that this standard is consistent with prevailing medical, ethical, and legal principles, and more specifically with the formal resolution passed on March 15, 1986 by the Council on Ethical and Judicial Affairs of the American Medical Association, entitled "Withholding or Withdrawing Life-Prolonging Medical Treatment."

B. This position is consistent with the medical community's clear support for the principle that persistent vegetative state patients need not be sustained indefinitely by means of medical treatment.

While the moral and ethical views of health care providers deserve recognition, they are in general secondary to the patient's and family's continuing right to grant or to refuse consent for life-sustaining treatment.

C. When the attending physician disagrees with the decision to withhold all further medical treatment, such as artificial nutrition and hydration, and feels that such a course of action is morally objectionable, the physician, under normal circumstances, should not be forced to act against his or her conscience or perceived understanding of prevailing medical standards.

In such situations, every attempt to reconcile differences should be made, including adequate communication among all principal parties and referral to an ethics committee where applicable.

If no consensus can be reached and there appear to be irreconcilable differences, the health care provider has an obligation to bring to the attention of the family the fact that the patient may be transferred to the care of another physician in the same facility or to a different facility where treatment may be discontinued.

D. The Academy encourages health care providers to establish internal consultative procedures, such as ethics committees or other means, to offer guidance in cases of apparent irreconcilable differences. In May 1985, the Academy formally endorsed the voluntary formation of multidisciplinary institutional ethics committees to function as educational, policy-making, and advisory bodies to address ethical dilemmas arising within health care institutions.

IV. It is good medical practice to initiate the artificial provision of fluids and nutrition when the patient's prognosis is uncertain, and to allow for the termination of treatment at a later date when the patient's condition becomes hopeless.

A. A certain amount of time is required before the diagnosis of persistent vegetative state can be made with a high degree of medical certainty. It is not until the patient's complete unconsciousness has lasted a prolonged period—usually 1 to 3 months—that the condition can be reliably considered permanent. During the initial period of assessment and evaluation, it is usually appropriate to provide aggressive medical treatment to sustain the patient.

Even after it may be clear to the medical professionals that a patient will not regain consciousness, it may still take a period of time before the family is able to accept the patient's prognosis. Once the family has had sufficient time to accept the permanence of the patient's condition, the family may then be ready to terminate whatever life-sustaining treatments are being provided.

B. The view that there is a major medical or ethical distinction between the withholding and withdrawal of medical treatment belies common sense and good medical practice, and is inconsistent with prevailing medical, ethical, and legal principles.

C. Given the importance of an adequate trial period of observation and therapy for unconscious patients, a family member must retain the ability to withdraw consent for continued artificial feedings well after initial consent has been provided. Otherwise, consent will have been sought for a permanent course of treatment before the hopelessness of the patient's condition has been determined by the attending physician and is fully appreciated by the family.

Initiating and Withdrawing Life Support
Principles and Practice in Adult Medicine

John Ruark, Thomas Raffin, and the
Stanford University Medical Center Committee on Ethics

Dr. Ruark is a clinical assistant professor of psychiatry at Stanford University Medical School and is involved in private practice as the consulting psychiatrist for Stanford's bone marrow transplantation program. Dr. Raffin is a professor and chair of the Division of Pulmonary and Critical Care Medicine at Stanford. These authors have shared the Stanford University Medical Center Committee on Ethics' reflections periodically. This sharing of policies and deliberations with the professional community and public is a model for permitting scrutiny and feedback to foster modifications and improvement. In this statement of principles and practice about initiating and withdrawing life support, the Committee provides valuable guidance to clinicians but also makes several statements that deserve critical reflection. First, the guidelines assert that a "basic principle of medical ethics is obviously the preservation of life." Second, the statement avers that "given the invasive and at times almost brutal nature of the procedure [cardiopulmonary resuscitation], it is hard to reconcile the relatively small chance of a successful outcome with the loss of a more dignified death." Third, "If no one knows the patient well enough to provide information about his or her quality-of-life values, professionals can establish a group composed of physicians, nurses, family or friends, and two patient advocates . . . to identify what it believes to be the most thoughtful substituted judgment. Only rarely is legal assistance necessary."

During the past century, dramatic changes have occurred in physicians' ability to prolong life. A hundred years ago, little more than rudimentary supportive care could be offered to most critically ill patients. Doctors now choose from a vast array of interventions that, when combined with effective therapies for underlying conditions, often greatly prolong survival. Unfortunately, the quality of the additional life so skillfully sought can range from marginally tolerable to positively miserable.

These considerations underscore the importance of a clear ethical framework for making decisions about the initiation and withdrawal of all medical treatments. This paper considers basic and advanced life support, controversial procedures with serious potential for causing more harm than good. It begins with a review of recent legal trends and precedents involving life support. Then it suggests general and specific principles for appropriate decision making. Finally, it applies these principles to four fundamental situations—initiating basic life support, initiating advanced life support, withdrawing advanced life support, and withdrawing basic life support.

Recent Legal Precedents

A number of California laws and judicial decisions illustrate the current legal framework in which life support may be initiated and withdrawn. Although they apply only locally, they typify legal opinion on these issues throughout the country. The right of competent adults to accept or refuse medical treatment on the basis of full information is defined as informed consent.[1] The right of competent adult patients with incurable but not immediately terminal illnesses to refuse treatment over the objection of physicians and hospitals was affirmed by the California Court of Appeals' 1984 decision in *Bartling v. Superior Court.*[2] Subsequently, *Bouvia v. Superior Court*[3] established the right to refuse even nourishment and hydration. However, some courts may treat withholding or withdrawing nutrition and hydration from incompetent patients differently from other treatments.[4]

Some legal criteria for the withdrawal of life support were identified in 1983 in *Barber v. Superior Court.*[5] This case involved murder charges against two physicians who, with the informed consent of the patient's spouse and children, withdrew intravenous nourishment and hydration from an irreversibly comatose man. In dismissing the charges, the court relied on the vital concept of proportionality as the criterion to be used in deciding whether to withdraw life support. The court stated, "Proportionate treatment is that which, in the view of the patient, has at least a reasonable chance of providing benefits to the patient which outweigh the burdens attendant to the treatment." The *Barber* court then addressed the central question of defining such terms as "benefits" and "burdens." It relied in part on the *Quinlan* decision, which examined "the reasonable possibility of return to cognitive and sapient life as distinguished from . . . biological vegetative existence."[6] The court suggested that a benefit exists when life-sustaining treatment contemplates "at very least, a remission of symptoms enabling a return toward a normal functioning, integrated existence."

The recent Massachusetts case of *Brophy v. New England Sinai Hospital*[7] also emphasized the outcome of proposed treatment. The court authorized the withholding of nutrition and hydration although they might have sustained the patient in a persistent vegetative state. It noted that this measure was appropriate because the patient would never "regain cognitive behavior, the ability to communicate, or the capability of interacting purposefully with his environment."

The *Barber* court also discussed who can appropriately decide for incompetent patients. In such cases, physicians must identify a surrogate to make a "substituted judgment" on the patient's behalf. The court found that, barring legislation to the contrary, it is legal to bypass formal conservatorship proceedings. It reasoned that the spouse and children are the most appropriate surrogates because they are in the best position to know the patient's feelings and desires regarding treatment, would be most affected by the treatment decision, are concerned for the patient's comfort and welfare, and have expressed an interest in the patient through visits or inquiries to the patient's physician or hospital staff.

In addition to court decisions, certain documents bear on the initiation and withdrawal of life support. The living will[8] is a nationally distributed document that expresses patients' wishes regarding medical care should they become incompetent to decide. Although this document has no binding force in some states,[9] it still stands as a clear expression of the patient's wishes. Currently, 38 states have enacted living-will or "natural death" legislation.[10] The more recent California "durable power of attorney for health care"[11] creates a simple and legally protected procedure whereby people can indicate treatment preferences in various situations and designate an "attorney in fact" who is empowered to make medical decisions should patients become unable to decide for themselves. However, the attorney in fact must be explicitly informed of the patient's wishes in order to make clear-cut decisions.

General Ethical Fundamentals

The fundamental principles underlying the ethics of medical intervention in all settings are discussed exhaustively in various books.[12] Therefore, although some basic principles are listed here, only the practical principles will be considered in detail. A basic principle of medical ethics is obviously the preservation of life, which is frequently tempered by the second principle, the alleviation of suffering. A third is the injunction that physicians "first do no harm" (*primum non nocere*). A fourth principle, respect for the autonomy of the individual patient, finds a lively expression in the current surge of medical consumerism. A fifth fundamental principle is the concept of justice, exemplified by the effort to ensure that medical resources are allocated fairly.[13] The final principle is truth telling, well discussed recently by Bok.[14] Because medical practice often brings these principles into conflict, resolving such conflicts is central to the art of medicine.

Underlying Practical Principles

Establishment of the Source of Authority

The most important key to appropriate ethical management of the initiation and withdrawal of life support is constant awareness of the true source of authority. Although physicians must often be authoritative about the options available to patients, all involved should recognize that the actual authority over the patient never resides with the physician. Patients alone, or their legal surrogates, have the right to control what happens to them. Many of the ethical dilemmas in critical care situations derive from overt or tacit violations of this principle. Physicians should act as consultants engaged to evaluate their patients' problems, present reasonable options for treatment in understandable language, and facilitate decision making. Except in emergencies, doctors should feel permitted to proceed with treatments only after those with the true authority have clearly decided.

Effective Communication with Patients and Families

The ability to communicate effectively with patients and families or legal surrogates is one of the most vital professional skills in appropriate decision making. Especially in critical care situations, stress, fear, intimidation, and unfamiliarity with the setting can overwhelm even sophisticated patients and families. Health professionals are responsible not merely for attempting to communicate, but for ensuring that effective communication takes place.

Certainly, some physicians communicate better than others. When physicians are made aware of communication problems by patients, families, or members of the health care team, they should promptly enlist a proven facilitator—a social worker, chaplain, or psychotherapist, for example. There are several reasons why communication in this setting is difficult for doctors. First, each case is stressful and emotionally wrenching, taking a major physical and psychological toll on physicians. Second, the cumulation of many such cases exacts a high price from physicians in terms of emotional fatigue and distance, personal fear of death, guilt, insecurity, and anxiety. Third, effective communication in catastrophic situations requires time, a scarce commodity among doctors. Outside facilitators can be valuable on the health care team because they have the communication skills and the time to exercise them.

The following are some guidelines for effective communication. First, create an environment that fosters communication. Rushed or chaotic settings such as a hospital corridor hinder effective decision making. Second, remember that stress often impairs the reasoning ability of patients and families. Keep communication simple until it is clear that more detail will be helpful rather than overwhelming. Third, encourage patients and families to ask questions and express feelings. This helps to counteract the intimidation that many people experience when dealing with physicians.

In addition, present information in the language and at the level of detail that best enables patients or surrogates to decide. It is not useful to speak honestly about a situation if you are intimidating people with an esoteric vocabulary, unnecessary details, or an inappropriate emotional tone. Ask patients and families to summarize what has been said in order to check the accuracy of vital communications, provide a chance to correct misunderstandings, and assess their level of sophistication and reasoning. Finally, make a specific effort to sharpen your communication skills. Ivey and Authier,[15] for example, describe a useful model for effective communication by physicians. Various resources[16] offer more detailed advice on communication in the presence of life-threatening illness.

Early Determination and Ongoing Review of Individual Quality-of-Life Values

The ethics of life support require physicians to ascertain, whenever possible, the views of each patient or representative on the balance between quality and mere prolongation of life—the concept of proportionality. Professionals should diligently avoid making assumptions in this area, especially with patients of different religious or ethnic backgrounds. The balance between the probable extension of life and the reduction in quality of life resulting from any treatment must be explicitly described and discussed with each patient. Absolute candor about the level of discomfort associated with any anticipated treatment is essential, but emotional coldness or brutal abruptness should be avoided.

On the other hand, there is no evidence that any worthwhile end is accomplished by painting an unduly optimistic picture. Physicians who do so may unintentionally appear untrustworthy at a time when the ability to trust one's doctor is particularly critical. Specific treatment options for probable complications should be explored as early as possible, to avoid unnecessary guilt in surrogates who are forced to decide for incompetent patients. With permission from patients, family members should be included in anticipatory decision making so that they have no doubt about the patient's wishes.

As an illness progresses, patients commonly reassess the relative costs and benefits of treatments as they gain familiarity with various therapies and as their energy wanes with advancing debilitation. Thus, at a minimum, every important change in a patient's condition demands that decisions about proportionality be reevaluated. Such reassessment requires carefully exploring the ambiguous feelings of families as they make decisions or attempt to influence those of the patient.

Any medical intervention should be oriented toward the patient's goals—for example, to spend some time at home—as well as toward solving a clinical problem. In many cases there is a critical point beyond which medical interventions may act less to prolong acceptable life than to extend a miserable dying process.[17] Professionals cannot expect patients or families to take the lead in raising these questions.

Recognition of Patients' Rights

The final basis for appropriate decision making about life support is the code of patients' rights as articulated by the American Hospital Association and enacted into law in many states. If these rights are observed in spirit as well as in letter, it is difficult to go wrong in initiating or withdrawing medical treatments. In many states, the law requires posting these rights in appropriate places within every hospital. The following patients' rights[18] are particularly relevant: to receive considerate and respectful care; to receive information about the illness, the course of treatment, and the prospects for recovery in terms that the patient can understand; to receive as much information about any proposed treatment or procedure as the patient may need in order to give informed consent or to refuse this course of treatment (except in emergencies, this information should include a description of the procedure or treatment, the medically important risks involved in this treatment, alternative courses of treatment or nontreatment and the risks involved in each, and the name of the person who will carry out the treatment or procedure); to participate actively in decisions regarding medical care (to the extent permitted by law, this includes the right to refuse treatment); and to have all patients' rights apply to the person who may have legal responsibility to make decisions about medical care on behalf of the patient.

Specific Applications

Initiation of Basic Life-Support Measures

Basic life-support measures—providing food, water, and supplementary oxygen—are among the most difficult to forgo in medical practice because of their high emotional content. Although few of us may know what it feels like to undergo cardiopulmonary resuscitation or heart transplantation, we all know what it is like to be hungry, thirsty, or short of breath. Health care professionals may provide these basics of care almost as a reflex, without fully considering whether they are performing a truly caring act.

In critical illness, thoughtful clinicians need to replace such impulses with a careful decision-making process that takes into account several major points. First of all, every medical intervention should serve what patients consider to be their best interests as determined in an active dialogue with their families and their physicians. Second, as in most cases involving the initiation or withdrawal of life support (or any major medical intervention), it is wise to include close family members in the decision-making process whenever possible. This enlists the family on the side of the eventual treatment course, minimizing the possibility of harrowing conflicts at times of great stress. Third, physicians should anticipate the likely medical course and elicit clearly—in advance—the specific choices the patient wishes to make for each possible situation.

Fourth, once any medical intervention is begun in grave illness, withdrawing it in order to avoid an agonizing dying process requires a direct action that may result in a death. However necessary and humane such an action may be, those forced to make such decisions and those who carry them out are inevitably left with disturbing feelings. Furthermore, medications need to be evaluated carefully. In particular, problems may arise from the use of antibiotics or steroids to treat infections or cerebral edema. Comatose, hopelessly ill people may be pulled back needlessly from a painless death to live out an extra few days or weeks in pain and indignity. Perhaps some physicians, frustrated by underlying illnesses that defy medical intervention, gain a sense of control by treating conditions they can treat. In addition, if those responsible for the patient want every possible measure taken to keep the patient alive, professionals should comply with this request at first. If the desire to persist in treatment seems inappropriate, a direct, logical challenge by the professional will often fail, whereas a nonjudgmental exploration of underlying feelings can result in sounder decision making.

Also, physicians need to clarify the purpose of placing intravenous lines. Unless a patient-oriented goal has been defined, it is not acceptable to begin intravenous therapy for "hydration and nutrition." Once an intravenous line is in place, it becomes harder to refrain from treating the infections and chemical imbalances that might provide a humane release. This same reasoning applies to ordering laboratory tests or assessing vital signs: once it is demonstrated that a treatable problem exists, it becomes much harder not to act. Finally, similar cautions apply to the placement of feeding tubes, especially in patients in chronic vegetative states.

Instituting Advanced Life-Support Measures

Cardiopulmonary resuscitation raises many ethical questions. A patient in cardiac or pulmonary arrest presents professionals with a medical emergency that requires a set of automatic responses if function is to be restored before severe organ damage occurs. Unless they are aware of the patient's previously expressed wishes about resuscitation, physicians must act first and evaluate later.

One recent study[19] of all the resuscitations at a major medical center in one year showed that only 14 percent of those who received cardiopulmonary resuscitation survived to leave the hospital. Only 19 percent of all patients discussed the procedure with their physicians, and in only 33 percent of the cases was the family consulted about resuscitation, even though more than 95 percent of the physicians claimed to believe such consultations appropriate. In a related study involving do-not-resuscitate orders,[20] 22 percent of patients and 86 percent of families were involved in decisions not to resuscitate. The families identified the attending physician as the best source of help with their decisions. Other useful factors included the presence of coma or brain death, indicating a hopeless prognosis; support and reassurance from physicians and nurses that the decision was appropriate; assurances from staff that care and comfort would be maintained; and previous conversations with the patient about resuscitation.

These studies underscore the ethical dilemma presented by cardiopulmonary resuscitation. Given the invasive and at times almost brutal nature of the procedure, it is hard to reconcile the relatively small chance of a successful outcome with the loss of a more dignified death—particularly in the setting of chronic, severely debilitating, or terminal conditions. In attempting to resolve this dilemma, there are some important points the physician should take into account. First, since cardiopulmonary arrest is likely to occur during the hospitalization of an elderly, chronically ill, or terminally ill person, there is little ethical justification for not discussing it in advance. This imperative also applies to similar patients who remain at home or in nursing homes. The code status of patients should be identified early and officially conveyed to patients, families, and all health care providers. Prominent signs on the front of medical charts or records are useful.

Attending physicians must take the lead in bringing up this matter. If they neglect to do so, family members or nurses (who are likely to be first on the scene) pay a high price. Physicians who feel uneasy with such decision making or who are poorly prepared to facilitate it have an obligation to seek education or counseling to prepare them to perform this duty effectively. When there is any doubt or a persistent lack of unanimity on the health care team, they should enlist the aid of a facilitator, as discussed above.

Finally, one aspect of this question that is seldom adequately considered is that successful resuscitation almost inevitably results in admission to an intensive care unit or a cardiac care unit. Few patients who have not received intensive care can comprehend the general unpleasantness of even the most humane intensive care unit—the invasive monitoring and treatment, the noise and activity around the clock, and the necessary restrictions on visitors. In particular, mechanical ventilators virtually preclude communication with family members at times when emotional support is most needed. These realities must be clearly communicated when physicians seek informed consent. Given that an average of less than 10 percent of patients with hematologic cancers who receive intensive care survive to leave the hospital,[21] special caution should be employed in deciding to intubate or resuscitate them.

Renal dialysis is another intensive treatment that is difficult to withdraw once it has been started. Its withdrawal, like that of mechanical ventilation, leads directly and observably to the death of patients dependent on it. Thus, in order to avoid the emotional distress and long-term guilt connected with "pulling the plug," careful informed consent, perhaps including a chance to talk to a patient on dialysis, should be obtained before dialysis is started. Similar reasoning can be applied to more aggressive interventions such as renal, cardiac, lung, and bone marrow transplantation.

Withdrawing Advanced Life Support

The decision to withdraw advanced life-support measures can be one of the most difficult for professionals and family members to face. Ideally, if such measures are initiated as outlined above, the guidelines for their withdrawal will have been well defined by patients or surrogates. In reality, such clear definition is more the exception than the rule. The following are some suggestions for physicians:

Exercise reasonable clinical judgment about the likelihood of medical benefit from further treatment. Studies such as APACHE (Acute Physiologic Assessment and Chronic Health Evaluation) II[22] provide valuable prognostic guidelines.

Assess the patient's competence. A sound evaluation of mental status is vital to decision making, and psychiatric consultation should be sought when the state of competence cannot be clearly identified.

Seek unanimity among members of the health care team. Problems may arise when any professional feels excluded from the decision-making process. Because nurses provide most of the intensive care, they often have information about patients and families that is available only to those who have spent hours at the bedside.

Vigorously solicit the patient's judgment regarding withdrawal of treatment. Although most persons on life support will be legally incompetent, any shred of evidence about what the patient wants will be enormously valuable to those who must decide. Competent patients who request that their life support be stopped must be carefully evaluated. Such patients have a legal right to control their health care, and professionals who do not comply may be committing battery.

Do not rush decision making with families. These negotiations must be regarded as delicate processes with their own timing. Facilitation by nonphysician experts, especially chaplains, is often invaluable. The health care team should work with the family toward unanimous decisions regarding the life support of incompetent patients.

Establish time-limited goals, based on clinical judgment and information such as the APACHE II data. After being advised that life support should be discontinued, families are often overwhelmed with confusion and guilt and may resist the advice. They can be helped in their decision making if concrete temporal milestones can be identified that herald improvement or failure. For example, the doctor might say to the adult children of a man who had been on a ventilator with respiratory and renal failure for two weeks, "If we see no signs that your father has improved over the next 72 hours, then we believe you should consider withdrawing life support. We believe your father is suffering and has essentially no chance to regain any reasonable quality of life, and to withdraw life support would allow him a more peaceful and dignified death."

The interlude provided by these time-based goals is a time for families to let go of the patient emotionally. Able facilitation of this process can be invaluable. Often, patients and family members have agreed to interventions on the basis of unrealistic expectations—of both eventual benefits and quality of life during the treatments. Before they can make rational decisions, they may need to express the anger and mistrust generated by suboptimal informed consent. Here physicians must tolerate expressions of hostility without becoming defensive, but anger usually subsides once patients and families feel that their doctors are truly understanding and supportive. Even if patients or families do not express this anger, look for it in situations where it should reasonably be present. Statements such as, "This may have turned out to be a lot more than you bargained for. It wouldn't surprise me if you were angry about it," can open the way to the expression and resolution of feelings.

An effective way of telling patients or families that you believe life support should be withdrawn is to say, "It is my best judgment, and that of the other doctors and nurses, that your relative has essentially no chance to regain a reasonable quality of life. We believe that life support should be withdrawn, which means that your relative will probably die." There are two important components to this statement. First, the statement is realistically qualified, in a way that implies that the decision must be shared. Second, it is made clear that death is the probable result of the recommended course. Without this knowledge, there is no true informed consent, and potential liability (both emotional and legal) looms.

Grief-stricken or guilty family members may attempt to relieve their distress at the patient's expense by pressing for disproportionate treatment. Such insistence usually dissolves once the underlying feelings are acknowledged and understood.

Professionals should avoid involving themselves with cases that are inconsistent with their ethical principles. The tension and resentment inevitably arising under such circumstances may compromise clinical judgment. If such involvement cannot be avoided, frequent ventilation of feelings with understanding colleagues will make optimal care more likely.

If patients are judged incompetent and no written or oral communication about withdrawal of treatment exists, the problem is greater. The most satisfactory resolution of such cases occurs when professionals and families painstakingly explore the quality-of-life values previously held by the patient. Once family members have agreed that the patient would not have wanted to go on, consent to withdraw treatment usually follows. If no one knows the patient well enough to provide information about his or her quality-of-life values, professionals can establish a group composed of physicians, nurses, family or friends, and two patient advocates (at least one of whom represents an organized religion, preferably that of the patient). This group identifies what it believes to be the most thoughtful "substituted judgment." Decisions should be made by family, friends, health care providers, and facilitators. Only rarely is legal assistance necessary.

Withdrawal of Basic Life Support

The withdrawal of basic life support, such as hydration or nutrition by intravenous lines or feeding tubes, is ethically controversial and complex. Although most people eventually feel at peace with stopping more technical medical interventions, these basic measures are regarded more as signs of caring than as treatment. No one is comfortable with the thought that a loved one may "die of thirst" or "starve to death." Indeed, legal sanction notwithstanding, families will feel guilty if these feelings are not explored and resolved.

The three states whose courts have addressed the question of withdrawal of nutrition and hydration from incompetent patients have treated it in the same manner as the withdrawal of advanced life support.[4,5,7] As additional cases are adjudicated, broader judicial support is expected for withdrawing these treatments when they are not clearly benefiting patients.

The key to resolving ethical problems in this area lies in clarifying the patient's interests. In the presence of truly informed consent and sensitive psychosocial management of decision making, most painful ambiguities can be resolved. The patient's wishes regarding withdrawal of the whole array of treatments should be detailed in writing. If possible, conflicts between the patient's wishes and those of the family should be mediated toward a consensus, although the patient's wishes must be controlling. Families need assurances that comfort and caring will be maintained and that doctors will not abandon them.

Conclusions

Most of the ethical dilemmas involved in life support can be avoided with careful attention to certain important points. Recognize that authority in medical care rests with patients or their legal surrogates. Support them in exercising this authority. Support patients' rights, particularly the right to give informed consent. Emphasize effective communication, and be aware of and avoid the circumstances that tend to impair it. Enlist a proven facilitator rapidly if communication becomes less than optimal. Review proportionality decisions early in each treatment course and with each major change in clinical status. Recognize that once an intervention is started, its withdrawal can cause problems; nevertheless, in many settings life support should be thoughtfully withdrawn. And finally, besides being aware of your own feelings, provide emotional support to the other members of the health care team in these difficult cases.

References

1. Cobbs v. Grant, 8 Cal. 3d 229, 1872.
2. Bartling v. Superior Court, 163 Cal. App.3d 186, 195, 1984.
3. Bouvia v. Superior Court, 179 Cal. App.3d 1127, 1986.
4. E.g., In re Conroy, 464 A. 2d 303 (N. J. Super. Ct., App. Div. 1983), rev'd, 486 A.2d 1209, N.J. 1985.
5. Barber v. Superior Court, 147 Cal. App.3d 1006, 1983.
6. In re Quinlan, 70 N.J. 10, 355 A.2d 647, 79 ALR3d 205, 1976.
7. Brophy v. New England Sinai Hospital, 497 N.E.2d 626, Mass. 1986.
8. Society for the Right to Die. Living will. New York, 1985.
9. Eisendrath SJ, Jonsen AR. The living will: Help or hindrance? JAMA 1983; 249:2054–8.
10. Jonsen AR. Dying *right* in California: the Natural Death Act. Clin Res 1978; 26:55–60.
11. Gilfix M, Raffin TA. Withholding or withdrawing extraordinary life support: optimizing rights and limiting liability. West J Med 1984; 141:387–94.
12. E g., Brody H. Ethical decisions in medicine. Boston: Little, Brown, 1976.
13. Fuchs VR. The "rationing" of medical care. N Engl J Med 1984; 311:1572–3.
14. Bok S. Lying: moral choice in public and private life. New York: Pantheon, 1978.
15. Ivey AE, Authier J. Microcounseling: innovations in interviewing, counseling, psychotherapy, and psychoeducation. 2nd ed. Springfield, Ill.: Charles C Thomas, 1978.
16. Gonda TA, Ruark JE. Dying dignified: the health professional's guide to care. Menlo Park, Calif.: Addison-Wesley, 1984.
17. Young EWD. Reflections on life and death Stanford MD 1976; 15: 20–4.

18. Title 22, Section 70707, California Administrative Code.
19. Bedell SE, Delbanco TL, Cook EF, Epstein FH. Survival after cardiopulmonary resuscitation in the hospital. N Engl J Med 1983; 309:569–76.
20. Bedell SE, Pelle D, Maher PL, Cleary PD. Do-not-resuscitate orders for critically ill patients in the hospital: How are they used and what is their impact? JAMA 1986; 256:233–7.
21. Schuster DP, Marion JM. Precedents for meaningful recovery during treatment in a medical intensive care unit: outcomes in patients with hematologic malignancy. Am J Med 1983; 75:402–8.
22. Knaus WA, Draper EA, Wagner DP, Zimmerman JE. Prognosis in acute organ-system failure. Ann Surg 1985; 202:685–93.

Ethics Committees and Decisions to Limit Care

The Experience at the
Massachusetts General Hospital

Troyen A. Brennan

Troyen A. Brennan is an internist and lawyer at Harvard Medical School. He received fellowship training in ethics through the Program in Ethics and the Professions at Harvard University. He reports on the experience of the Optimum Care Committee's (OCC) experience with 73 case consultations between 1974 and 1986. Dr. Brennan classifies the cases into six categories. The five useful categories included (1) OCC defers to the competent patient; (2) OCC recommends limited care, referring physician defers to family wishes for resuscitation and unlimited care; (3) OCC supports a family's wish that care be withdrawn; (4) patient accorded DNR status at family's wish; (5) OCC recommends DNR order despite family's wishes; and (6) OCC's advice had little impact on the patient's case. Over time, there were increasing numbers of cases, especially from the medicine service and in the first and fifth categories. The OCC's approach to cases in category #5 is controversial, and this publication permits the professional reader and public the opportunity to criticize the approach.

To make available more information on clinical ethics and consultative ethics committees, I have reviewed the experience of the OCC of the Massachusetts General Hospital. Its four members currently include a nurse, a surgeon, an internist who is also a lawyer, and the chairperson, a psychiatrist with a divinity degree. From 1974 through 1986, the committee's 73 full consultations represented a very broad experience with the ethical problems that arose when care for terminally ill patients was limited. A review of that experience and a comparison with cases in which care was limited without OCC input illustrate some of the ethical problems that arise in the care of critically ill patients, as well as the evolution of the committee's role within the hospital.

A physician who wishes to consult the OCC may contact its chairperson. The OCC is generally consulted when an ethical problem arises that presents especially sensitive issues or that is a source of disagreement among the treating physicians. When a request is received, one of the physician members of the OCC interviews the physicians caring for the patient and, if appropriate, dis-

cusses matters with the patient and available family members. The OCC nurse
gathers information on patient status, the attitudes of family members, and the
opinions of the nursing staff about the limitation or withdrawal of care. The
physicians requesting the consultation must record their prognosis for the patient. The committee members then consult with one another, sometimes as a
group and sometimes by telephone, and discuss the case. They are guided mainly
by a principle of beneficence, asking what would be the best thing to do for the
patient. Finally, one committee member writes a note in the chart with some
suggestions and the ethical and medical rationale for any limitations of care.

Unlike some other consultative ethics committees, only physicians may
consult the OCC, although the nursing staff can, and often does, advise the
attending physician that an OCC consultation would be helpful. The OCC role
is advisory. . . .

Classification of Cases

Each OCC case was classified into one of six broad categories on the basis of
type of decision made by the OCC and the attending physician. The categories,
which are my own and therefore were not used by the OCC members, are as
follows:

Type 1: The OCC found the patient to be competent and supported the
patient's wish that full treatment be maintained. (The OCC respected completely
the autonomy of the competent patient.)

Type 2: The attending physician declined to accept OCC advice that care
be limited. (The OCC's role was to provide advice, not to dictate policy.)

Type 3: The OCC and attending physician supported the family's wish that
an incompetent patient's care be withdrawn or withheld. In these situations, the
OCC consultation was requested to reaffirm the decision reached by the family
and the attending physician.

Type 4: The OCC and attending physician supported the family's wish that
an incompetent patient be accorded DNR status.

Type 5: The OCC and attending physician decided that an incompetent
patient be accorded DNR status independent of or despite the family's wishes.

Type 6: In a small number of cases, the OCC advice had little impact on
the patient's care . . . because of a change in the clinical status of the patient.

Results

. . . Comparing the OCC experience with data obtained from a three-month
study of patients accorded DNR status without OCC input demonstrates that
the OCC reviews only a very small percentage of all the cases with limited-care
orders. In the last three months of 1986, 113 patients had DNR or other limited-
care orders written, but only six of these patients were interviewed by the OCC.
Thus, in the great majority of cases, the physicians, patients, or patients' families
were in agreement that the care be limited.

. . . Patients tended to be in the intensive care unit more frequently than "control limited-care" patients. In addition, the OCC patients, who were younger than the control patients, were more likely to die during hospitalization. The OCC patients were thus a relatively young, very sick group of patients and might be expected to produce more controversial decisions about limiting care. . . .

Comment

. . . I have noted that the OCC provides advice on five different types of cases. Each presents different problems and reflects a different aspect of the OCC's reasoning and function. Type 1 cases demonstrate that when patients are competent, the OCC always defers to their wishes. Type 2 cases highlight the fact that the OCC's function is advisory: the physician seeking guidance is always free to accept or reject it.

The other three types of situations encountered by the OCC involve decisions to limit care. In type 3 cases the OCC supported the wishes of the family that care be withdrawn. It appears that more families are now requesting that care be withdrawn when there is no hope of recovery. Many physicians hesitate to defer to the family's wish that mechanical ventilatory support or hydration be stopped. The OCC often reassures caregivers that withdrawal of care is ethically defensible once it is clear that the disease process is irreversible and the patient moribund. Moreover, the OCC can help physicians and patients' families clarify the types of care that can be withheld and the nature of care that provides comfort.

Type 3 cases also reflect the OCC's emphasis on ethical rather than legal imperatives. For instance, the OCC recommended removal of nasogastric feeding tubes at patients' families requests in 1985 even though the Massachusetts courts were then considering this issue in the Brophy case.[1] The committee's notes made clear that it would continue to be informed by ethical principles, especially the principle of beneficence.

The committee appears to pay close attention to case law that is developing in the area of limited treatment for terminally ill patients. Indeed, in 1978 and 1979, the OCC reviewed fewer cases, perhaps because of the confusion created by the Saickewicz decision with regard to whether a court order was required before a DNR order could be written.[2,3] Nonetheless, the committee maintains a separation from the hospital's general counsel's office, which both parties feel is appropriate.

Type 4 cases are those in which the OCC and the attending physician agreed with a family's request for DNR status. These cases were relatively more frequent in the 1970s than they are at present. The evolution of type 4 cases indicates the degree to which physician and patient thinking about limited care has evolved in the past ten years. Even so, there remain physicians uncomfortable with limiting care in cases in which communication problems develop. The committee pays close attention to the psychodynamics of health care workers' relationships with patients and families and helps overcome the problems that are prevalent in discussions about DNR status.[4] Including the nursing staff in the discussions is an important aspect of the OCC approach. In addition, the OCC's clinical expertise reassures the health care team.[5]

Type 5 consultations, those in which the OCC recommended a DNR order for an incompetent and moribund patient independent of the wishes of the patient's family, were clearly its most controversial recommendations. In many cases there was no family, or the family members were far away and would not make a decision for the patient. In others, the family was divided. Still other families wanted no limitations on care despite the fact that the patient was clearly not going to recover. In these cases, the OCC wrote comprehensive notes in the chart, detailing its thinking and its interpretation of the clinical situation. The consultation was never concealed, as has occurred elsewhere (*New York Times*, March 24 1984, p. 17). In addition, the OCC carefully and fully discussed its reasoning with the family.

In type 5 cases the OCC applied a consistent set of ethical principles. It argued that the physicians had fulfilled their duty to the patient by doing everything possible to restore health, a task now judged impossible. Since the primary medical goal for the patient in this situation was relief of suffering, the committee argued that further heroic therapy, such as cardiopulmonary resuscitation, would be useless and would detract from the dignity of the patient's death. The OCC also stated that the patient's dignity and integrity outweighed whatever psychological benefit the family would gain from knowing that further invasive, yet useless, procedures would be pursued. Thus the OCC emphasized the principle of beneficence in its reasoning.[6] In all cases, the families either ultimately accepted this reasoning or ceased insisting that invasive procedures be used. The OCC is unaware of any suits filed with regard to cases on which it consulted.

Although rational and consistent with ethical principles, the OCC's approach to type 5 cases must be considered controversial. The number of type 5 consultations has increased, perhaps reflecting an increased willingness on the part of physicians to act in what they believe to be the best interests of an incompetent patient. As I have argued elsewhere, the ethical issues that arise in type 5 consultations are extremely complex.[7] The major question that arises is the extent and nature of the duty of physicians to defer to family wishes, especially when those wishes are unrealistic.[8]

Some would argue that deference is always due the family's wishes because the family is best placed to speak for the patient. The OCC reasoning was that the family wishes should be overruled when they were inconsistent with a rational patient's wishes. From a chart review, it was difficult to tell if the families in type 5 cases were stating an explicit wish of the patient. Nevertheless, the OCC placed a duty to act according to an ethical principle of beneficence before a duty to follow a family's wishes when those wishes were based on unrealistic or irrational expectations.

Type 5 decisions are controversial from other perspectives as well. For instance, the law concerning these situations is not definitive.[9] In Massachusetts, an appeals court opinion has allowed physicians and family to decide on DNR status for an incompetent patient without court intervention. However, the court deferred judgment on the issue of DNR status when the family and physicians disagree.[10] Thus the legal importance of family agreement is still open. Moreover, the role of ethics committees in making these decisions is not clear.[11,12] It is not easy to say whether an ethics committee should recommend that physicians overrule family wishes on the assumption that a rational person would opt for DNR status if terminally ill and incompetent.

The argument that physicians should not be allowed to usurp the family's decision-making role is powerful, particularly at a time when many feel that physicians have long been too powerful. On the other hand, one risks degrading physicians if they are forced to provide aggressive but useless therapy for terminally ill, incompetent patients only because a family insists on it. Indeed, this process may contribute to the inhumane appearance of some deaths in hospitals and the perception of physicians as uncaring.[13] One can hardly foster in physicians a sense of morality and ethical behavior if they are forced to provide aggressive care even when they consider it unethical. . . .

References

1. *Brophy v New England Sinai Hospital*, 398 Mass 417, 497 NE2d 626 (1986).
2. Relman A: The Saikewicz decision: Judges as physicians. *N Engl J Med* 1978;298:508–509.
3. Annas G: Reconciling Quinlan and Saikewicz: Decision-making for the terminally ill incompetent. *Am J Law Med* 1979;4:110–136.
4. Bedell S, Delbanco T: Choices about cardiopulmonary resuscitation in the hospital. *N Engl J Med* 1984;310:1089–1093.
5. Siegler M: Ethics committees: Decisions by bureaucracy. *Hastings Cent Rep* 1986;16:22–24.
6. Beauchamp R, Faden R: *A Theory and History of Informed Consent*. Baltimore, The Johns Hopkins University Press, 1985, pp 11–17.
7. Brennan T: Do-not-recuscitate orders for the incompetent patient in the absence of family consent. *Law Med Health Care* 1986;14:13–19.
8. Jonsen A, Siegler M, Winslade W: *Clinical Medical Ethics*. University of Chicago Press, 1985, chap 4.
9. Mooney CA: Depending not to resuscitate hospital patients: Medical and legal perspective. *Univ Illinois Law Rev* 1986;1986:1025–1118.
10. *In re Dinnerstein*, 380 NE2d 134, 139 n11.
11. Levine C: Hospital ethics committees: A guarded prognosis. *Hastings Cent Rep* 1977;7:25–27.
12. Veatch R: Hospital ethics committees: Is there a role? *Hastings Cent Rep* 1977;7:20–25.
13. Cohen C: The operation of an ethics committee. *Crit Care Med* 1982;10:42–43.

Questions for Discussion
Part III, Section 2

1. According to some analyses, physicians who refuse to abide by the Baby Doe regulations (which are described in "Child Abuse and Neglect Prevention and Treatment") are practicing a responsible form of civil disobedience; in your opinion, are physicians who commit voluntary active euthanasia doing the same thing?

2. According to Greco and others, what questions about advanced care planning should the federal government have addressed prior to implementing the Patient Self-Determination Act?

3. Does the President's Commission identify any ethical basis for distinguishing between withholding and withdrawing life-sustaining treatment? Do you agree or disagree with the Commission's opinion?

4. Why are Living Will statutes in many states written to apply only to people with terminal illness under circumstances where treatment merely prolongs the dying process? How did California's Natural Death Act shape this development?

5. What are the positive and negative ramifications of providing partial or complete legal immunity to ethics committee members? Do you agree or disagree with the New York State Task Force's recommendation in this matter?

6. Why does the American Medical Association assert that physicians cannot ethically refuse to treat HIV-positive patients just because of their seropositive status? Is this reasoning persuasive?

7. The American Academy of Neurology maintains that patients in a persistent vegetative state should not receive treatments that provide no benefit to the patient or family. Do they include in this guideline the medical provision of artificial nutrition and hydration? Do you think nutrition and hydration are similar to or different from other medical treatments? What do Ruark and others have to say about this question?

8. Why does Brennan oppose providing useless medical treatment to an incompetent patient if the family requests it?

SECTION 3

CULTURAL ASSUMPTIONS IN THE PRACTICE OF BIOETHICS

Western Bioethics on the Navajo Reservation Benefit or Harm?

Joseph A. Carrese and Lorna A. Rhodes

Joseph Carrese is a general internist and assistant professor of medicine at the Johns Hopkins University School of Medicine. He practiced medicine for four years in the U.S. Public Health Service on the Navajo Indian reservation in Northeast Arizona. Lorna Rhodes is an anthropologist and associate professor of anthropology at the University of Washington in Seattle. This paper examines traditional Navajo perspectives regarding discussion of negative information in order to identify the limits of Western bioethical analysis in dealing with patients of non-Western cultures.

The United States is a pluralistic society, consisting of people from many different traditions and from diverse cultural backgrounds. Accordingly, not all patients share the values and moral perspectives of dominant society as currently reflected in mainstream Western biomedicine and bioethics.[1,2] Surprisingly, little research has been done on the variability of patients' values and moral perspectives by community as compared with prevailing societal, biomedical, and bioethical views. Yet, as demonstrated by two recent studies, one comparing Mexican-American and Anglo-American attitudes toward autopsies[3] and the other comparing attitudes about end-of-life care among African Americans, Hispanics, and non-Hispanic whites,[4] there are important differences to be appreciated. . . .

Joseph A. Carrese and Lorna A. Rhodes. "Western Bioethics on the Navajo Reservation: Benefit or Harm?" Abridged from *The Journal of the American Medical Association*, Volume 274, 1995, pp. 826–829.

In the culture of Western biomedicine[5] and bioethics, the principles of autonomy and patient self-determination are centrally important.[6] Consequently, explicit and direct discussion of negative information between health care providers and patients is the current standard of care. For example, informed consent requires disclosing the risks of medical treatment, truth telling requires disclosure of bad news, and advance care planning requires patients to consider the possibility of a serious future illness. Physicians have been criticized for failing to meet these standards.[7]

In traditional Navajo culture, it is held that thought and language have the power to shape reality and to control events. Discussing the potential complications of diabetes with a newly diagnosed Navajo patient may, in the view of the traditional patient, result in the occurrence of such complications. . . .

In this study we were interested to learn how health care providers should approach the discussion of negative information with Navajo patients. Achieving a better understanding of the Navajo perspective on these issues might result in more culturally appropriate medical care for Navajo patients in Western hospitals and clinics. Finally, this inquiry provided the opportunity to consider the limitations of dominant Western bioethical perspectives.

Methods

Design

The study was a focused ethnography.[8] Ethnography is helpful in understanding the differences between various cultures and systems of meaning.[9] As a set of qualitative research methods, ethnography uses techniques such as participant observation and in-depth interviewing to generate, rather than test, hypotheses[10]; the intent of these approaches is to minimize the possibility that the nature and conduct of the inquiry itself will miss or exclude relevant information.[11]

Study Site and Population

Fieldwork was conducted between February 1993 and March 1994 on four trips to the Navajo Indian reservation, which is located primarily in northeast Arizona, but also includes portions of southern Utah and northwest New Mexico. The Navajo reservation is approximately 25,000 square miles, about the size of West Virginia; it is the largest Indian reservation in the United States.[12] . . .

Historically, the Navajo relationship with dominant society has been marked by conflict. Prominent examples include the military campaign of Kit Carson in 1863, the 300-mile Long Walk and subsequent incarceration of tribal members at the Bosque Redondo in New Mexico from 1864 to 1868, and the livestock reduction program of the 1930s.[13]

Sampling

Two sampling strategies were used in this study. First, purposeful or judgment sampling was used in the recruitment of several key informants, such as public health nurses, community health representatives, a Veterans Affairs representative, a social worker, and mental health workers. Judgment sampling was also used by the key informants, who were primarily responsible for the selection of study informants. Second, in a few cases informants themselves identified others who should be interviewed; this represents network or snowball sampling.[14]

These approaches generated a group of informants from different tribal clans and having different locations of residence and medical problems.

Informants

Thirty-four Navajo informants were interviewed, 16 men and 18 women. The age range was 26 to 87 years, with a median of 58.5 years and a mean of 60 years. We deliberately included a subgroup of eight Navajo biomedical health care providers because they were in a unique position to comment on the traditional Navajo culture as well as the Western biomedical culture.

Of the remaining 26 informants, at least six functioned in some capacity as traditional diagnosticians or healers, and all had received traditional medical services. Seventeen (65%) spoke only Navajo during the interviews, requiring the use of an interpreter. . . .

Data Sources

In-depth, open-ended interviews were conducted by the principal investigator (J.A.C.), primarily in the homes of the informants. The interviews, which averaged 1 to 2 hours each, were audiotaped and then transcribed. Second interviews were conducted if informants were willing and if the first session indicated that more could be learned from an additional meeting; this was the case for six informants.

Informants were asked to talk about their experiences with Western biomedical providers and institutions. Particular attention was paid to informants' views about the disclosure of risk and bad news as these issues emerged in the context of their stories. Probe questions were asked to clarify and further explore confusing or seemingly contradictory information.

We solicited the views of 22 of the 34 informants about the idea of advance care planning. The 12 informants who were not asked included seven patients, four (of eight) Navajo biomedical health care providers, and one traditional provider. The decision to ask patients and traditional providers about advance care planning was made after the first five interviews were conducted. These interviews included four patients. Subsequently, the decision was made to ask Navajo biomedical health care providers about advance care planning as well, because the data we were gathering from informants led us to ask not only how information about advance care planning should be discussed, but whether it should be discussed at all. The traditional health care provider was not asked about advance care planning because an interpreter was not available for the entire interview. Finally, three patients who had cancer or who were being evaluated for a diagnosis of cancer were not asked to comment on advance care planning because the investigators felt that this line of inquiry might be too upsetting.

Non-interview-related observations and reflections were recorded in a journal on a daily basis during fieldwork. Finally, Indian Health Service, federal government, and state of Arizona advance directive documents and policies were reviewed.

Data Analysis

As the transcripts were read, observations and reflections about ideas in the text were written in the margins of the transcripts, a process referred to as coding. Text with similar codes was examined and compared across interviews, leading to the identification of several major themes. Throughout the period of data analysis emerging themes were continually reviewed, alternative interpretations considered, and revisions made. Also, comments discordant with dominant themes were identified and examined.

Trustworthiness

Several steps were taken to ensure trustworthiness of the findings, a concept in qualitative research comparable to validity and reliability in quantitative research.[15] Briefly, these included (1) conducting four group feedback sessions with a total of 24 Navajo informants, three of whom were part of the original sample, to verify that the information we obtained and its interpretation made sense; (2) independent review of interpreter performance by three other Navajo speakers; (3) independent coding of a small sample of transcripts by two other physicians with fellowship training in qualitative research; (4) review of analysis with an anthropologist who is an expert in Navajo culture and with a Navajo graduate student in anthropology; (5) comparing our findings with the work of others on the Navajo; and (6) soliciting peer review in a variety of settings, such as formal work-in-progress sessions, graduate seminars, and invited presentations. . . .

Results

Transcript analysis identified several themes; only a portion of the findings will be presented here. First, we describe two themes that emerged from the open-ended interviews, followed by data regarding informants' opinions about advance care planning.

Think and Speak in a Positive Way:
Hózhoojí Nitsihakees/Hózhoojí Saad

Informants commented often that it was important to "think and speak in a positive way." This theme is encompassed by the Navajo phrases *hózhoojí nitsiha-*

kees and *hózhoojí saad.* The literal translations are "think in the Beauty Way" and "talk in the Beauty Way." The prominence of these themes reflects the Navajo view that thought and language have the power to shape reality and control events.

A public health nurse referred us to a woman who had resisted attending a prenatal clinic. In the woman's experience the risks of pregnancy were discussed at the clinic, a practice she found troubling. She made the following remarks:

> I've always thought in a positive way, ever since I was young. And even when the doctors talked to me like that, I always thought way in the back of my mind: I'm not going to have a breech baby. I'm going to have a healthy baby and a real fast delivery with no complications, and that's what has happened.

This theme of thinking and speaking in a positive way often emerged when informants reflected on how doctors should communicate with patients; it reflects the Navajo view that health is maintained and restored through positive ritual language. A traditional diagnostician, commenting on how she counsels her own patients on matters of health and illness, said the following:

> In order to think positive there are plants up in the mountains that can help you. Also there are prayers that can be done. You think in these good ways, and that will make you feel better and whatever has stricken you in the deadly manner will kind of fall apart with all these good things that you put in place of it. . . . The doctor may say, "You're not going to live," but I say, *"Hózhoojí nitsihakees"*; that means "think in the Beauty Way."

Avoid Thinking or Speaking in a Negative Way: Doo'ájiniidah

Informants made a related point of requesting that providers "avoid thinking or speaking in a negative way." This theme is approximated by the Navajo phrase, *"Doo'ájiniidah."* The literal translation is "Don't talk that way!"

Often this theme was expressed as informants recounted interactions with medical providers that upset them, the idea being that negative thoughts and words can result in harm. A middle-aged Navajo woman who is a nurse, speaking about how the risks of bypass surgery were explained to her father, said the following:

> The surgeon told him that he may not wake up, that this is the risk of every surgery. For the surgeon it was very routine, but the way that my Dad received it, it was almost like a death sentence, and he never consented to the surgery.

A second example of this theme comes from a highly regarded medicine man commenting about the special care required when healers communicate with patients:

> In my practice, when I'm working with the patient, I am very careful of what I say, because any negative words could hurt the patient. So, with Western medicine, a doctor could be treating a patient, and he can mention death, and that is sharper

than any needle. Therefore, with the tongue that we have, we have to be very careful of what we say at the time and point we're treating the patient.

Advance Care Planning

Given the Navajo discomfort with negative information, we were interested to learn how informants regarded the idea of advance care planning. Advance care planning requires competent patients to leave instructions (living will) or designate an agent to speak for them (durable power of attorney) to guide decisions about medical treatment in case the patient becomes unable to communicate his or her wishes owing to mental incapacity. Advance care planning requires patients to contemplate and plan for a future state characterized by profound illness.

The Patient Self-determination Act was passed into federal law effective December 1, 1991.[16] A major goal of this legislation was to increase patient participation in end-of-life decision making by encouraging adults to complete advance directive documents.[17] To facilitate this goal, two of the law's major requirements are (1) providing all adult patients admitted to hospitals with written material, at the time of admission, summarizing state law and hospital policies addressing the patient's right to formulate an advance directive, and (2) educating staff and the surrounding community about issues concerning advance directives.

In March 1992, the Indian Health Service fully adopted the requirements of the Patient Self-determination Act. Indian Health Service policy also states: "Tribal customs and traditional beliefs that relate to death and dying will be respected to the extent possible when providing information to patients on these issues."[18]

Nineteen (86%) of the 22 informants who were asked about advance care planning stated or implied that it was a dangerous violation of traditional Navajo values and ways of thinking. Nine informants stated this explicitly. For example, a 76-year-old man with chronic pain said:

> That's *doo'ájíníidah*, you don't say those things. And you don't try to bestow that upon yourself, the reason being that there are prayers for every part of life that you can put your trust on. The object is to live as long as possible here on earth. Why try to shorten it by bestowing things upon yourself?

Ten informants would not even discuss the issue because they felt that it was too dangerous. An 87-year-old male World War II veteran's response was characteristic of this group:

> In my opinion, I wouldn't recommend it, wouldn't want to talk about it, or want to comment about it.

Of the 22 informants whose opinions about advance directives were sought, only three (14%) found the idea somewhat acceptable. All of these Navajo informants were trained as Western biomedical health care providers and employed by the Indian Health Service, and their responses were consistent with Indian Health Service policy. The following comment was characteristic of this group:

> One of our responsibilities here is to work on these living wills and the power of attorney. In the Navajo philosophy you don't say these things, you don't discuss these things. But this is something that is new to the hospital, and we need to discuss it with every patient.

Comment

Our study sought to understand the perspective of Navajo informants regarding the discussion of negative information. Two closely related themes emerged from the interviews. Informants explained that patients and health care providers should think and speak in a positive way and avoid thinking or speaking in a negative way.

Ethnographers and anthropologists who have studied the Navajo people[19-21] identify *hózhó* as the central concept in Navajo culture. Its meaning is approximated by combining the concepts of beauty, blessedness, goodness, order, harmony, and everything that is positive or ideal.[22] *Hózhó* defines the traditional Navajo way of thinking, speaking, behaving and relating to other people and the surrounding world.

It is clear that these Navajo informants have their own way of thinking about and coping with issues related to safety and danger, health and sickness, and life and death. It is a way of thinking and using language that reflects the Navajo concept *hózhó* and the Navajo view that thought and language shape reality. Discussing negative information conflicts with the Navajo view of language and its relationship to reality and with our informants' expectation that communication between healers and patients embodies the concept of *hózhó*. . . .

Hospital policies complying with the Patient Self-determination Act, which are intended to expose all hospitalized Navajo patients to the idea, if not the practice, of advance care planning, are ethically troublesome. For Navajo patients like our informants, an advance care planning discussion may not be viewed as beneficial, and in fact it is more likely to be regarded as potentially harmful. The study's findings question whether it is possible to comply with an Indian Health Service policy that requires providing information to all patients about advance care planning while respecting traditional views. In light of these findings, health care providers and institutions caring for Navajo patients should reevaluate their policies and procedures regarding advance care planning.

This study further demonstrates that the concepts and principles of Western bioethics are not universally held.[23-26] In our pluralistic society there are communities of patients who do not identify dominant values as their own, a fact that health care providers and institutions need to appreciate. Providers interested in understanding their patients' values and perspectives should "practice an intensive, systematic, imaginative empathy with the experiences and modes of thought of persons who may be foreign to [them] but whose foreignness [they come] to appreciate and humanly engage."[27] A deeper understanding of patients' perspectives should follow, and this in turn should be used to inform clinical interactions, research and educational activities, and institutional policies.

Finally, additional research should be done among communities of patients whose views depart from prevailing moral perspectives. We have studied one population for whom dominant Western bioethical concepts and principles are problematic. This challenges us to consider other populations for whom the routine application of these concepts and principles may pose difficulties.

References

1. Carrese J, Brown K, Jameton A. Culture, healing and professional obligations. *Hastings Cent Rep.* 1993;23:15–17.
2. Jecker NS, Carrese JA, Pearlman RA. Caring for patients in cross cultural settings. *Hastings Cent Rep.* 1995;25:6–14.
3. Perkins HS, Supik JD, Hazuda HP. Autopsy decisions: the possibility of conflicting cultural attitudes. *J Clin Ethics.* 1993;4:145–154.
4. Caralis PV, Davis B, Wright K, Marcial E. The influence of ethnicity and race on attitudes toward advance directives, life-prolonging treatments, and euthanasia. *J Clin Ethics.* 1993;4:155–165.
5. Rhodes LA. Studying biomedicine as a cultural system. In: Johnson TM, Sargent CE, eds. *Medical Anthropology: Contemporary Theory and Method.* New York, NY: Praeger; 1990:159–173.
6. Jonsen AR, Siegler M, Winslade WJ. *Clinical Ethics.* 3rd ed. New York, NY: McGraw-Hill Inc; 1992:37–38.
7. Katz J. *The Silent World of Doctor and Patient.* New York, NY: The Free Press; 1984.
8. Muecke MA. On the evaluation of ethnographies. In: Morse J, ed. *Critical Issues in Qualitative Research Methods.* Beverly Hills, Calif: Sage Publications; 1993:198–199.
9. Agar MH. *Speaking of Ethnography.* Beverly Hills, Calif: Sage Publications; 1986.
10. Spradley JP. *The Ethnographic Interview.* New York, NY: Harcourt Brace Jovanovich College Publishers; 1979.
11. Muecke MA. On the evaluation of ethnographies. In: Morse J, ed. *Critical Issues in Qualitative Research Methods.* Beverly Hills, Calif: Sage Publications; 1993:203.
12. Goodman JM. *The Navajo Atlas.* Norman: University of Oklahoma Press; 1982.
13. Locke RF. *The Book of the Navajo.* Los Angeles, Calif: Mankind Publishing; 1976.
14. Bernard HR. *Research Methods in Cultural Anthropology.* Beverly Hills, Calif: Sage Publications; 1988:97–98.
15. Lincoln YS, Guba EG. Establishing trustworthiness. In: *Naturalistic Inquiry.* Beverly Hills, Calif: Sage Publications; 1985:289–331.
16. Omnibus Budget Reconciliation Act of 1990. Pub L No. 101–508, §§4206, 4751.
17. Wolf SM, Boyle P, Callahan D, et al. Sources of concern about the Patient Self-determination Act. *N Engl J Med.* 1991;325:1666–1671.

18. US Dept of Health and Human Services, Public Health Service, Indian Health Service. *Patient Self-determination and Advance Directives Policy.* Indian Health Service Circular 92-2, March 1992:1–5.

19. Wyman LC. *Blessingway.* Tucson: University of Arizona Press; 1970.

20. Reichard GA. *Navaho Religion: A Study of Symbolism.* New York, NY: Bollingen Foundation; 1950.

21. Kluckhohn CK. The philosophy of the Navaho Indians. In: Northrop FSC, ed. *Idealogical Differences and World Order.* New Haven, Conn: Yale University Press; 1949.

22. Witherspoon G. *Language and Art in the Navajo Universe.* Ann Arbor: University of Michigan Press; 1977:24.

23. Beyene Y. Medical disclosure and refugees: telling bad news to Ethiopian refugees. *West J Med.* 1992;157:328–332.

24. Meleis AI, Jonsen AR. Ethical crises and cultural differences. *West J Med.* 1983;138:889–893.

25. Surbone A. Truth telling to the patient. *JAMA.* 1992;268:1661–1662.

26. Swinbanks D. Japanese doctors keep quiet. *Nature.* 1989;339:409.

27. Kleinman A. *The Illness Narratives: Suffering, Healing, and the Human Condition.* New York, NY: Basic Books Inc; 1988:230.

Gender, Race, and Class in the Delivery of Health Care

Susan Sherwin

Susan Sherwin is a professor of philosophy and women's studies at Dalhousie University in Halifax, Nova Scotia, Canada. Most of her research and teaching efforts are concentrated in the areas of health care ethics and feminist theory. Her chapter in *No Longer Patient: Feminist Ethics and Health Care* provides a forceful account of the relationship among gender, race, and class in the delivery of health care. Despite the error of attributing causation from associations, she articulates a line of argument that has not been sufficiently appreciated. In America (and many other places) dominant oppressive social and political structures have maintained power relationships to the disadvantage of women (gender), people of color (race), and people of lower socioeconomic status. The author argues that the medical models for understanding disease, health care delivery, and medical research perpetuate the patterns of oppression that shape society in the United States. Bioethicists have a responsibility to consider how existing institutions can be modified to provide a more egalitarian distribution of health and well-being.

Oppression and Illness

It is widely recognized throughout the field of biomedical ethics that people's health care needs usually vary inversely with their power and privilege within society. Most bioethical discussions explain these differences solely in economic terms, observing that health and access to health resources are largely dependent on income levels. Poverty is an important determining factor in a person's prospects for health: being poor often means living without access to adequate nutrition, housing, heat, clean water, clothing, and sanitation, and each of these factors may have a negative impact on health (Lewis 1990). . . . And the poor suffer higher rates of mental illness and addiction than do other segments of the population. Financial barriers also often force the poor to let diseases reach an advanced state before they seek professional help; by the time these individuals do receive care, recovery may be compromised.

It is not sufficient, however, just to notice the effects of poverty on health; it is also necessary to consider who is at risk of becoming the victim of poverty. In a hierarchical society such as the one we live in, members of groups that are

---

Susan Sherwin. "Gender, Race, and Class in the Delivery of Health Care." Abridged from *No Longer Patient: Feminist Ethics and Health Care*, 1992, pp. 222–240. Reprinted by permission of Temple University Press.

oppressed on the basis of gender, race, sexuality, and so forth are the people who are most likely to be poor. Moreover, not only does being oppressed lead to poverty and poverty to poor health but being oppressed is itself also a significant determining factor in the areas of health and health care. Those who are most oppressed in society at large are likely to experience the most severe and frequent health problems and have the least access to adequate medical treatment.[1] One reason for this vulnerability is that oppressed individuals are usually exposed to high levels of stress by virtue of their oppressed status, and excessive stress is responsible for many serious illnesses and is a complicating factor in most diseases. Another important factor to consider, as we shall see, is that the same prejudices that undermine the status of the oppressed members of society may affect the treatment they receive at the hands of health care workers.

North American society is characteristically sexist, racist, classist, homophobic, and frightened of physical or mental imperfections; we can anticipate, then, that those who are oppressed by virtue of their gender, race, class, sexual orientation, or disabilities—and especially, those who are oppressed in a number of different ways—will experience a disproportional share of illness and will often suffer reduced access to resources. Moreover, the connection between illness and oppression can run in both directions; because serious or chronic illness is often met with fear and hostility, it may also precipitate an individual's or family's slide into poverty and can therefore lead to oppression based on class.

The damaging connections between oppression and illness are profoundly unfair. Because this situation is ethically objectionable, bioethicists have a responsibility to consider ways in which existing medical institutions can be modified to challenge and undermine these connections, rather than contribute to them. Ethical analyses of the distribution of health and health care must take into consideration the role that oppression plays in a person's prospects for health and well-being.

Patients as Members of Oppressed Groups

. . . Women are the primary consumers of health care, but the care they receive does not always serve their overall health interests. In a report presented to the American Medical Association, Richard McMurray (1990) reviewed recent studies on gender disparities in clinical decision-making; he found that although women are likely to undergo more medical procedures than do men when they present the same symptoms and condition, they have significantly less access than men do to some of the major diagnostic and therapeutic interventions that are considered medically appropriate for their conditions. In some cases the discrepancies were quite remarkable: for example, despite comparable physical needs, women were 30 percent less likely than men to receive kidney transplants, 50 percent as likely to be referred for diagnostic testing for lung cancer, and only 10 percent as likely to be referred for cardiac catheterization. The studies were unable to identify any biological difference that would justify these discrepancies. In addition, even though biological differences are sometimes significant in the course of various diseases and therapies, McMurray found that medical researchers have largely ignored the study of diseases and medications in women; for instance, cardiovascular disease is the leading cause of death in women in the United States, but research in this area has been almost exclusively conducted on men.

Therefore, as a group, it appears that women are particularly vulnerable to poor health care. Although they receive a great deal of medical treatment, the relevant research data are frequently missing, and specific treatment decisions seem to be biased against them. When women are medically treated, they are often overtreated, that is, subjected to excessive testing, surgery, and prescription drugs (Weaver and Garrett 1983). . . .

In the United States the poor usually have (at best) access only to inadequate health services. Many people who find themselves employed full time but receiving annual incomes well below established poverty lines fail to qualify for Medicaid support. Those who do receive subsidized health care must confront the fact that many physicians and hospitals refuse to accept Medicaid patients. . . .

Canadians have so far avoided the two-tiered system of private and public health care. In Canada poor women are not turned away from hospitals or doctors' offices,[2] but they may not be able to afford travel to these facilities. Rural women are often restricted from access to needed health care by lack of transportation. . . .

In bioethics literature the issue of justice is often raised, but most discussions focus on whether or not everyone has a right to health care and, if so, what services this right might entail. Accessibility is viewed as the principal moral concern, but even where there is universal health insurance (for example, in Canada), the system is not designed to respond to the particular health needs of many groups of women. Being subject to violence, at risk of developing addictions to alcohol or other mood-altering drugs, and lacking adequate resources to obtain a nutritious food supply are all factors that affect peoples' prospects for health and their ability to promote their own well-being. Such threats to health are a result of the social system, which promotes oppression of some groups by others. Health care alone will not correct all these social effects, but as long as the damage of oppression continues, it is necessary to help its victims recover from some of the harms to their health that occur as a result of their oppressed status.

Bioethicists share with health care professionals and the rest of the community an ethical responsibility to determine how the health needs generated by oppressive structures can best be met. Medical care per se will not always be the most effective means of restoring or preserving the health of oppressed persons. Investigation of how best to respond to these socially generated needs is a topic that must be added to the traditional agenda of health care ethics.

The Organization of Health Care

Much of the explanation for the different ways in which health care providers respond to the needs of different social groups can be found in the very structures of the health care delivery system. The dominance structures that are pervasive throughout society are reproduced in the medical context; both within and without the health care delivery system, sex, race, economic class, and able-bodied status are important predictors in determining someone's place in the hierarchy. The organization of the health care system does not, however, merely mirror the power and privilege structures of the larger society; it also perpetuates them.

Within existing health care structures, women do most of the work associated with health care, but they are, for the most part, excluded from making the policy decisions that shape the system. They are the principal providers of home health care, tending the ill members of their own families, but because this work is unpaid, it is unrecorded labor, not even appearing in statistical studies of health care delivery systems; it carries no social authority, and the knowledge women acquire in caring for the ill is often dismissed by those who have power in the system. Furthermore, support is not made available to provide some relief to women carrying out this vital but demanding work.

In the formal institutions of health care delivery, women constitute over 80 percent of paid health care workers, but men hold almost all the positions of authority.[3] Health policy is set by physicians, directors, and legislators, and these positions are filled overwhelmingly by men. Despite recent dramatic increases in female enrollment in medical schools, most physicians are men (78.8 percent in Canada and 84.8 percent in the United States as of 1986)[4]; further, female physicians tend to cluster in less influential specialties, such as family practice and pediatrics, and they are seldom in positions of authority within their fields. Most medical textbooks are written by men, most clinical instructors are men, and most hospital directors are men.[5] The professional fields that women do largely occupy in the health care system are ones associated with traditionally female skills, such as nursing, nutrition, occupational and physical therapy, and public health. Women who work in health administration tend to be situated in middle-management positions, where their mediating skills may be desirable but their influence on policy is limited. . . .

When we focus directly on issues of race and economic class, the isolation of health care provider from consumer becomes even more pronounced. Although many members of minority races and plenty of poor people are involved in the delivery of health care, very few hold positions of authority. Working-class and minority employees are concentrated in the nonprofessional ranks of cleaners, nurses' aides, orderlies, kitchen staff, and so forth. Women from these groups generally have the lowest income and status in the whole health care system. They have no opportunity to shape health care policy or voice their concerns about their own health needs or those of persons for whom they are responsible. One result of this unbalanced representation is that there has been virtually no research into the distinct needs of minority women (White 1990). . . .

The gender and racial imbalances in the health care system are not accidental; they are a result of specific barriers designed to restrict access to women and minorities to the ranks of physicians. Regina Morantz-Sanchez (1985) documents how the medical profession organized itself over the last century to exclude and harass women who sought to become doctors, and Margaret Campbell (1973) shows that many of these mechanisms are still with us. Blacks, too, have been subject to systematic barriers, which keep them out of the ranks of physicians. For example, it is necessary to serve as an intern to become licensed to practice medicine, but until the 1960s, few American hospitals would grant internship positions to black physicians; those blacks who did manage to become qualified to practice medicine often encountered hospitals that refused to grant them the opportunity to admit patients (Blount 1990). Because black women must overcome both gender and race barriers, they face nearly insurmountable obstacles to pursuing careers as physicians (Weaver and Garrett 1983; Gamble 1990). Therefore, although blacks make up 12 percent of the population of the United States, they account for only 3 percent of the population of practicing doctors, and black women constitute only 1 percent of the nation's physicians; further, blacks represent only 2 percent of the faculty at medical schools (Gamble 1990). . . .

Gender, Race, and Class as Ideological Influences in Health Care

Beyond the basic injustice apparent in the differential opportunities and care that result from an unequal health care system, indirect moral costs are also created. The hierarchical organization of our health care system not only reflects the sexist, racist, and classist values of society but also lends support to them.

That the demographic patterns of the health care system are reflections of those found in the larger society compounds their effect. When the patterns of gender, race, and class distribution that are found in health care are repeated in most other major social institutions—including universities, the justice system, the business community, and the civil service—they appear inevitable. In health care, as throughout society, the most prestigious, rewarding, and powerful positions are occupied by privileged white males, who are supported by a vast pyramid of relatively undervalued, white, professional women; unskilled laborers of color have been relegated to the realm of "merely physical" work.[6]

This arrangement is of moral concern not just because of its obvious unfairness but because it provides an ideological foundation for maintaining a hierarchically structured, stratified society.[7] Within the realm of health care, authoritarian structures are rationalized as necessary to the goals of achieving good health. The metaphors that structure participants' experiences within the system appeal explicitly to models of dominance: doctors "command" health care teams, "battle" illnesses, and "lead campaigns" against dangerous life-styles. Their expertise entitles them to give "orders" to workers in the affiliated health professions (nurses, physical therapists, pharmacists, and so forth) and to patients. These arrangements are justified in terms of their end, health. Because the end is of unquestionable value, the means are usually considered acceptable to the degree that they achieve this goal. Thus medicine's worthy goals and remarkable accomplishments are said to demonstrate the benefits of retaining power and privilege for a socially vital elite. That numerous critics have questioned the success of this model in the actual achievement of health has done little to dissuade the medical establishment from encouraging the public to accept its structures as necessary (York 1987). When feminists and other critics challenge the legitimacy of social hierarchies, the medical model can be held up as evidence of the value of hierarchical structures in achieving important social goals.

Moreover, when the physicians are overwhelmingly male, white, able-bodied, and upper- or middle-class, social messages about the appropriate holders of authority are delivered with the technical medical information they control. When predominately white, female nurses accept the authority of mostly male doctors and follow their directions, they convey gender messages to patients and health care workers alike. When these nurses assume professional superiority and authority over nonprofessional hospital workers of other races, the patterns of racial oppression are also sustained. In these ways, the role patterns of the health care system rationalize society's sex and race inequalities and confirm the existing stereotypes that maintain these inequalities.

There are further reasons for concern over the close correspondence between system and social power in an oppressive society. Decisions about illness in members of oppressed groups may be tainted by the social expectations that accompany discriminatory practices. Such decisions often reflect cultural stereotypes, which themselves derive from unjust social arrangements. At the same time, those decisions may serve to legitimize particular damaging stereotypes and the social divisions that depend on them.

For example, white health care experts (and others) have identified alcoholism as a pervasive problem in the native American community; they have preached abstinence as a response. Generally, these judgments are made without examining the devastation that white culture has wrought on native community values and without extending any support for traditional, native healing options as alternative paths to recovery. Often health care workers have uncritically accepted the stereotypical view of "drunken Indians" and suggested that natives are either weak-willed or have some genetic propensity to alcohol dependency; either way, their misfortune is a reflection of some deficiency within them, not society. Most health professionals are committed to the individualistic medical model, which views diseases as belonging to individuals; although they may acknowledge a role for genetic or sociological factors, they believe that the individual is the proper site for health care treatment.

Other conceptions are available, however, and it is useful to reflect on alternatives in these circumstances. Some native healers suggest that alcoholism in their communities is really a social disease of the community, which should be understood as connected to the brutal separation of their people from their culture. Their account leads to an alternative strategy for recovery and a distinct form of health care; where the medical model treats the individual, native healers believe it is necessary to heal the community.[8] Nevertheless, only the medically authorized response receives approval and support from those with the power to allocate health care resources.

The social harms extend further. Because the authority of health care deci-sion-making is concentrated in nonnative hands, native people who identify themselves as alcoholics are required to adapt to treatment programs that have been designed for a white, urban population. They are deemed to be failures if the programs do not succeed in curing them. Because the problems usually continue, native people are seen to fulfill their culturally generated stereotypes; their severely disadvantaged economic and social position is then explained away by experts who speak authoritatively of native peoples' "natural" propensity to alcohol abuse. As long as health care decision-making resides in the hands of an elite, nonnative few, we can anticipate its continued failure to recognize and address the real needs of the native community.[9] These failures, in turn, support the cultural prejudices that view natives as inferior members of modern society who cannot hope to rise above their designated status on the socioeconomic scale. . . .

The power and authority that society has entrusted to doctors give them the opportunity to destroy many of the patriarchal assumptions about women collectively and the racist, classist, homophobic, and other beliefs about various groups of women that are key to their oppression. Few physicians, however, have chosen to exercise their social power in this way. Many doctors have accepted uncritically the biases of an oppressive society, and some have offered evidence in confirmation of such values. As a group, physicians have held onto their own power and privilege by defending the primacy of the authoritarian medical model as a necessary feature of health care. Most have failed to listen honestly to the alternative perspectives of oppressed people who are very differ-ently situated in society.

The medical model organizes our current attempts at defining and re-sponding to health needs. It has been conceived as a structure that requires a hierarchically organized health care system, in which medical expertise is privi-leged over other sorts of knowledge. It grants license to an elite class of experts to formulate all matters of health and to determine the means for responding to them. As we have seen, however, there are several serious moral problems with this model. First, it responds differently to the health needs of different groups, offering less and lower-quality care to members of oppressed groups. Second, its structures and presuppositions support the patterns of oppression that shape our society. Finally, it rationalizes the principle of hierarchy in human interactions, rather than one of equality, by insisting that its authoritarian struc-tures are essential to the accomplishment of its specific ends, and it tolerates an uneven distribution of positions within its hierarchy.

Some Conclusions

We need, then, different models to guide our thinking about ways to organize the delivery of health care. In addition to the many limits to the medical model that have been named in the bioethics literature, the traditional model reflects and perpetuates oppression in society. I conclude by summarizing some feminist suggestions that I believe should be incorporated into alternative models, if they are to be ethically acceptable.

A model that reflects the insights of feminist ethics would expand its conceptions of health and health expertise. It would recognize social as well as physiological dimensions of health. In particular, it would reflect an understanding of both the moral and the health costs of oppression. Thus it would make clear that those who are committed to improving the health status of all members of the population should assume responsibility for avoiding and dismantling the dominance structures that contribute to oppression.

Such a model would require a change in traditional understandings of who has the relevant knowledge to make decisions about health and health policy. Once we recognize the need to include oppression as a factor in health, we can no longer maintain the authoritarian medical model, in which physicians are the experts on all matters of health and are authorized to respond to all such threats. We need also to recognize that experiential knowledge is essential to understanding how oppression affects health and how the damage of oppression can be reduced. Both political and moral understandings may be necessary to address these dimensions of health and health care. Physiological knowledge is still important, but it is not always decisive.

Therefore, a feminist model would resist hierarchical structures and proclaim a commitment to egalitarian alternatives. Not only would these alternatives be more democratic in themselves and hence more morally legitimate, they would also help to produce greater social equality by empowering those who have been traditionally disempowered. They would limit the scope for domination that is available to those now accustomed to power and control. More egalitarian structures would foster better health care and higher standards of health for those who are now oppressed in society; such structures would recognize voices that are now largely unheard and would be in a position to respond to the needs they express.

The current health care system is organized around the central ideal of pursuing a "cure" in the face of illness, wherein "cure" is interpreted with most of the requisite agency belonging to the health care providers. A feminist alternative would recommend that the health care system be principally concerned with empowering consumers in their own health by providing them with the relevant information and the means necessary to bring about the changes that would contribute to their health. The existing health care system, modeled as it is on the dominance structures of an oppressive society, is closed to many innovative health strategies that would increase the power of patients; a feminist model would be user-controlled and responsive to patient concerns.

Such a change in health care organization would require us to direct our attention to providing the necessities of healthy living, rather than trying only to correct the serious consequences that occur when the opportunities for personal care have been denied. Moreover, as an added benefit, a shift to a more democratized notion of health needs may help to evolve a less expensive, more effective health care delivery system; most patients seem to be less committed than are their professional health care providers to a costly high-tech, crisis-intervention focus in health care (York 1987).

A health care system that reflects feminist ideals would avoid or at least lessen the contribution that the system of health care makes in the maintenance of oppression. It would be significantly more egalitarian in both organization and effect than anything that we are now accustomed to. This system not only would be fairer in its provision of health services but would also help to undermine the ideological assumptions on which many of our oppressive practices rest. Such an alternative is required as a matter of both ethics and health.

To spell out that model in greater detail and with an appropriate understanding, it is necessary to democratize the discipline of bioethics itself—hence, bioethics, as an area of intellectual pursuit, must also recognize the value of incorporating diverse voices in its discussions and analyses. Like medicine or any other discipline, bioethics is largely defined by the perspective of its participants. If we hope to ensure a morally adequate analysis of the ethics of health care, then we should ensure the participation of many different voices in defining the central questions and exploring the promising paths to answers in the field. . . .

Notes

1. Writers who are concerned about oppression are likely to make the connection prominent; for example, Beverly Smith states: "The reason that Black women don't have good health in this country is because we are so oppressed. It's just that simple" (quoted in Lewis 1990, 174).
2. Nevertheless many provinces would like to reinstitute a "small" user fee. Quebec has recently announced plans to proceed with a five-dollar charge for each visit to a hospital emergency room.
3. Canada census data statistics for 1986 list 104,315 men and 418,855 women employed in the areas of medicine and health. Brown (1983) reports that over 85 percent of all health-service and hospital workers in the United States are women.
4. The Canadian figure is from Statistics Canada census figures; the American figure is taken from Todd (1989).
5. To correct the apparently systematic gender bias in the provision of health care McMurray (1990) recommends that efforts be made to increase "the number of female physicians in leadership roles and other positions of authority in teaching, research and the practice of medicine."
6. Fortunately, there is now widespread social agreement that all social institutions should be transformed to reflect fairer selection procedures and to challenge the pervasive stereotypes that nurture oppression; many institutions have affirmative action programs in place to bring about such structural changes. Until such redistributions occur, however, the organization of the health care system will continue to promote attitudes that foster oppression.
7. I use the term "ideology" in its simplest sense: "a body of ideas used in support of an economic, political, or social theory" (*Webster's* 1989).
8. For alternative therapies developed within native culture, see Hodgson (1990).

For a discussion of the special needs of black, female alcoholics, see Battle (1990). For an African discussion of alternative therapy in general, see Minh-ha (1989), 135–41.

9. For a clear explanation and detailed description of the cultural changes required to provide helpful health services to native Americans, see Hagey (1989).

References

Blount, Melissa. 1990. "Surpassing Obstacles: Pioneering Black Women Physicians." In *The Black Women's Health Book: Speaking for Ourselves*, ed. Evelyn C. White. Seattle: Seal Press.

Campbell, Margaret. 1973. "Why Would a Woman Go into Medicine?" *Medical Education in the United States: A Guide for Women*. Old Westbury, N.Y.: Feminist Press.

Gamble, Vanessa Northington. 1990. "On Becoming a Physician: A Dream Not Deferred." In *The Black Women's Health Book: Speaking for Ourselves*, ed. Evelyn C. White. Seattle: Seal Press.

Lewis, Andrea. 1990. "Looking at the Total Picture: A Conversation with Health Activist Beverly Smith." In *The Black Women's Health Book*. See Battle 1990.

McMurray, Richard J. 1990. "Gender Disparities in Clinical Decision-making." Report to the American Medical Association Council on Ethical and Judicial Affairs.

Morantz-Sanchez, Regina Markell. 1985. *Sympathy and Science: Women Physicians in American Medicine*. New York: Oxford University Press.

Weaver, Jerry L., and Sharon D. Garrett. 1983. "Sexism and Racism in the American Health Care Industry: A Comparative Analysis." In *Women and Health*. See Brown.

White, Evelyn C., ed., 1990. *The Black Women's Health Book: Speaking for Ourselves*. Seattle: Seal Press.

York, Geoffrey. 1987. *The High Price of Health: A Patient's Guide to the Hazards of Medical Politics*. Toronto: James Lorimer and Company.

Questions for Discussion
Part III, Section 3

1. To what degree is the concept of informed consent culturally shaped?

2. According to Carrese and Rhodes, how should Western physicians discuss a medical problem and possible treatment with a patient whose culture forbids discussion of possible negative outcomes?

3. In addition to the groups Sherwin identifies (ethnic minorities, the poor, and women), what other groups have received unfair treatment in health care delivery and treatment?

4. How would the field of bioethics benefit by including more diverse voices in ethical debates and analysis? How would the practice of medicine benefit?

Index